COMPLETE
FIRST AID

EVERYTHING YOU NEED TO KNOW TO DEAL
WITH ACCIDENTS, EMERGENCIES & ILLNESSES

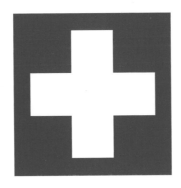

DR DAVID BASS, PROF. MAURICE KIBEL & ROD BAKER

NH
NEW
HOLLAND

Published in 2007 by New Holland Publishers Ltd.
London • Cape Town • Sydney • Auckland
86 Edgware Road, London W2 2EA, United Kingdom
80 McKenzie Street, Cape Town 8001, South Africa
Unit 1, 66 Gibbes Street, Chatswood, NSW 2067, Australia
218 Lake Road, Northcote, Auckland, New Zealand
www.newhollandpublishers.com

Publishing Managers: Claudia Dos Santos and Simon Pooley
Commissioning Editor: Alfred LeMaitre
Editors: Di Kilpert, Roxanne Reid & Gill Gordon
Designers: Lyndall du Toit, Richard MacArthur &
Glyn Bridgewater
Photographers: Lisa Trocchi, Isabel Koorts and Luke Calder
Illustrators: Ian Lusted, Stephen Felmore
Picture Research: Karla Kik, Tamlyn McGeean
Production: Myrna Collins
Proofreader/indexers: Sylvia Grobbelaar, Elizabeth Wilson
Consultants: Dr Malcolm Henry, Sarah Colles (Home Safety
Adviser, RoSPA)

ISBN 978 1 84537 883 7

Reproduction by Resolution Colour (Pty) Ltd., Cape Town, SA
Printed and bound in Malaysia by Times Offset (M) Sdn. Bhd.

10 9 8 7 6 5 4 3 2 1

The life-support techniques and sequences in this book are
modelled on those devised and advocated by the Advanced
Life Support Group (ALSG) in the United Kingdom. They
have been used extensively for the training of healthcare
professionals in Europe, South Africa and Australia.

DISCLAIMER

The advice contained in this book is intended for
reference only and cannot replace the advice of a
qualified physician. A licensed physician should be
consulted for the diagnosis and treatment of any and all
medical conditions and emergencies. The publisher
assumes no liability for any consequences, loss, injury
or inconvenience sustained by any person using this
book or the advice given in it.

FOREWORD

'My mother had a great deal of trouble with me, but I think she enjoyed it.'
Mark Twain

The joy of seeing children grow and develop is inevitably marred on occasion by minor mishaps and illnesses, which cause the parent or care-giver considerable anxiety. A health professional is not often on the spot at such times, and it is up to you to cope. This book will not give a detailed account of injuries and medical conditions that affect children. It is intended to help you manage the injury or illness yourself in an emergency, and will give guidance on whether and when further professional help is needed. Such help varies greatly according to circumstances. It might be a general practitioner who knows the whole family well, a paediatrician, or a nurse. It might be a clinic down the road, or a health centre many miles away. Guidance will also be given as to how soon such help is needed – next week will do, or should it be tomorrow? An emergency call for an ambulance, or a rushed journey to hospital by car will occasionally be required, and these unpleasant situations are described. Stick a list of important phone numbers at the back of this book – your doctor, an ambulance service, the local hospital, the police. And make sure the book is readily available!

Prevention is the name of the game! A lot of discomfort, worry and money can be saved by preventing the problem in the first place. So space has been allocated to the important fields of injury prevention in and outside the home. Immunization is one of the most cost-effective measures we have to prevent certain illnesses – not only in your own child but in the community at large. There are many misconceptions about immunization, and you will find answers to commonly asked questions on this subject on pages 146–148.

CONTENTS

FIRST AID FOR BABIES AND CHILDREN

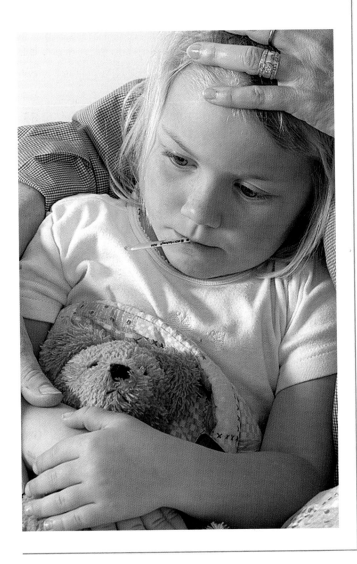

FIRST AID FOR FAMILY EMERGENCIES

FIRST AID

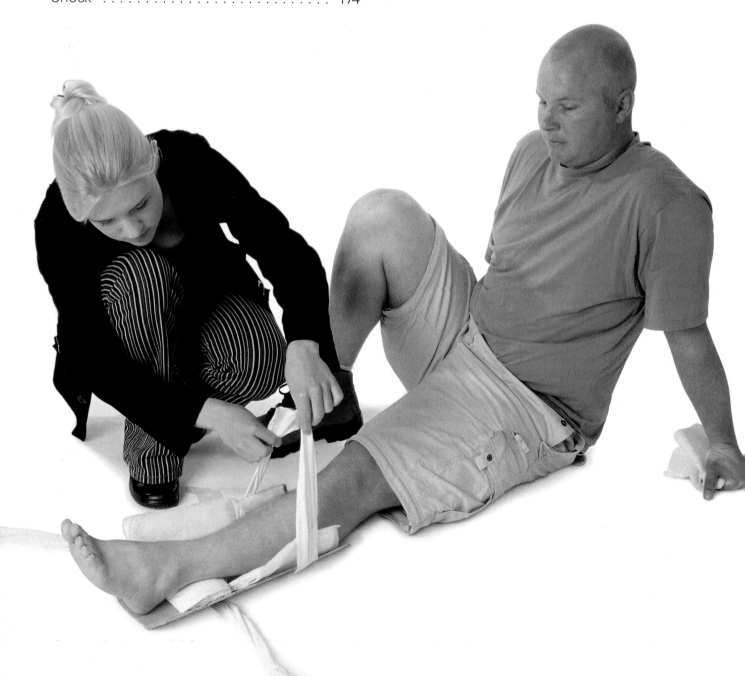

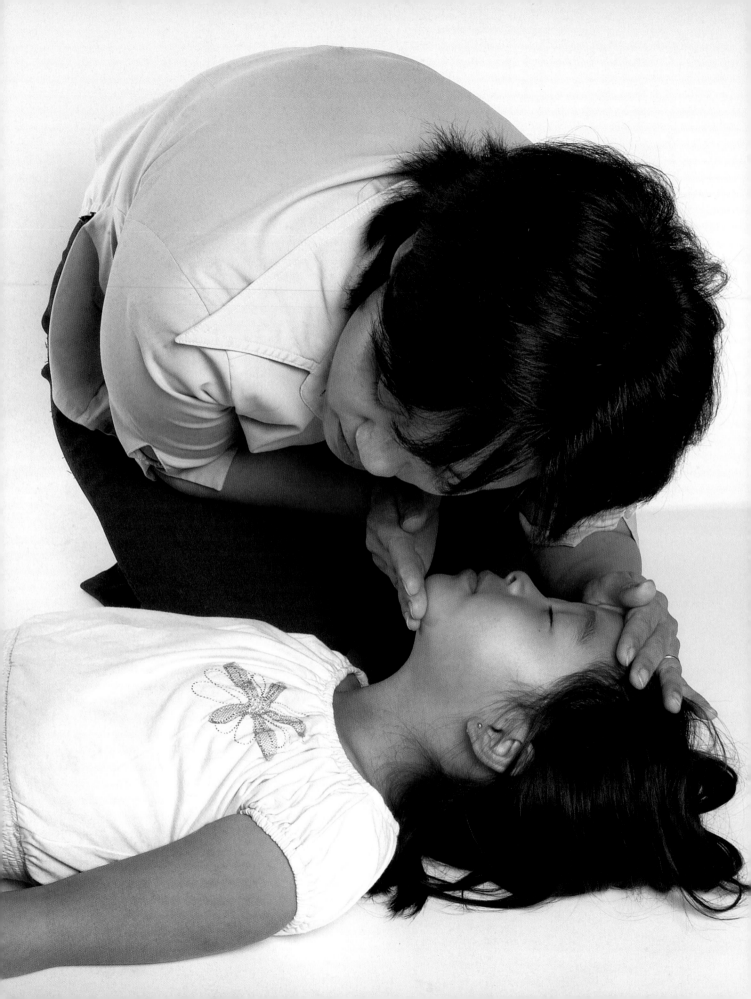

Part 1

First Aid
& Home Safety

COPING IN AN EMERGENCY

We all hope that we will never be called upon to assist in a situation requiring us to provide first aid, but by preparing yourself beforehand you will know what to do. A knowledge of basic first-aid procedures will help you to be calm and efficient. The individual procedures in this book offer a range of specific instructions, but be sure to learn the basics at least and attend a recognized first-aid course.

In an emergency situation, a desire to provide meaningful care and comfort can easily dissolve into blind panic unless you have certain basic skills and a systematic approach to resuscitation procedures. This is well within anyone's capabilities! A little knowledge, insight and hands-on training in basic first aid will give you confidence in yourself. You will be amazed at how useful – and even heroic – you can be when the occasion demands.

This manual is not designed to turn you into an expert. What we offer you is a set of skills any responsible person can apply in a wide variety of emergencies involving children. In many respects, your role in a medical emergency may be the most vital of all. As a parent, guardian or child minder you are likely to be the first person on the scene when a child is injured or suddenly becomes ill. Equipped with the basic tools and practical skills covered in this book, you should be in a position to do your bit as the first responder, and perhaps avoid a visit to the local doctor or the hospital.

You may even save a life by applying basic life-support measures to a choking or unconscious child.

Once you have read the guidelines provided in this book you should go one step further and become a fully-fledged life-support provider. We recommend that you register for a lay person's course available in your area, which is endorsed by the national council or first aid service operating in your country. Most recognized courses will not only teach you valuable life-support sequences designed to deal with almost any medical emergency, but will allow you to practise and fine-tune your skills on lifelike manikins.

Note:
To simplify, we refer to the 'child' (aged one to eight years) throughout this book, though of course infants (under one year of age) are included. If treatments or first-aid procedures differ for an infant this is specified.

Please remember
Not only is prevention always better than cure – it can also save your child pain and you much heartache. We sincerely believe that almost every injury can be prevented, and you should believe this too. For that reason we have included some practical hints and measures aimed at reducing the risk of accidents in and around the home (*see* pages 35–41). Putting these simple measures into practice will cost you time, effort and perhaps even money, but just consider the alternative. Do you really want to tempt risk, fate or disaster? Of course not!

ROLE OF THE FIRST RESPONDER
Most serious injuries and medical emergencies occur without warning. Trained medical personnel may not be able to get to the scene of an accident in time and so the outcome – sometimes the difference between life and death – often depends on just two factors:
* how quickly basic life support is provided

- whether anyone at the scene can assess nature and severity of the situation, call for appropriate assistance and, if necessary, commence resuscitation procedures (*see* pages 22–31) until help arrives.

Particularly in life-threatening emergencies such as near drowning (*see* pages 100–103), choking (*see* pages 32–34) and severe bleeding (*see* page 13), survival often depends upon whether the first responder can initiate effective resuscitation while waiting for help. As a parent, grandparent, teacher, child-minder or sports coach you should have the skills necessary to take decisive action.

Call for help

Call for assistance before you commence first aid if the infant or child is:

- unconscious, drowsy or disoriented
- having difficulty breathing or is not breathing at all
- suffering from multiple injuries, or burns
- bleeding heavily from one or more wounds
- suspected of having ingested a poisonous substance.

If you are unsure of the cause of the collapse or injury, another reliable person should phone for assistance while you commence first aid. If you are alone, phone for help first before you start resuscitation procedures. Whom you call depends on the services that are available in your area.

What to say on the phone:
Calm down and speak clearly so that you do not have to repeat yourself unnecessarily. You must provide basic information:

- your **name and contact telephone number**
- your **location** (physical address), and possibly directions as well
- a brief **description of the incident**

Do not hang up until you are told to do so. The dispatcher may be able to give you helpful assistance.

EMERGENCY NUMBERS

Keep a record of emergency contacts next to your telephone, in your diary and in the directory of your mobile phone. *See* page 304 for an emergency list. Also inform your children – even toddlers can memorize their home address and the (usually simple) numbers to dial for emergency response.

Assess the injured child

Temper your enthusiasm with good judgement: look before you leap in, regardless of the seeming severity of the emergency. Any situation you encounter should be calmly and objectively assessed before you decide on your best course of action.

Protect yourself and the injured child from further danger

In a potentially dangerous environment, good judgement is essential to ensure everyone's safety including your own. Even if you are the only one who is able to provide help you must never put your own life at risk.

Giving first aid

If a child is unconscious, in shock, or breathing with difficulty, the speed with which you restore normal breathing and blood circulation is the single most important factor. In many instances, the care required from you as first responder may be fairly straightforward; no outside help may be necessary. At other times the extent and severity of the condition may not be clearly apparent and your quick response will give the casualty the best possible chance of recovery.

FIRST-AID KITS

You should always have a first-aid kit handy in your home and vehicle, and whenever you engage in outdoor pursuits, such as hiking or camping with your children. Many commerically available ready-made kits suit the most basic of needs, but consider making your own one or supplementing a bought kit, so that it takes into account the ages and specific requirements of your family members.

Check on expiry dates from time to time to ensure that your supply is not out of date and ensure that all first-aid kits and their contents are safe from small, enquiring hands and stored in a safe, lockable place.

Putting a kit together

If you decide to design your own first-aid kit, choose a container that is durable, preferably waterproof, and big enough to contain all the items so that you can see and get at them easily without having to tip them all out. Carry-alls for fishing tackle, or small toolboxes are ideal because they have convenient compartments.

On the lid of your first-aid kit, stick a list of useful telephone numbers (*see* page 304) – such as your family doctor, local clinic or hospital, poison centre, ambulance service, next-door neighbour and neighbourhood security patrol.

When you decide what to include, do not overstock. Simply remember to replace whatever you use, and check the kit at least once a year to ensure that nothing is lacking to cater for the changing needs of your growing children.

An inexpensive plastic lunchbox makes an ideal container for a small basic first-aid kit.

Your first-aid shopping list

- One sturdy container

Instruments

- 1 small pair of sharp stainless steel scissors
- 1 large pair of dressmaker's scissors, for cutting bandages and plasters
- 1 pair of fine tweezers for removing dirt, thorns and other foreign bodies
- A few 19–21 gauge sterile injection needles for teasing out splinters
- A few sterile 5ml (1 teaspoon) syringes or measuring spoons, for giving oral medication to infants and toddlers
- An oral mercury thermometer or temperature strips (*see* Fever, page 107)
- A few paperclips, for draining blood from under nails
- A couple of large safety pins for keeping slings in place
- Two pairs of disposable surgical gloves
- Two small eye droppers

LATEX ALLERGY

Approximately 1% of adults may be allergic to gloves made from natural rubber latex. They usually get skin rashes or symptoms similar to hay fever, and sometimes wheezing and other severe reactions. You may be sensitive to latex if you are allergic to kiwi fruit, tomato, avocado, bananas or water chestnuts. If you think you may be at risk of latex allergy, rather use gloves made from synthetic latex or vinyl.

FIRST-AID KIT

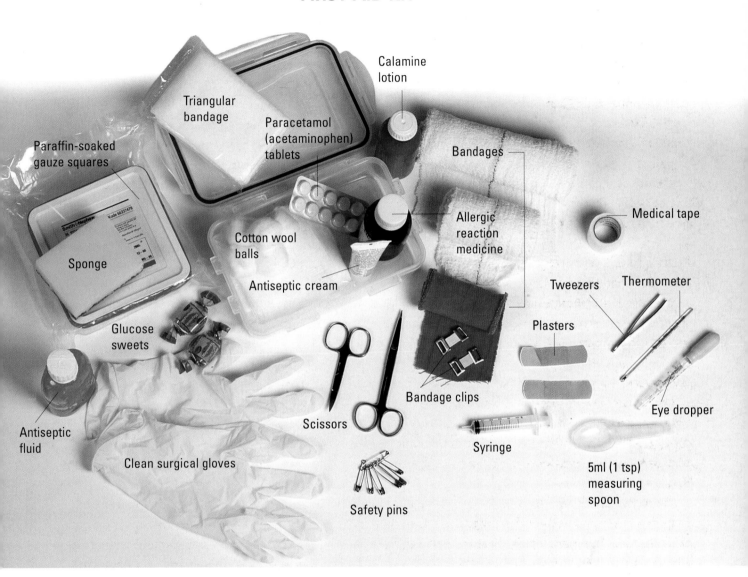

- Calamine lotion
- Triangular bandage
- Paracetamol (acetaminophen) tablets
- Bandages
- Paraffin-soaked gauze squares
- Medical tape
- Sponge
- Cotton wool balls
- Allergic reaction medicine
- Antiseptic cream
- Tweezers
- Thermometer
- Glucose sweets
- Plasters
- Bandage clips
- Eye dropper
- Antiseptic fluid
- Scissors
- Syringe
- Clean surgical gloves
- 5ml (1 tsp) measuring spoon
- Safety pins

Oral medications
- Paracetamol (acetaminophen) in liquid or chewable tablet form for pain relief (do not give aspirin or anti-inflammatory medication to children under 12 years of age)
- Promethazine hydrochloride in syrup or tablet form for mild allergic reactions
- Glucose water or sweets

Topical medications
- Antiseptic solution (chlorhexidine) for cleaning wounds and instruments
- Povidone-iodine ointment for dressing wounds
- Calamine lotion for sunburn, rashes and minor skin irritations
- Cream or gel containing the local anaesthetic benzocaine, for insect bites and stings

Dressings

- 2 packs of sterile cotton wool balls or swabs
- 2 packs of sterile gauze pads
- 2 small dishwashing sponges for cleaning wounds
- 1 roll of hypoallergenic medical tape for securing dressings
- Gauze bandages – 2cm and 5cm width (³/₄in and 2in)
- Elastic bandages with clips
- Adhesive tape and bandages – 2.5cm and 5cm width (1in and 2in)

- 1 tin of paraffin-impregnated gauze squares
- Cotton sheeting and 1m (3ft) flannel strips for slings
- 2 eye protectors, made by cutting the bottom half off two polystyrene cups (*see* Eye Injuries, page 61)

To keep in your freezer

- A bag of frozen peas to use as a cold compress (*see* Bumps and Bruises, page 42)

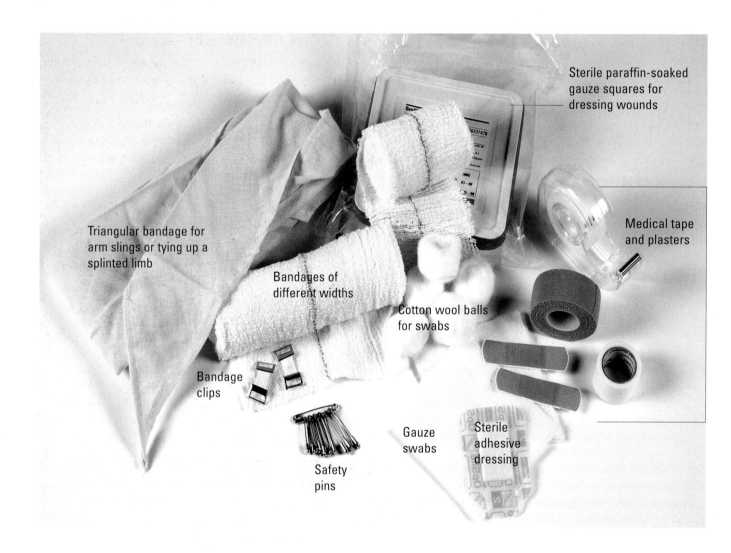

Sterile paraffin-soaked gauze squares for dressing wounds

Medical tape and plasters

Triangular bandage for arm slings or tying up a splinted limb

Bandages of different widths

Cotton wool balls for swabs

Bandage clips

Gauze swabs

Sterile adhesive dressing

Safety pins

Additional items for travel

- Sunscreen with a sufficiently high SPF
- Insect repellent
- Medicines prescribed and taken for chronic conditions (insulin, bronchodilators, and so on)
- Blankets for conserving warmth, particularly in cold weather
- Paper and pen or pencil for taking down telephonic instructions from the doctor

Some important tips

Accidents can happen next door or at the local playground and you may need to grab your kit and do a 'housecall'. So, even if you already have some of the listed items in your medicine cupboard, it is worth having duplicates in your first-aid kit as well.

Clean all non-disposable instruments with detergent and water after use, and dry them well (so they will not rust) before putting them back in the first-aid kit.

Use medicines only in the prescribed doses; check with your family doctor or local clinic that they are safe for your child.

Store your kit in a cool place, away from direct sunlight, and where it is out of the reach of small children but easily accessible to adults.

For reasons of hygiene, disposable gloves must never be reused.

STANDARD PRECAUTIONS

If you have completed a recognized basic first-aid course, and are ready to volunteer your skills in a medical emergency, always carry a few pairs of light surgical gloves around with you (*see* Latex Allergy, page 14). The main purpose of the gloves is to protect you from infection, so they need not be sterile, just clean and unbroken. Particularly if the person you are resuscitating is a stranger, always consider the possibility of communicable infectious diseases. This is especially important if you risk coming into contact with the subject's blood or other body fluids, for example:

- when performing mouth-to-mouth resuscitation, or if the person is bleeding from any site;
- you have a fresh skin wound of any size on your own hands or face;
- you live in a country or region where there is a high prevalence of infectious hepatitis or human immunodeficiency virus (HIV).

If you are obliged to administer life support without gloves, and even if it appears to your naked eye that no contamination with body fluids has occurred, always wash your hands thoroughly with soap and water as soon as possible afterward.

ACCIDENTS HAPPEN

There is nothing worse for a parent, teacher, grandparent, or caregiver than to see a child injured and in pain, or, worse yet, in dire need of medical attention. Children are adventurous and enthusiastic in their explorations of the world around them, and accidents are bound to happen some time. Luckily, serious mishaps are relatively rare, but it helps to be prepared in any case of emergency.

If you are first to arrive on the scene of a serious injury, you need to be able to take charge and direct additional helpers until medical support arrives. To be effective you must remain calm, and concentrate on what you have to do. The sooner effective treatment can begin, the better the potential for a positive outcome. The most urgent situation occurs when breathing ceases and the heart stops beating. This emergency takes precedence over anything else – any other injury.

WHAT YOU CAN DO TO HELP

Time is critical, so remain focused and follow the guidelines given below. Details of the rescue breathing procedure can be found on pages 22–31.

Determine the priorities
- Check the child's level of responsiveness (*see* Are you alright? on this page).
- As soon as possible check the child's airway and breathing (*see* pages 22–24).

- If the child is unconscious but breathing, place her in the recovery position (*see* page 27). Unconscious infants should be held in the recovery position as shown on page 30.
- Check if there is any visible bleeding; control the bleeding by applying pressure on the wound.

Are you alright? (*See also* page 21)
A child lying motionless on the ground may not be unconscious. However, if she does **not** respond to you, establish whether she is conscious and breathing.

Children between one and eight years old
Squeeze the child's hand, call her name if you know it, ask 'Are you alright?' or give a command such as 'Open your eyes!' If the child responds and speaks to you it indicates that the airway is clear and that the child is able to breathe – she is not unconscious.

If the child is drowsy, move her into the recovery position and stay with her until the emergency service arrives. A child who is in shock, or is bleeding, may be covered with a blanket to conserve body heat. If the child does not respond to you, call for help, open the airway and begin rescue breathing (*see* page 23).

Infants under one year old
Place the infant on his back directly in front of you, on a firm surface. Tap the sole of his foot and call his name. If the infant responds take him with you while you telephone for medical assistance.

If the infant fails to respond open his airway and begin rescue breathing (*see* page 31).

Monitor the child's responsiveness
An injured child may progress from being conscious to unconsciousness, her condition either improving or deteriorating fairly rapidly. A fully conscious child will be able to respond to your questions anything less is a cause for concern.

Watch out for the following signs which indicate depressed consciousness in a child:
- drowsy or difficult to arouse
- clearly disoriented (not able to tell you their name, which day it is, or where they are)
- slurred speech
- unable to answer easy questions correctly.

MOVING AN INJURED CHILD

As a general rule, resuscitation and first aid should be administered right where you have found the child, to ensure the quickest possible restoration of vital functions and reduce the serious risk of complications such as shock and the aggravation of injuries. While you commence first aid procedures on the spot, another reliable and responsible person should be sent to call for medical assistance immediately.

Severe injuries

Due to the risk of aggravating a possible spinal injury a seriously injured child should not be moved, though there are exceptions to this rule (*see* SAFE approach on page 20). Neck and spine injuries are very difficult to detect during a routine first-aid assessment, and any attempts to move someone with an injured spine can convert the condition from a relatively harmless to disastrous. It is advisable always to assume spinal injury in the following cases:
- an unconscious child
- obvious signs of a head injury
- sporting injuries (as a result of playing a contact sport, or a fall from a horse)
- in a child who complains of a painful neck or back
- if a child is unable to move arms or legs.

If you have reason to suspect a neck or spinal injury, ensure that the child lies still on a flat surface and that its head and neck are aligned (not bent forwards, backwards or sidewise, but kept in a neutral position).

Immobilize the neck with whatever you have to hand. Some stiffly rolled up towels or T-shirts can serve as handy subsitutes to prevent movement. Ensure that you stabilize the sides of the head and neck only – the throat must not be obstructed in any way, to prevent depressing the child's airway.

Exceptions to the rule
No matter what the injury, you must move a casualty to safety if:
- it is near a fire (*see* pages 76–80)
- it is in water (*see* pages 100–103)
- there is a toxic substance or gas nearby.

Minor injuries

Once first aid has been provided, a child with a minor injury can safely be moved to a more convenient or sheltered location. Bear in mind that fainting is quite common when an injured person (who has been lying on the ground) suddenly gets up. This is due a combination of factors such as emotional shock, pain and minor blood loss. It is best to stay with the child and guide its steps as it walks.

Injury in remote places

In a remote location the decision to move an injured child (apart from the exceptions above) depends on how far you are from the nearest telephone, and how long it will take before medical assistance can get to you. Children weighing under 20kg (44lbs), whose injuries consist of fractures below the knee, may be carried for short distances provided the limb has been splinted and the patient experiences no discomfort.

ASSESSING THE SITUATION

Infants are particularly prone to choking and viral infections; toddlers and older children are prone to injuries received during play and as a result of their unstoppable fascination with the world around them. Whatever the situation in which you find yourself, the key to being an effective first responder is to follow the basic guidelines in the sequences recommended in this section.

Upon arrival at the scene of any accident, the competent first responder will endeavour to calmly sum up the situation by establishing the following vital facts in the shortest amount of time possible. Not only will this information guide your immediate course of action, it must also be relayed to any medical personnel that are called to the scene:

- What happened and how did it happen?
- How many persons (children) are injured?
- Is everyone, including the first responder and/or any other helpers, free from danger?
- Is medical assistance necessary?

THE 'SAFE' APPROACH

The **SAFE** acronym (below) summarizes the correct sequence in an easy-to-remember fashion. Whenever you approach a child that has collapsed, for any reason whatsoever, you should always:

- summon help immediately – either by yourself or by sending another reliable and responsible person to call for medical assistance while you begin to attend to the child.
- ensure your own safety as well as that of the child. This applies especially when attending to someone who has been injured in a traffic accident, fire or as a result of inhaling a toxic substance, as well as due to electric shock, or any other situation where the risk of injury persists in the vicinity.

WHEN A CHILD HAS COLLAPSED

Various injuries as well as medical conditions can cause a child to become confused and dazed in the more extreme cases he may even lose consciousness. If you are the first responder at a scene where a child has collapsed for unknown reasons, it is your duty to test the casualty's responsiveness (*see* opposite and page 18) to establish whether he is fully, or partly conscious

 Shout for help: Summon medical assistance or the emergency services immediately.

 Approach with care: Check for surrounding hazards that may also be a danger to yourself.

 Free from danger: Even though we recommend that casualties should not be moved, this precaution must be weighed against any obvious risk, e.g. if a child has been knocked down on a busy street you must move him or her – with all possible care, of course – to a safe place before commencing resuscitation.

 Evaluate the ABC (see page 22–25)**:** Having taken the above precautions, you are now ready to assess vital functions and commence resuscitation if required.

or not. A temporary loss of consciousness occurs when the blood flow to the brain is decreased as a result of a sudden slowing of the heart rate. The condition commonly occurs when someone is feeling very hot, not eating enough, or as the result of emotional upset. Usually, the only first aid required is reassurance and something sweet to drink once consciousness returns.

The unconscious child

Check the responsiveness of a child lying motionless on the ground (*see* page 18 'ARE YOU ALRIGHT?') to establish that his airway is clear and that breathing and circulation are satisfactory. If the vital signs check out alright, then stay with the child to keep him calm until medical assistance arrives. If the child is very drowsy, position him in the **recovery position** (for children: *see* page 27; for infants: *see* page 30).

WHAT TO DO

- Check the response (as described above and on page 18). If there is no response, **call for help**.

- Your priority is to **check the ABC** (*see* page 22). If the airway is blocked the child will be unable to breathe so your aim is to **open the airway** (for children: *see* page 28; for infants: *see* page 31), check the breathing again.

- If the child is breathing and displays signs of life, such as coughing and movement, position him in the **recovery position** (for children: *see* page 27; for infants: *see* page 30).

- If the child has stopped breathing and shows no signs of life, administer **chest compressions** and **rescue breaths** (for children: *see* page 29; for infants: *see* page 31).

Unconsciousness as a result of a near-drowning incident

Near-drowning victims (*see also* pages 100–103) may be unconscious and will probably be unable to breathe as a result of having been under water.

WHAT TO DO

- Get the child out of the water immediately.

- Call an ambulance. It is imperative that you get help in all cases of near-drowning.

- If the child is not breathing **commence rescue breathing** without delay (for children: *see* page 28; for infants: *see* page 31).

- When the child is breathing again, position him in the **recovery position** (for children: *see* page 27; for infants: *see* page 30).

UNCONSCIOUS WITH A SUSPECTED NECK INJURY

If there is ANY possibility of a neck injury in an unconscious child who is not breathing, you must restore breathing without moving the head. To do this you must apply the jaw-thrust method: if the child is breathing, kneel behind him and gently cup its head between your palms, thumbs resting on the cheek bones and fingers touching the jaw, keeping head, neck and body aligned. Stay with the child, reassure and calm him if he is frightened, and ask the child not to move. Continue to gently support the head in alignment with neck and body, until medical assistance arrives.

PROCEDURES FOR RESUSCITATION

To be really useful and effective, first aid procedures must adhere to certain rules and be performed in a specific sequence. This section outlines the basic skills and proven step-by-step techniques that you must follow. To become adept at these you should join a recognized first aid course in your area, so that you can gain practical experience and become comfortable in the knowledge that you know what to do.

Normal breathing and blood circulation supply the body with oxygen and nutrients. These vital functions may become impaired, or fail completely during injury or acute illness, creating a serious condition that calls for immediate action.

Cardiopulmonary resuscitation (CPR) is a combination of rescue breathing and chest compressions designed to re-establish respiration and heartbeat. It consists of a practical set of skills that enable you to:
- ensure a clear airway
- assess adequacy of breathing and circulation
- provide oxygen to a child who is not breathing
- re-establish a heartbeat.

ESTABLISHING THE ABC

The ABC is what we focus on during all life-support procedures, and always in this sequence. It is very easy to remember this, the common purpose in life-support manoeuvres, as it ensures:

- **A**irway – the child has a clear anatomical channel through which to breathe.
- **B**reathing – oxygen can flow through the airway and into the lungs.
- **C**irculation – the blood carries oxygen from the lungs to all parts of the body.

Checking the airway

The airway extends from the mouth and nose down to the windpipe. A child's airway is narrower than an adult's – the smaller the child, the greater the risk of choking or suffocation. A child's airway may become obstructed by mucus; enlarged tonsils; food or solid matter that cannot be swallowed; and abnormal positioning of the head (as can happen if the child is unconscious).

The nerve reflex that stops food 'going down the wrong way' in adults is not completely developed in infants and toddlers, which is why they are so prone to **choking** (*see* page 32) and aspiration (that is, foreign objects going into the lungs).

A child's airway is also softer and more pliable than an adult's – therefore avoid compressing any part of the airway with your hands during resuscitation. Keep

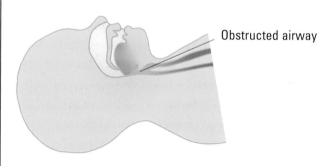

Obstructed airway

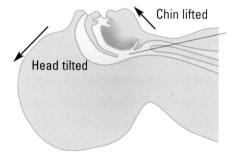

Chin lifted

Head tilted

Tilt head back and lift the chin to create an unobstructed passage to the lungs the child's head in a neutral position so that no part of the airway becomes stretched or kinked.

WHAT TO DO
- Open the airway (*see* **chin lift** page 22).

- Check that there is no obstruction by a foreign matter (*see* **choking** page 32).

Restoring breathing
Children breathe faster than adults – their bodies burn up oxygen at a faster rate. A child struggling to breathe will run out of energy sooner than an adult and may stop breathing quite suddenly when exhausted.

WHAT TO DO
- Restore the normal position of the tongue and the airway by using a combination of the **chin-lift and head-tilt** (for children: *see* page 28; for infants: *see* page 31).

- Carefully and gently feel in the mouth for foreign bodies and remove what you see (for children: *see* page 32; for infants: *see* page 34).

- When you have opened the airway the child may start breathing unaided. All that is necessary is to turn the casualty into the recovery position (for children: *see* page 27; for infants: *see* page 30) and ensure that the airway remains open until help arrives. If the casualty does not begin breathing normally, you should assume that the heart has stopped beating and commence resuscitation as described below.

- In children: give **30 chest compressions** (*see* page 29) followed by **2 rescue breaths** (*see* page 28). Repeat this sequence until the casualty begins breathing or help arrives.

- In infants: give **5 rescue breaths** (*see* page 31) followed by **30 chest compressions** (*see* page 31). Repeat this sequence for one minute. If by then, the child has not begun to breathe unaided, call for help, and continue the sequence. If there is another person present to assist, you can alternate cycles of **15 chest compressions** followed by **2 rescue breaths**.

BREATHING DIFFICULTIES
The following are possible indicators that a child with breathing difficulty is in need of urgent medical attention:
- increasing rate of breathing;
- noisy breathing or wheezing;
- visible flaring of the nostrils each time the child breathes in (in an infant, the use of these muscles may cause the head to bob up and down with each laboured intake of breath);
- sucking in of the muscles between the ribs each time the child breathes in;
- visible contraction of the neck muscles each time the child breathes in;
- the child's skin loses its healthy colour, turning mottled, dusky or pale;
- the skin, and fingers in particular, feel cold to your touch;
- the child has no interest in food or is too tired to eat or drink;
- the child becomes drowsy;
- rapid breathing suddenly slows, or becomes shallow.

• If the child begins to breathe unaided, place it in the recovery position (for children: *see* page 27; for infants: *see* page 30). Monitor its vital signs.

Assessing the circulation

The smaller the child, the faster the normal heart rate. Normally, the rate should fall within the ranges shown in the table below.

Measuring the heart rate by feeling the pulsation

NORMAL HEART RATE IN CHILDREN	
Age (in years)	Heartbeats per minute
under 1 year	110 – 160
2 – 5 years	95 – 140
5 – 12 years	80 – 120
over 12 years	60 – 100

of the transmitted heartbeat is the most objective and reliable means of assessing the state of the circulation in children and adults. However, it may be particularly difficult to locate the arterial pulse in small children, and we suggest that only trained health care providers rely on this technique in a child who has collapsed or is not breathing. Other physical signs which may indicate poor circulation or shock are listed in the box on the opposite page.

Regardless of whether you are able to feel a pulse or not, any child who is not breathing or shows no signs of life should receive chest compressions together with rescue breaths as described in detail on pages 26–31.

The most common cause of a raised pulse rate is fever, usually as a result of infection. a fast pulse rate in a child who has been injured should alert you to the possibility of blood loss or shock.

In babies with breathing difficulties, a pulse rate

below the normal range may indicate a severe lack of oxygen. Call a doctor or ambulance immediately and prepare to start basic life support.

WHAT TO DO

• In infants and small children the pulse is easily felt in the **brachial artery** (crook of the arm), in older children in the **carotid artery** (side of the neck). In a healthy child, you can feel the pulse of the **radial artery** (inside of wrist). In a sick child, the pulse here is often too weak to be reliable.

• The rhythm of the pulse should be regular and strong enough for you to feel easily.

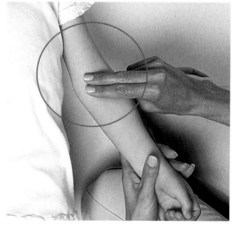

Location of the brachial artery inside the elbow.

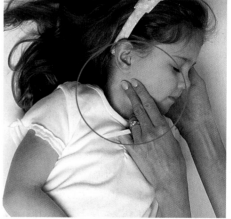

Location of carotid artery at the side of the neck.

PHYSICAL SIGNS THAT MAY INDICATE POOR CIRCULATION OR SHOCK

- The heart rate is faster or slower than the ranges indicated in the table on page 24.
- The pulse rhythm is irregular.
- The arterial pulse is weak or difficult to feel.
- The lips, tongue and mouth lining are pale or dusky instead of a healthy pink colour.
- The child's fingers are cold to your touch.
- The child becomes increasingly drowsy even in the absence of head injury.
- There is active bleeding from an injury to any part of the body.

- If you cannot detect a pulse at all and the heart has stopped beating restore circulation without delay using rhythmic chest compressions (for children: *see* page 29; for infants: *see* page 31).

What is 'shock'?

In medical terminology, 'shock' refers to any disorder of the blood circulation which interferes with the normal supply of oxygen and nutrients to the rest of the body, and in particular to the vital organs – the brain, kidneys, heart and lungs.

Bleeding and shock

Shock due to loss of blood requires urgent medical attention. In children, it most frequently results from injury to larger bones – particularly the pelvis – or to the liver and spleen, in which case bleeding may not be obvious at first glance. It is therefore vital that you assess the circulation to establish whether shock is developing, or already present.

Replacing fluid in shock: 'Mom, I'm thirsty!'

As a general rule, every injured child will complain of a dry mouth. This is part of the body's natural response to any form of injury – minor or major.
- If the child has a minor injury, offer him something to drink as a comfort rather than a necessity.

- If the child has been seriously injured, do not give him anything at all to eat or drink before he is assessed by a doctor.

WHAT TO DO

- Always call for help.

- Assess the child's ABC (by pulse rate and volume, skin colour and temperature).

- Exert firm pressure over bleeding wounds, using a sterile or clean dressing fixed in place with sticking plaster. Covering open wounds helps to reduce the risk of infection.

- Splint fractured bones (*see* pages 53–55). Splinting reduces pain and the risk of sharp bone fragments damaging blood vessels and nerves.

- To divert blood to the vital organs, raise the child's legs higher than the rest of the body using a firm cushion or a rolled-up blanket.

- Keep the child covered to reduce heat loss.

RESUSCITATION FOR CHILDREN 1–8 YEARS

The resuscitation procedure can be broken down into three major scenarios that you may encounter. It is important that you first assess which category the child falls into before you begin treating it.

For each of the 'What to do' scenarios on the following pages it is assumed that you have classified into the relevant and correct scenario. They may be categorized as follows:

(1) Unconscious - breathing - sign of life

(2) Unconscious - not breathing - no sign of life

Condition	Children 1–8 years of age
Unconscious breathing (*see* below)	Place in **recovery position** (*see* opposite) Call an ambulance Ensure airway remains open and that normal breathing continues
Unconscious not breathing no signs of life/ no circulation (*see* page 28)	Call an ambulance **Open the airway** (chin lift and head tilt – *see* page 28) Look, listen and feel for signs of breathing for 10 seconds If the child is not breathing normally, give 1 minute of CPR **Give 5 rescue breaths** Give **30 chest compressions** (*see* page 29) followed by **2 rescue breaths** (*see* page 28) Continue cycles of **2 breaths to 30 compressions** until breathing resumes or help arrives

SCENARIO 1 unconscious   breathing   signs of life/circulation

WHAT TO DO

• Place the child in the **recovery position** (*see* opposite).

• Call an ambulance.

• Ensure the airway remains open and that normal breathing continues.

UNCONSCIOUS CHILD (RECOVERY POSITION)

An unconscious child who is breathing unaided and has normal circulation should be placed in the recovery position. You need to put the child on her side to prevent the tongue from falling back, minimize the risk of vomit being sucked into the lungs and allow you to monitor her breathing and circulation as you wait for help. For treatment in case of suspected neck or spinal injury see page 59.

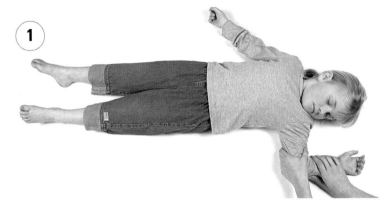

1 Angle the left arm next to the child's head at approximately 90°.

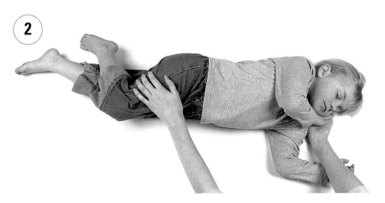

2 Position the left hand as shown and bring the right across her chest towards you to, palm showing out and the back of the hand resting against the right cheek. Bend the right leg at the knee as shown.

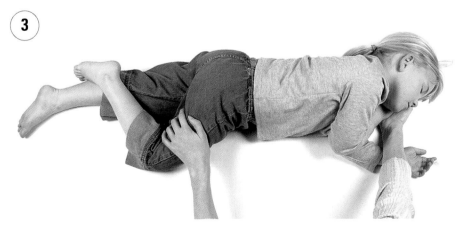

3 You can now move the child into the recovery position, your one hand stabilizing her head to protect her neck, while you use the other to bend her knee. Gently roll the trunk over. Ensure that her airway remains open and she continues to breathe normally.

SCENARIO 2   unconscious   not breathing   no signs of life/no circulation

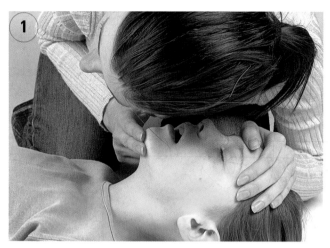

Gently lift the chin using two fingers of one hand while the other holds the head steady. Listen and feel for signs of normal breathing for 10 seconds.

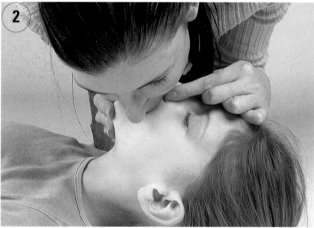

Maintaining the position of the head, gently pinch the child's nose shut. Place your mouth over the child's mouth and give 5 rescue breaths.

WHAT TO DO

- **Open the airway** (*see* step 1).

- Listen and look for **signs of normal breathing.** If the child is not breathing normally, give one minute of CPR (*see* below), then call an ambulance. If there is another person present then ask them to call an ambulance immediately.

- CPR: Open the airway. Remove any visible obstructions from the mouth and nose. Pinch the child's nose. Place your mouth over the child's mouth and attempt **5 initial rescue breaths** (*see* steps 2 and 3).

- Position your hand on the centre of their chest. Press down one third of the depth of the chest sing one or two hands, depending on the size of the child and your own size (*see* step 4).

- After every **30 chest compressions** give **2 breaths**.

- Continue with cycles of **30 chest compressions** and **2 rescue breaths** until emergency help arrives or the child begins to breathe normally.

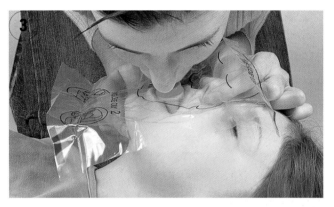

To use a **face shield**: place it over the child's face, filter in the mouth. Pinch its nose shut and breathe directly through the filter.

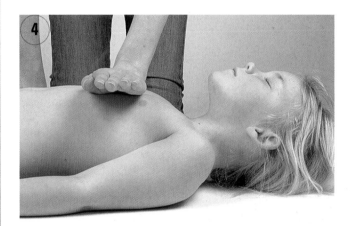

Using the heel of one hand, compress the chest to a depth of about 3cm (1in) in a quick movement. For every 30 chest compressions, give 2 rescue breaths. Do 100 compressions per minute, alternating with rescue breaths as described. Do this until the child is breathing normally, or until medical help arrives.

RESUSCITATION FOR INFANTS UP TO 12 MONTHS

The resuscitation procedure can be broken down into three major scenarios that you may encounter. It is important that you first assess which category the infant falls into before you begin treating it.

RECOVERY POSITION

Cradle the infant in your arms. Your one hand should support his head, holding it slightly below the rest of the body, while the other hand firmly supports the infant's back.

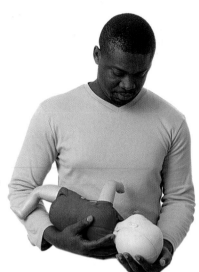

Condition	Infants 0–12 months of age
Unconscious breathing (*see* below)	Hold in **recovery position** (*see* above) Call an ambulance Ensure airway remains open and normal breathing continues
Unconscious not breathing signs of life/ circulation (*see* opposite)	Call an ambulance **Open the airway** (*see* opposite, step 1) and remove any visible obstruction from the mouth and nose Look, listen and feel for signs of breathing for 10 seconds Give **5 rescue breaths** Check the **circulation** (*see* page 24) – refer to Scenario 3 (*see* opposite) if necessary
Unconscious not breathing no signs of life/ no circulation (*see* opposite)	If no circulation or response to rescue breaths, give **30 chest compressions** (*see* opposite, step 4) Continue cycles of **2 breaths to 30 compressions** until breathing resumes or help arrives If normal breathing resumes place in **recovery position** (*see* above) and monitor carefully

SCENARIO 1   unconscious   breathing   signs of life/circulation

WHAT TO DO

• Place the infant in the **recovery position** (*see* top).

• Call an ambulance.

• Ensure the airway remains open and that normal breathing continues.

SCENARIO 2 unconscious · not breathing · signs of life/circulation

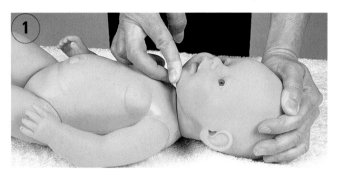

With one hand stabilize the infant's head. Tilt his chin up with the index finger of your other hand to open the airway.

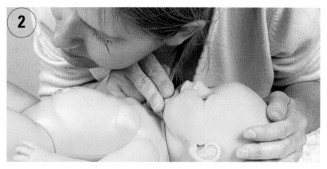

Listen for sounds of breathing for 10 seconds.

WHAT TO DO

- Call an ambulance.

- Open the airway and remove any visible obstruction from the mouth and nose. Give **5 rescue breaths** (*see* right) followed by **30 chest compressions** (*see* step 4).

- Continue with cycles of **30 chest compressions** and **2 rescue breaths** until emergency help arrives or the infant begins to breathe normally.

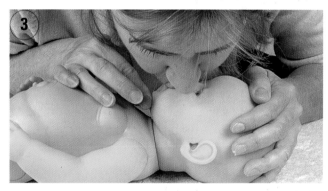

Then cover mouth and nose with yours and gently exhale.

SCENARIO 3 unconscious · not breathing · no signs of life/no circulation

WHAT TO DO

- Call an ambulance.

- Open airway and **give 5 rescue breaths**.

- **Using 2 fingers do 30 chest compressions** (at a rate of 100 per minute) to a depth of about 2cm (¾in).

- Give **2 rescue breaths for every 30 compressions** until breathing resumes or help arrives.

- If you are alone, do cycles of 2 breaths per 15 compressions for one minute. Call ambulance, taking the infant with you.

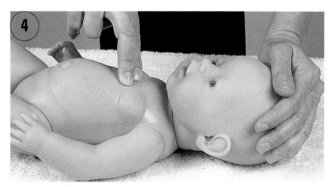

Position the infant on a firm flat surface. Trace a line between the infant's nipples and put your two fingertips on a spot about a finger below that line.

CHOKING

Choking results when the upper airway is obstructed, commonly as a result of food or a small object becoming impacted. In some cases, a coughing spell may be enough to expel the foreign body and clear the airway. However, even small objects can lodge firmly in the narrow airway of an infant or small child, in which case you may have to use the techniques described on these pages.

Common sites of airway obstruction

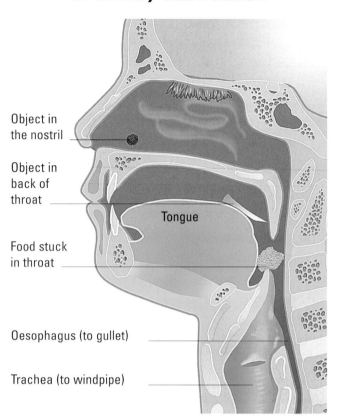

Object in the nostril

Object in back of throat

Tongue

Food stuck in throat

Oesophagus (to gullet)

Trachea (to windpipe)

FIRST AID FOR CHOKING CHILDREN 1–8 YEARS

Condition	Children 1–8 years of age
Suspected choking	If coughing, encourage cough and monitor carefully Up to 5 back blows – check the mouth and remove any obstruction Up to 5 abdominal thrusts – check the mouth and remove any obstruction Do 3 cycles of back blows and abdominal thrusts If breathing: **open airway** and remove visible foreign matter (*see* page 28) place in **recovery position** (*see* page 27) If unconscious or not breathing, commence **resuscitation sequence** (*see* page 28)

Use a combination of back blows and abdominal thrusts for small children who show signs of choking and are unable to breathe or cough up the foreign body themselves. **Do 3 cycles of the entire procedure then call an ambulance if there is no improvement**. If still unsuccessful, begin resuscitation (*see* pages 26–29). You can stand, sit or kneel behind the child to perform these procedures.

BACK BLOWS – WHAT TO DO

- Stand or knee behind the child.

- Give up to five sharp back blows between the shoulder blades with the heel of your hand.

- Check the mouth for any obstructions and remove without probing blindly.

- If there is no relief, do 5 abdominal thrusts.

ABDOMINAL THRUSTS – WHAT TO DO

- If back blows are ineffective in clearing the obstruction, do up to 5 abdominal thrusts.

- Place one fist on the child's abdomen, cover it with your free palm and then thrust firmly inwards and upwards up to five times.

- If the casualty begins to breathe again unaided, carefully check the mouth and clear away any visible foreign object.

- If there is no relief after 3 cycles of back blows and abdominal thrusts **call an ambulance**.

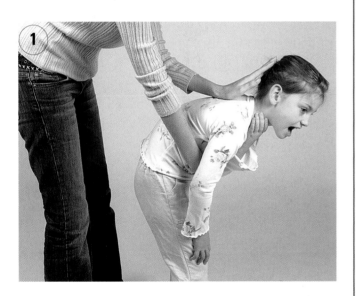

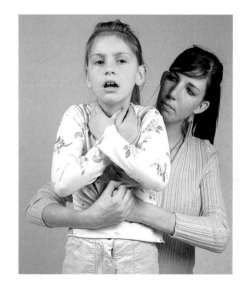

FIRST AID FOR CHOKING INFANTS 1–12 MONTHS

Condition	Infants 0–12 months of age
Suspected choking	If coughing, encourage cough and monitor carefully Up to 5 back blows – check the mouth and remove any obstruction Up to 5 chest thrusts – check the mouth and remove any obstruction Do 3 cycles of back blows and chest thrusts If breathing: **open airway** and remove visible foreign matter (*see* page 30) hold in **recovery position** (*see* page 30) If unconscious or not breathing, commence **resuscitation sequence** (*see* page 31)

Use a combination of back blows and chest thrusts for choking infants. **Do 3 cycles of the entire procedure, then call an ambulance if there is no improvement**. If unsuccessful, begin resuscitation (*see* pages 30–31). **NOTE: NEVER DO ABDOMINAL THRUSTS ON AN INFANT.**

BACK BLOWS – WHAT TO DO

• Hold the infant face down on your forearm, and tilted head-down. Rest your arm on your thigh for extra support.

• Using the flat palm of your free hand, deliver up to 5 back blows on the infant's back.

• Turn the infant over onto your other arm. Carefully and gently check his mouth and remove any foreign object.

• If this does not help, do chest thrusts.

CHEST THRUSTS – WHAT TO DO

• Turn the infant face-up, with his head lower than his hips, supported on your forearm.

• With the tips of two fingers, give 5 chest thrusts over the breastbone (depress about 2cm; ¾in). Thrusts should be aimed downwards and be about three seconds apart.

• Check the mouth. If the infant does not breathe after 3 cycles, call an ambulance immediately.

NEVER DO ABDOMINAL THRUSTS ON AN INFANT

SAFETY IN THE HOME

Your home should be a place of happiness, your sanctuary, a shelter from the elements and a place where your personal history will unfold as your family grows. Accidents can – and do – happen, but you can lower the odds considerably by applying a few general safety precautions. No hi-tech equipment is needed; all you need to safeguard the happiness and health of your family is dedication, vigilance and some common sense.

The majority of childhood accidents occur in and around the home – the place we think is safest. This is hardly surprising. Home is where children spend most of their early lives, begin to move about and discover the world around them – finding out how it looks, feels, tastes, smells and sounds. This incredible journey of discovery is one that even the most docile child must undertake. The little rascal who scurries around the living room grabbing, tugging and sticking everything into his mouth is often labelled 'naughty', but this behaviour is a vital part of his normal development.

We cannot stop our children from finding things out for themselves – and of course we should not. This section will help you see your home with new eyes and recognize common hazards for the developing child. It discusses some basic safety devices and strategies for minimizing the risk of injury while still allowing your growing child the much-needed freedom to explore.

Your adventurous child needs supervision to keep him out of trouble. For all children, particularly infants and toddlers, the most important safety device is the one you cannot buy – the watchful eye of a responsible adult. Think of it as SUPER VISION – your eye always on the child, whatever tasks you may be juggling, even if the doorbell chimes, the phone rings and the pot on the stove boils over all at the same time. Never leave your infant or child alone anywhere.

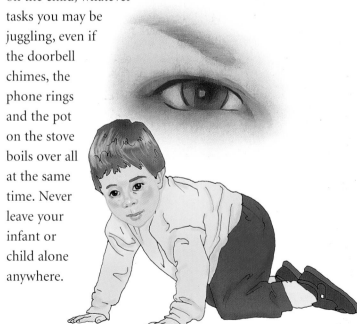

If you are still planning your family, the quickest way to identify safety hazards in your home is to invite a friend or family member to bring her own one-year-old bundle of joy over and let her loose. Within an hour you will know exactly where the problems areas are. But if your nerves are not made of tempered steel, following these 10 suggestions might be less harrowing.

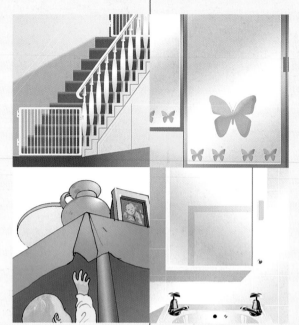

Do not throw anything that might be harmful to your child into an open bin or container. Assume that your child, particularly when he is at the crawling stage, will be fascinated by whatever the bin holds and want to shove it directly into his mouth.

Store poisonous substances in locked cupboards or on high shelves that cannot be reached – in the lounge (liquor cabinets), kitchen, bathroom and garage or workshop.

Make sure that all poisonous or harmful substances are packaged in bottles or containers which are clearly labelled with stickers. Never decant poisons into old food or drink containers while there are small children in the home. Ask your pharmacist to dispense all medicines and tablets in childproof containers, and keep these in a wall-mounted medicine chest out of children's reach.

Avoid table covers that a toddler may tug, bringing everything on the tabletop crashing down.

Keep sharp items such as scissors, letter openers and metal kitchen utensils out of sight and out of reach, preferably in locked drawers.

Prevent infants and toddlers from gaining access to solid foodstuffs, toy parts or any objects small enough to fit into their mouths, noses or ears. The smaller the child, the less able she is to spit or cough them out, so there is a high risk of airway obstruction, choking and suffocation. For this reason too the toddler's toys should be the right kind for her age, with no small parts that come off, and not made of materials that might be poisonous if chewed. Only buy toys tested and approved by the national standards bureau operating in your country.

Keep matches, lighters and burning cigarettes well away from children. (And keep unlit cigarettes away from them too.)

Block off all staircases by installing safety gates at the top and bottom. These should comply with national standards for their height and the spacing of their bars – not more than 6cm (2½ in) apart. These gates can be removed once your youngest child is walking confidently enough to negotiate stairs without danger.

Mark large panes of glass in windows or doors with bright stickers. Small children at play may become so absorbed in chasing each other around the house that they will not notice the difference between glass and fresh air.

Never carry a cup of tea or any other hot liquid in one hand while using the other hand to hold, carry or nurse a baby or small child. The time you save by 'multi-tasking' is not worth the risk of stumbling and scalding the child.

SETTING A GOOD EXAMPLE

Like all other habits (good and bad), children learn safe behaviour from their significant role models – older siblings, teachers and, most of all, you, the parent. If you wear a seat belt without fail you will have no trouble getting your children to do the same. To punish children for taking the same risks they have seen you take regularly is not only counterproductive, it confuses them, and eats away at the trust which is such an important element of family relationships. So try to set a good example.

Electrical safety

Particularly if your house is more than 25 years old, ask an electrical contractor to check the wiring and to ensure that the circuit-breakers are functioning properly. In addition, ask your electrician to install as many power points as you need in any room or space, rather than mounting multi-plug adaptors on top of one another. Keep exposed wiring and extension cords to a minimum, and ensure that the insulation layer is not frayed or cracked at any point.

Do not buy any electrical appliances that have not been approved by the testing authority in your country. These are seldom properly tested, or adapted for the electrical supply in your country. As a result, they may overheat, or damage the electrical circuits in your home. What appears at first to be a bargain may cost a lot more in the long run, as well as being hazardous to your family.

Make sure that supply cords from table lamps, kettles and other appliances are only as long as is

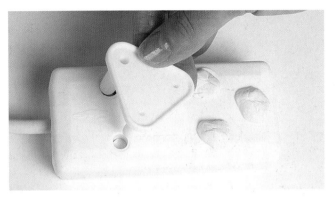

Whether you use two- or three-pronged plugs, cover unused points to deter prying fingers.

necessary, and that they are well concealed. Small children just love to give these a yank. Why? To see what will happen, of course!

Cover all unused electric power points. Inexpensive safety covers are available from child safety organizations and electrical retailers. Alternatively, unconnected two-point or three-point plugs secured in place with a blob of mouldable non-toxic adhesive will do just as well.

Unplug any household electric appliance that is not in use and store it in a safe place. Switch off all electric power points not in use.

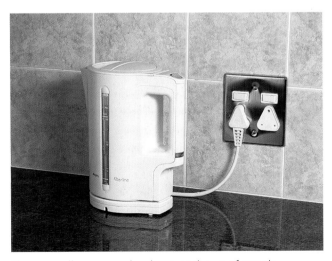

Keep appliance cords short and out of reach.

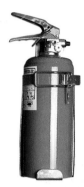

Fire safety

Fire in the home is one of a parent's greatest fears, and so it should be. It threatens life and limb of the entire family and has the power to destroy everything you hold dear, in an instant. It can start at any point in the home where enough heat is generated – from unprotected flames, defective or overloaded electrical circuits, the stove, leaking gas that ignites, or heaters standing too close to flammable materials. Besides this, non-flammable materials that do not actually ignite when heated can still generate enough smoke to cause serious injury or death from inhalation of smoke or toxic chemicals.

Safety tips: dealing with fire hazards at home

- Install a wall-mounted fire extinguisher in your kitchen, at a level where children cannot reach it, and get it serviced regularly.
- Install fireguards (below) around open wood, coal or gas fires. Do not hang clothing or anything else on the fireguard – this only creates another fire hazard.
- Fit at least one approved smoke detector per level in a multi-storey house. In a single-level house, install the detector just outside your kitchen. Check the batteries at least once a year.

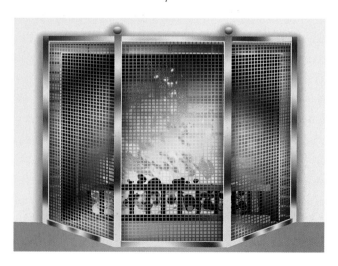

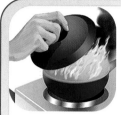

POTS ON FIRE

If hot oil on your stove bursts into flame, do not move the pot or pour water over it, and do not attack it with the fire extinguisher – this will just cause burning oil to splash everywhere. Cover the pot with a snug-fitting lid or wooden breadboard to kill the flames by starving them of oxygen, and switch off the gas or power supply. Do not disturb the pot until it has completely cooled. Consider baking potato chips in the oven instead – it is healthier and safer!

- Avoid electric bar heaters and space heaters, which are difficult to child-proof. Closed-system heaters fuelled by gas, anthracite or oil are safer.
- Clean ovens regularly so there is no old dripped food in them that might catch fire.
- Ban smoking in bedrooms (and preferably everywhere indoors).
- Train children to keep their distance from heaters and open fires, particularly if their night clothes are made of flammable materials.
- Do not light outdoor fires closer than 5m (15ft) to your house. Avoid open outdoor fires when the wind is blowing, particularly in dry weather. Never coax a smouldering fire by pouring lighter fuel or any other flammable liquid over it.
- Designate one outside door as the best escape route in the event of fire. If the worst happens, grab your children, cover their mouths and noses with handkerchiefs or other material to reduce smoke inhalation, and get out.

Water safety

Children love playing with water – it attracts them like a magical force. Next time you enjoy a summer's day at the beach, look out for any young mother with a toddler. You will see how she battles to keep her little bundle of energy from charging off toward the water's edge again and again – and you will understand that where water is concerned, the cardinal safety rule is SUPERVISION. Nothing substitutes for an adult's watchful eye.

Never leave small children alone near water – a fish pond, splash pool, lake or the sea – or even a full washing bucket. It does not matter if the water is shallow at all points. Small children can drown in water no deeper than 2.5cm (1in) – just enough to cover the mouth and nose.

Even children who have been taught to swim should be closely supervised in water until the age of eight. Smaller children should never enter a swimming pool enclosure without a flotation device, even if you are holding them in the pool. Whatever device you prefer to use should be snug-fitting, age-appropriate, and approved by your national standards authority. Children under 12 months of age lose heat very quickly in unheated water and should not be in a pool for more than 15 minutes at a time.

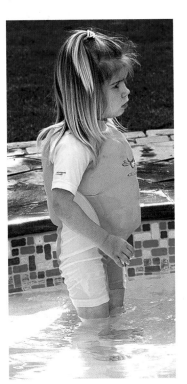
Flotation devices are essential for small children.

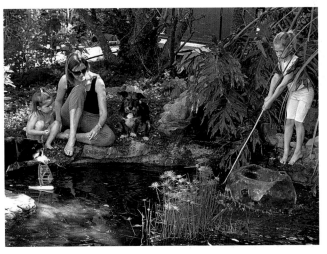
Never leave small children alone near water.

Swimming pool safety

In most countries it is a legal requirement to provide secure fencing around domestic swimming pools, and to ensure that the enclosure satisfies set measurements and other criteria. The following specifications are common to legislation in almost all countries where such laws are in place, but please check with your local authority or county council that your fence is 100% in keeping with the regional or national laws or by-laws.

- All swimming pool fences should be 1.2m (4ft) in height at all points, with no gaps of more than 10cm (4in) above ground level.
- Gaps between vertical poles should be no more than 10cm (4in).
- Gates should be the same height as the fence, automatically self-closing and self-latching, and open outward (away from the pool) to prevent children pushing their way through an unlatched gate.
- Gate latches should be a minimum of 1.2m (4ft) from the ground if on the inside of the gate and 1.5m (5ft) from the ground if on the outside.
- Gates should always be closed.
- There should be nothing near or leaning against the pool fence to tempt children to climb over.

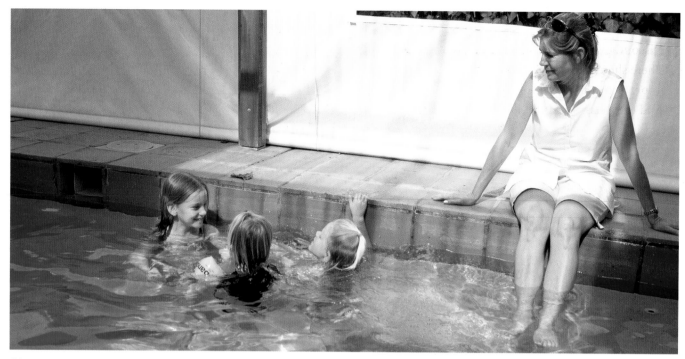

Always ensure an adult is present when children are playing in and around a swimming pool.

- Pool nets and covers are not a substitute for adult supervision or proper fences. Non-permeable pool covers collect rainwater and may themselves become drowning hazards.
- Do not permit children to play games inside a fenced swimming pool enclosure.
- Inflatable pools should be emptied immediately after use and deflated. All other portable pools should be stored upside down when not in use.

Buy only pool chemicals with childproof lids. Store them in a secure cupboard or tool shed, and not next to the pool. All pool chemicals are highly concentrated and lethal if swallowed.

If you install a swimming pool or a spa in your home, be prepared to deal with water accidents. Read the chapters on basic life support (*see* pages 20–34), and take a recognized CPR (cardiopulmonary resuscitation) course. Remember, quick action saves lives. If your child goes missing from the house, check the pool first.

Bathroom safety

The bathroom can be a very risky place, especially for small children whose inquisitive natures can lead to all sorts of unforeseen mishaps and disasters. Follow these sensible tips to protect your child against scalding, falls on hard, slippery surfaces, and drowning.

- Fill bath tubs only as deep as necessary in order to wash the child.
- When you are filling the bath tub, run the cold water before the hot, not hot first or both at the same time.
- Always check the bathwater temperature carefully before placing the child in the tub.
- Set the hot water thermostats of your hot water geyser to a maximum of 54°C (120°F) to prevent the risk of scalding.
- Position your child so that you can wash him at the end furthest away from taps – to prevent hot water dripping onto the child.

- Place a non-slip rubber mat in the tub.
- Discourage toddlers from standing in the tub.
- There should be no portable electrical appliances or unprotected electrical sockets in the bathroom.
- And once again, do not leave small children alone in the bath tub, not even for a second.

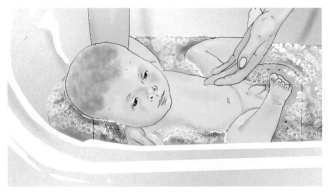

To prevent accidents, always place a non-slip rubber mat in a bath for babies or small children.

Kitchen safety

For many families, the kitchen is the heart of the home, particularly in the colder months. You may often have to prepare food or wash dishes while keeping an eye on children. If you follow these recommendations your child will be able to share the aromas and excitement of kitchen activity without being exposed to risk.

- High chairs keep infants and toddlers out of danger while allowing them to remain close to you in the kitchen. Ensure the child is securely harnessed in the chair to prevent him slipping under the tray and falling out.
- When cooking food, keep pot and pan handles turned away from the edge of the stove (right), and if possible use the back rings or plates.
- Store knives and other sharp cutlery and glass and breakable crockery in cupboards that are well out of a small child's reach. Any floor-level cupboards which contain dangerous or poisonous items should be self-locking or fitted with secure child-proof latches.
- Keep plastic shopping bags, garbage bags and any other plastic sheeting collected for recycling locked away well out of children's reach to prevent accidental suffocation.
- Kettles should ideally be cordless or have the shortest possible cords, which are less likely to droop over the edge of the kitchen counter.

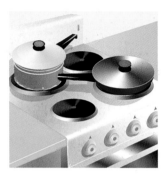

Be cautious about using microwave ovens, or allowing children to use them, to heat food or drinks. If unsure of how long to heat the food, or what power setting to use, always err on the side of caution. Lukewarm food may not be all that palatable, but a burnt mouth is agony! Always use appropriate containers that do not absorb too much heat. Before serving the food, stir it well to distribute heat evenly, and taste a mouthful yourself before serving it to your child.

SKIN AND SOFT-TISSUE INJURIES

Many minor injuries can be treated at home and require little more than a first-aid kit. Minor skin wounds that are correctly treated usually heal quickly, and with hardly any scarring. Cuts, scrapes and bruises are common as long as there are children of any age in the home, leading healthy, active lives. These injuries may be caused by sharp objects (kitchen equipment, tools, and so on), bites, falls, or bumps against solid objects.

BUMPS AND BRUISES

A bruise (or haematoma) can occur from a fall onto a hard surface, bumps against walls or furniture, or the blow of a cricket bat or ball. Although the skin is not broken, the blunt, high-energy impact ruptures small veins, causing mild bleeding – the greyish-brown blotch you see under the skin. As the dead blood cells are broken down by the body's natural defences, the bruise changes colour from brown to green and yellow over five to seven days, before disappearing completely within seven to 10 days.

➕ **FIRST AID** Limit bleeding and swelling by immediately applying a cold compress (ice blocks wrapped in a cloth, or a bag of frozen peas) to the injured area. Give a mild painkiller such as paracetamol (acetaminophen) if the bruise begins to throb. Unless the overlying skin is broken, bruises rarely become infected, and dressings are of little benefit.

MAKING A COLD COMPRESS

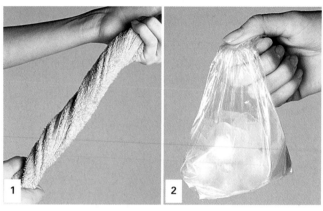

Wet and wring a towel.   Put ice in a plastic bag.

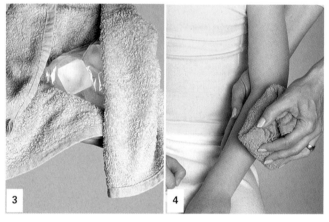

Wrap ice in the towel.   Apply to injured area.

Dark-skinned children may be more prone to the formation of keloid scars, which are prominent, and often out of proportion to the extent of the injury, even where treatment has been faultless. It is usually not possible to prevent keloid formation, but steroid injections or cosmetic surgery may be helpful for scars which are very large or unsightly.

A black eye

This is most often caused by a sporting injury or a punch. The blunt impact causes rapid bruising around the eye, particularly in the eyelid, which often swells to obscure the eye completely.

✚ FIRST AID The bruising may be reduced by immediately applying a cold compress to the eye socket for a few minutes. However, it is more important to ensure that the eye and the surrounding bone are not damaged. Any child with bruising covering up the eye should be examined by a doctor. (*See also* Eye Injuries, pages 61–63.)

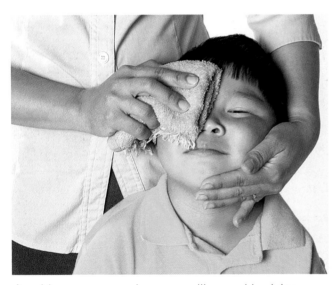

A cold compress reduces swelling and bruising.

Bruised fingernails

Bruising can occur under a fingernail or toenail (subungual haematoma) crushed between hard surfaces or objects. Blood collects under the nail, which turns an unsightly blue-black colour. Because the blood supply to the base of the nail is often disturbed, the nail will usually fall off over time and be replaced by a new one.

Treating a bruised fingernail

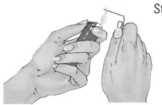

Straighten a paperclip, leaving one right-angle bend. Heat one end over a flame until it glows red-hot.

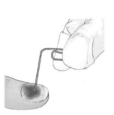

Press the hot end of the clip gently on the middle of the blackened nail. When you feel the nail 'give', remove the clip and allow blood to escape through the hole.

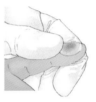

Massage the nail gently to improve drainage. Note: there is no value in performing this procedure more than once.

✚ FIRST AID Bruised fingernails do not usually need medical attention. However, you can reduce the chance of the nail being lost by draining the blood out, using the easy, painless method shown above. The sooner you drain the blood, the more likely the nail is to survive.

Children who bruise easily

Few perfectly healthy children survive childhood without some bruises. However, be concerned about any child who seems to bruise very easily or often, or where the bruise is bigger than you would expect from the injury. A small number of children have inherited bleeding disorders or skin abnormalities that predispose to easy or excessive bruising, even after minor injuries. If your child fits this description, seek a medical opinion as soon as possible. (*See also* Blood Spots under the Skin, page 139.)

Always seek medical attention for:

- scalp bruises in babies and small children, as there is a possibility of underlying skull fracture;
- bruises with severe pain on movement, suggesting a possible underlying fracture;
- a black eye (bruising around the eye socket);
- straddle injuries, with bruising to the thighs and genital area (the bruise can become quite large, compressing the bladder outlet and making it difficult for the child to urinate);
- children who appear to bruise easily or excessively after a minor injury.

OPEN WOUNDS

Open wounds are ones where there is a break in the skin. Once the skin barrier is disturbed, bacteria can invade and there is a risk of infection. To prevent infection, you need to clean germs and dirt out of the wound, and keep them out, so your first-aid priority is to treat all open wounds as quickly and thoroughly as possible with simple hygienic measures: washing, cleaning and dressing.

FIRST AID **Step 1: Washing**

Bleeding is the body's own way of washing germs and dirt out of a fresh wound. The first-aid provider's task is to continue the good work by washing with water and a dilute antiseptic solution (for example, Savlon™, Dettol™ or similar). Even if you cannot see dirt particles in the wound, assume they are there and need to be washed out. Injured arms, legs, hands or feet can be washed easily and adequately under a cold-water tap. Simply let the running water wash freely over the wound for two minutes. Wounds on all parts of the body can be washed with cotton wool, or a clean cloth dipped in weak antiseptic solution.

Pure concentrated antiseptic is very painful when applied to raw wounds; it should always be diluted according to the manufacturer's instructions.

Bear in mind that the red pigment inside blood cells (haemoglobin) acts like a strong dye, so that even 5ml (a teaspoonful) of blood will colour a basin of water red. Unless blood is pumping quickly out of the wound, try not to let this dramatic picture worry you or your child too much. If the wound continues to bleed briskly after washing, apply direct pressure to it for two minutes with one or two clean gauze pads before proceeding to the next step.

Step 2: Cleaning

Each tiny particle of dirt or foreign matter increases the risk of infection in an open wound. Dirt left in it may also cause permanent 'tattooing' underneath the new layer of skin. So your second task is to carefully remove all dirt or foreign matter visible in the wound after washing.

First wipe the wound gently but firmly with a clean soft kitchen sponge dipped in dilute antiseptic solution. Then, using a clean pair of tweezers from your first-aid kit, pick out any ingrained dirt which remains. Scan the entire wound carefully – particularly if it is a large abrasion – for bits of soil, clothing or any foreign matter which can be easily removed without tugging or causing the child excessive pain.

Wounds with deeply ingrained soil or dirt which is difficult to remove in this way might require cleaning under a general anaesthetic. In such cases, cover the wound with a clean dressing and take the child to the nearest clinic or hospital.

Cleaning and dressing a wound

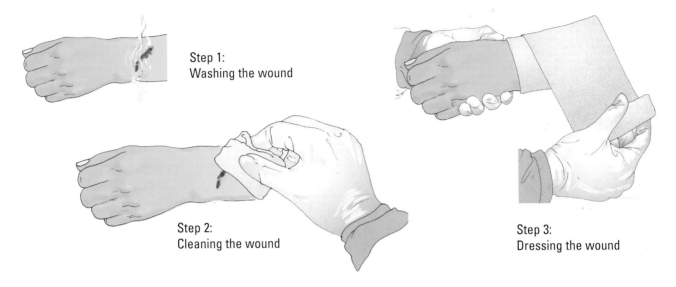

Step 1:
Washing the wound

Step 2:
Cleaning the wound

Step 3:
Dressing the wound

Step 3: Dressing

The main purpose of a dressing is to protect a fresh wound from re-injury, or becoming dirty or infected as the child resumes a normal level of activity. Tiny cuts and abrasions that are not actively bleeding may safely be left open, lightly dabbed with mercuro-chrome (no longer approved by the Food and Drug Administration in the United States) or antiseptic ointment or cream (for example, Savlon™, Dettol™ or Betadine™). But your child may insist you cover it with an adhesive plaster (for example, Band-Aid™) which will promptly be shown off to friends as proof of immense courage!

What to use

Most dressings have two components: a non-sticky pad or swab to cover the wound, and a secure bandage or adhesive plaster to keep the pad in place. Paraffin-impregnated gauze (Jelonet™) is a versatile dressing for any raw surface of skin. It conforms to the shape of the body surface, and comes away easily when removed. A single layer of paraffin gauze is sufficient to cover most wounds.

Do not use cotton wool to dress raw wounds because the fibres will become embedded in the scab, and removal may be very painful.

Do not encircle a finger, arm or leg with any tight plaster or bandage which could interfere with the blood supply. If the child complains of persistent pain, this could indicate that the dressing is too tight and it should be removed immediately.

Persistently brisk bleeding may be caused by a torn artery. If bleeding does not stop with direct pressure, cover the wound with a thick dressing secured with adhesive plaster, and take the child to your family doctor, or to hospital.

What size should the dressing be?

The dressing need only be big enough to cover the wound, and thick enough to remain dry (free of blood) on the surface. The bulkier the dressing, the more likely it is to come loose and need replacing within minutes or hours.

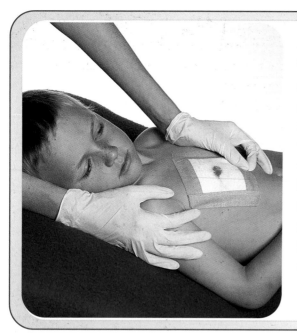

Whether you manage to clean a wound as described on page 44 will depend on how co-operative the child is. All soft-tissue injuries hurt, but each child experiences pain in his own individual way. Never feel obliged to try to cope on your own with a child who cannot be consoled, or struggles against you. It is better for all concerned to cover the wound with a clean dressing, and seek the assistance of a doctor or nurse. Let them deal with the injury, while you focus your energy on providing reassurance and comfort to the child.

Lotions

Spread a layer of antiseptic cream or ointment over abraded or raw skin before applying the dressing, which will prevent it sticking to the wound and make removal easier. If you have no medicated creams or ointments, a dab of plain petroleum jelly (Vaseline™) will do as well.

Never apply any powdered substances, foodstuffs or household cleaning agents to an open wound. Use only what is recommended here, or else nothing at all.

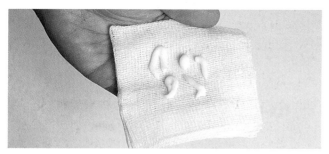

Apply antiseptic ointment to the dressing to help prevent infection.

Keeping the wound dry

Do your best to keep a fresh wound free of moisture for at least 48 hours.

How long do I leave the dressing on?

There is no hard-and-fast rule about how long a dressing should remain in place. You need not change it every day; doing so will disturb the scab, causing unnecessary discomfort and bleeding and delaying healing. However, a dressing that becomes wet, dirty, blood-soaked or tattered should be replaced. Dressings that remain clean and intact can be removed after seven days, and only replaced if the wound still appears raw.

How do I remove the dressing?

Many children dread this more than anything else. Your child may insist on removing the dressing herself. Let her do it if she wants to – even if it takes her a long time. If a dressing sticks fast to the wound, simply let her soak it in the bath tub for about 15 minutes. It will probably float off, or come away with a gentle tug.

SCRAPES AND ABRASIONS

An abrasion is a scrape that has shaved off some outer layers of the skin, and is deep enough to cause bleeding. Because tiny nerve endings just under the skin are damaged by the injury, abrasions can be particularly painful, depending on their size and depth.

 FIRST AID Wash and clean abrasions as described on page 44 to reduce the chance of infection and 'tattooing'. If the scrape occurred through the child's clothing, or on a sandy or grimy surface, fabric or dirt will be embedded in the damaged skin.

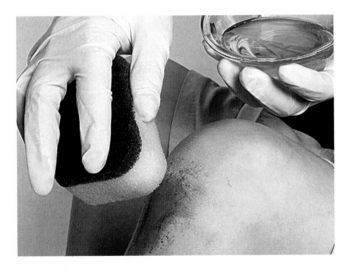

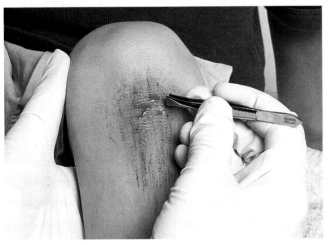

 Always seek medical attention if:

- the child requires an anti-tetanus booster (*see* Tetanus, page 50);
- there is excessive bleeding;
- there is deeply ingrained dirt in the wound;
- the wound is too painful for you to clean adequately.

Lacerations

A child's skin is delicate and can easily be lacerated (cut or torn) by sharp objects or blunt impact.

 FIRST AID Wash and clean the wound as indicated on page 44. If a flap of skin has been lifted over the cut, wash and clean well underneath the flap. If necessary, reduce or stop bleeding by applying pressure with a clean gauze pad for a few minutes. Clean, superficial cuts can be dressed with a small adhesive plaster as described in Step 3: Dressing, on page 45.

Always seek medical attention if:

- the child requires an anti-tetanus booster (*see* Tetanus, page 50);
- the wound gapes and may need stitches;
- there is a lot of dirt or other foreign matter visible in the wound;
- the laceration involves the hand;
- the laceration involves the scalp, an eye or the lips;
- there is a deep laceration on the chest or abdomen.

Left top: Gently clean the graze with a sponge dipped in a diluted antiseptic solution.

Left: Use tweezers to remove any pieces of dirt and grit from the wound.

PUNCTURE WOUNDS

These deserve special mention because of the higher risk of infection, particularly if they occur on the hand. Any domestic tools, cutlery or similar sharp objects that puncture the skin with force may cause considerable damage to the flesh, as well as injecting dirt deep under the skin. These wounds need to be washed out and possibly opened under anaesthetic to ensure all foreign matter is cleaned out.

Puncture wounds on the chest or abdominal wall may have damaged an underlying organ and should always be assessed by a doctor.

FIRST AID Wash the wound under an open tap for two minutes before covering it with a clean dressing. Puncture wounds should be examined by a doctor as soon as possible as they carry a risk of tetanus infection (*see* Tetanus, page 50).

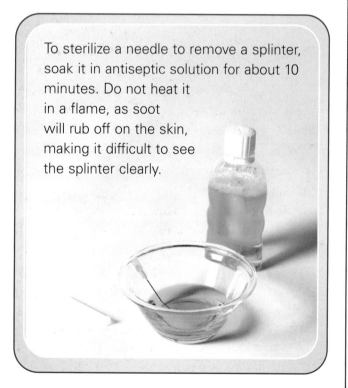

To sterilize a needle to remove a splinter, soak it in antiseptic solution for about 10 minutes. Do not heat it in a flame, as soot will rub off on the skin, making it difficult to see the splinter clearly.

SPLINTERS, FOREIGN OBEJCTS

Thorns or fine splinters of wood, metal or glass can easily become embedded in the soft skin of the soles of little feet, or fingertips. Even the tiniest splinters will sting, particularly if they get into the weight-bearing part of the foot. The discomfort and the risk of infection are two good reasons to do your best to remove the objects.

FIRST AID Only try to remove splinters or foreign bodies you can see. Those projecting outside the surface of the skin can be gripped with a pair of tweezers and pulled out. Wash and clean the skin well afterward with antiseptic solution.

Tiny splinters or thorns that poke out of the skin but are difficult to grip can be removed by wetting the skin and gently rubbing it with a pumice stone. Do not rub back and forth but only in the direction the splinter appears to be pointing.

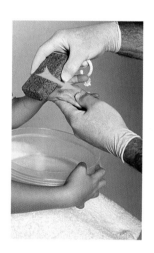

If the object is completely embedded under the skin, but still visible, soak the area in dilute antiseptic solution for at least 10 minutes to soften the outer layer of skin, making it easier to tease the splinter out. Using a steril-

Gently rub in the direction the splinter is pointing.

ized sewing needle, gently scratch away at the softened skin over the splinter. Once you can grip the end of the splinter with your tweezers, gently pull it out, taking care not to bend or break it. This method is not very painful, but requires the child's cooperation. If she is very anxious, or struggles against you, rather seek medical assistance.

Do not try to remove larger penetrating objects such as twigs, shards of glass or metal fragments which become deeply embedded in the soft tissues. Take the child to hospital immediately, as it may be necessary to take X-rays, or remove the object under a general anaesthetic. Deep penetrating wounds usually require an anti-tetanus booster as well.

BITES

Animal and human bites break the skin, crush underlying tissues and inject saliva, which always contains bacteria. This combination of factors creates a high risk of infection, particularly with bites by rodents, cats and humans, and especially with any bite to the hand.

+ FIRST AID   The key to preventing infection is rapid and thorough cleaning of the wound. Wash the wound as described on page 44. Then cover it with a clean dressing and take the child to a doctor or your nearest hospital immediately. The risk of tetanus and other infections rises with each hour of delay before treatment, so all bites that break the skin must be treated by a doctor without delay. If the wound is a large one, it may have to be cleaned under a general anaesthetic, so do not give the child anything to eat or drink after the injury.

An anti-tetanus booster may be necessary. Antibiotics may be prescribed to combat other bacterial infections, so make sure you tell the doctor if you know your child has an allergy, particularly to penicillin or other drugs.

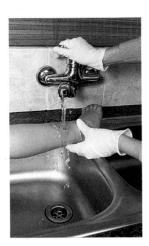

Run tap water over a bite wound to clean it.

Rabies

Bites caused by stray or wild animals, or domestic animals that are acting strangely, might carry a risk of rabies. Make sure to tell the doctor who treats the bite if you have any suspicions about the animal.

Preventing animal bites

Having a domesticated animal for a pet is one of the great joys of childhood. However, make sure your choice of pet is suitable for your child's age, the size of your home and how much time you have to care for the animal. Dogs, cats and domesticated rodents such as rabbits, hamsters and guinea pigs obtained from reputable pet shops or dealers will seldom act aggressively as long as they are disease-free and properly cared for. Dogs, however, particularly larger breeds, need regular exercise, and will become aggressive if kept indoors or restricted to a small garden all day.

Follow these guidelines to decrease the risk of bites and other injuries.

- Some classes and breeds of dogs are more suitable than others for families with small children. To help you make an appropriate choice, seek the advice of a reputable breeder recommended by a kennel club. Ensure pets are vaccinated against common diseases as recommended by your vet or the breeder.
- Unless you have experience in training animals, take your new dog to an obedience class with a professional trainer. Learn to control the dog instead of having him control you.
- All dogs should be neutered, unless bought specifically for breeding purposes.
- Never leave babies or toddlers unsupervised with any animal – even your own pets.
- Consult your veterinary surgeon about any animal that seems to be ill or behaves abnormally.
- A child with a fresh wound on any part of the body should not have physical contact with pets until the wound is properly healed.

- Encourage children to wash their hands after playing with the pet.
- Teach them to keep away from stray animals, and never to provoke dogs – especially those restrained on leads, in cages, or behind fences.

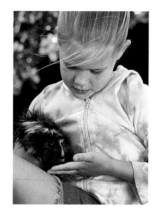

Tetanus

Always wash hands after handling animals.

Tetanus (lockjaw) is a life-threatening infection. The bacterial organism responsible (*Clostridium tetani*) is found in all types of dirt and soil and is particularly widespread in manure and other animal waste. Once it enters the human body through an open wound it targets the spinal cord, releasing a toxin that causes severe muscle spasms and breathing difficulty. Death can occur from heart or lung failure.

Tetanus is very difficult to treat as it does not respond to antibiotics once symptoms appear. Children are routinely immunized against it by standard vaccination schedules (*see* Immunization, pages 146–148.) Wash and clean all open wounds within six hours of injury to reduce the risk of infection.

Your child needs an anti-tetanus booster if:

- he did not get one as part of the routine childhood immunization schedule;
- he has not yet had all his routine childhood immunizations (three doses of the triple vaccine) or you are not sure what he has had so far;
- he is fully immunized, but it has been more than five years since he last had a tetanus booster;
- he has a dirty wound, a puncture or bite wound, a burn wound (*see* Burn Injuries, pages 76–80), or any wound that may be contaminated with manure or other animal waste.

MORE SERIOUS INJURIES

Minor scrapes, cuts and bruises can be adequately and easily dealt with at home. Proper washing, cleaning, and dressing as recommended in these pages will ensure they heal quickly without infection or other complications. However, wounds that carry a high risk of infection or other complications should be examined by a doctor or nurse as soon as possible.

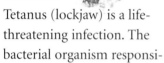 **Always seek medical attention for:**

- wounds that have not been washed and cleaned within six hours of injury;
- infected wounds – the surrounding skin is red and puffy, and there is a yellowish discharge and increasing pain;
- wounds contaminated with visible dirt, soil or other foreign matter;
- animal or human bites that have broken the skin;
- deep lacerations of the chest or abdominal wall;
- all puncture wounds;
- wounds that need stitches;
- wounds that continue to bleed through the dressing, despite adequate pressure;
- any penetrating wound below the wrist – because of the risk of tendon or nerve injury;
- open wounds involving the lip or the eye;
- any wound associated with painful movement of the underlying bone or joint (*see* Bone and Joint Injuries, pages 51–56);
- scalp wounds associated with symptoms of brain injury (*see* Head and Neck Injuries, pages 57–60);
- any wound that carries a risk of tetanus.

BONE AND JOINT INJURIES

Young, growing bones are more elastic and flexible than those of adults. They often bend rather than snap under force, so fractures are uncommon before a child begins to engage in outdoor activities and games. Fractures before the age of two, repeated fractures, or fractures that occur without significant trauma may be due to an inborn disorder of bone formation (brittle bones). If your child suffers fractures of these kinds, consult an orthopaedic surgeon who specializes in children's diseases.

The bones of the arm and shoulder may fracture when the child falls on an outstretched hand, but the larger bones of the leg require much more force to be broken – the type of impact that occurs in falls from a height or road traffic accidents. Fractures of the hand and foot are mostly caused by crush injuries, as when the hand is caught in a closing door, or something heavy falls on the foot. Injuries to any part of the skeleton may occur in team sports – particularly in contact sports. Joint dislocations are less common in childhood than fractures, and usually occur in association with a fracture.

SPRAINS AND STRAINS

Injuries to the ligaments around joints occur in older children, particularly at the knee and ankle, but usually together with bony injury. The actively growing bones

of younger children are more susceptible than the ligaments to injury, and fractures may be missed unless the injured child is carefully assessed by a doctor. Before you decide it is just a sprain or a strain, see the doctor to have X-rays taken so that bone injury can be ruled out.

Depending on the extent and angle of the force applied, a child's bones may fracture completely, or splinter so that part of the bone remains intact (the greenstick fracture). Any force applied along the length of the bone may cause a compression or buckle fracture, where the bone is distorted, but not broken.

Three types of bone fractures

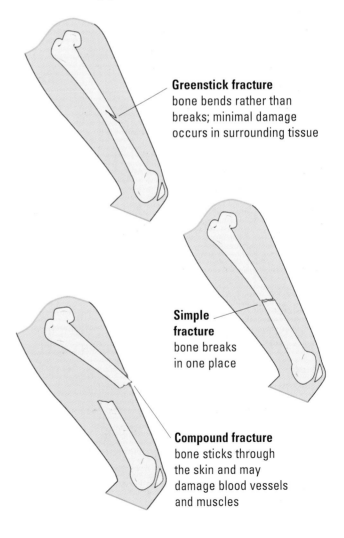

Greenstick fracture
bone bends rather than breaks; minimal damage occurs in surrounding tissue

Simple fracture
bone breaks in one place

Compound fracture
bone sticks through the skin and may damage blood vessels and muscles

GROWTH PLATE INJURIES

Near one end of each bone in the developing child's upper and lower limbs is a growth plate – a soft cartilaginous disc containing specialized cells that produce new bone tissue essential for growth. They continue to produce new bone tissue until the mid to late teens, when circulating hormones cause the growth plate to 'close' and skeletal growth ceases.

Fractures involving the 'open' growth plate are particularly common at the wrist, shoulder, and around the knee. Any swelling and tenderness at those parts of the skeleton should be regarded as a possible growth plate injury until shown otherwise on X-ray.

Failure to diagnose and treat these injuries quickly and correctly may result in permanent damage to the bone-producing cells, and the possibility of abnormal growth, even a complete cessation of growth in that particular bone. The cartilaginous growth plate is the most vulnerable part of the developing skeleton, more prone to injury than even ligaments and tendons. For this reason, 'sprains' and 'strains' are rare in children, and should only be diagnosed by exclusion when X-rays show no evidence of a fracture.

COMPOUND FRACTURES

In severe crush injuries, sharp bone fragments can pierce the skin from inside. Compound fractures carry serious risk of bone infection, which may prevent normal healing unless treated in hospital within six hours.

Nerves and blood vessels near a fracture or dislocation may be compressed by a blood clot that forms around a damaged bone, or lacerated by bone fragments. This is more likely with injuries around the elbow and knee where arteries and nerves lie close to the bone. There is a risk of tetanus infection (see Tetanus, page 50) in skin wounds contaminated with soil or dirt.

Signs of bone and joint injury

The four main signs of fracture or dislocation are:

- pain;
- swelling caused by bleeding from the damaged bone and muscle;
- deformity because bone ends are displaced or twisted at an angle;
- loss of movement – when the child immediately stops moving the affected arm or leg.

Other signs are:

- punctured or lacerated skin, which together with the signs above may indicate a compound fracture;
- numbness or pins and needles below the fracture, which may indicate nerve injury;
- pale, cold skin below the fracture, which may indicate blood vessel injury. Even if you are able to feel arterial pulses below the fracture site, this does not necessarily mean there has been no arterial injury. Check for other signs of poor circulation (see The ABC of Life Support, pages 22–31).

Injury, infection or inflammation?

Because healthy children run, bounce and jump through life, our first response to any complaint of pain in an arm or leg is understandably to treat it as minor injury. But, although far less common than injury, acute infection or inflammation of a bone or joint does occur in childhood, and can be very difficult to distinguish from a bump, bruise or fracture. Bacterial infection of bones and joints carries a high risk of spreading to other parts of the body and can lead to chronic infection unless it is treated urgently by an orthopaedic specialist.

Seek medical opinion urgently for any child who complains of limb pain without a clear history of injury, especially if she feels unwell or has a fever.

FIRST AID   A fracture or dislocation may be painful but is seldom life-threatening. If a child sustains severe or multiple injuries from any cause, always focus on the ABCs and provide basic life support if necessary (*see* The ABC of Life Support, pages 22–31) before paying attention to the bone injury. Then proceed as follows:

- Call an ambulance if the child is unable to walk.
- For lower limb injuries, give first aid where the injury happened. Do not move the child unless absolutely necessary.
- Do not move or try to straighten a bent limb as you may do further damage. Instead, leave it in whatever position you found it.
- Cover any skin wounds near the fracture with a clean gauze dressing.
- For crush injuries, apply ice or a cold compress for 15–20 minutes to reduce swelling.
- Immobilize the injured limb by splinting it as shown in the next few pages. This will help to reduce pain and bleeding, as well as the risk of injury to nerves and blood vessels.

SPLINTING FRACTURES BELOW THE ELBOW
(including the hand)

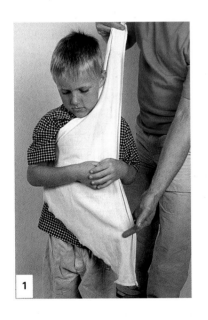
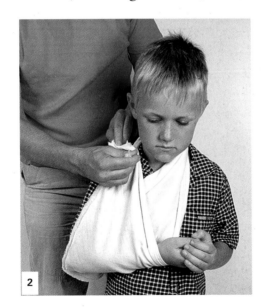
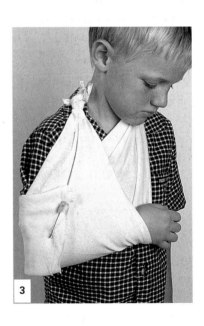

1. Prepare a triangular bandage while the child supports the injured arm.
2. Position the sling so the ends are away from his neck, to reduce movement and minimize keep pain. If the elbow joint itself is injured, do not try to move it. Tie the ends securely so the knot is positioned away from the neck.
3. Always apply the sling to the arm in whichever position you find it. Do not bend the elbow beyond 90 degrees; bone fragments can press on nerves and vessels that run in front of the elbow and may interfere with blood flow. For the same reason, never apply any sling or dressing that encircles the arm tightly at any point.

SPLINTING FRACTURES ABOVE THE ELBOW
(including shoulder and collarbone)

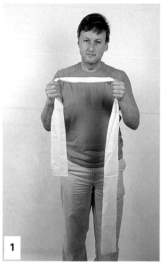 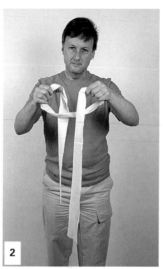 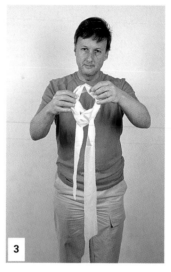 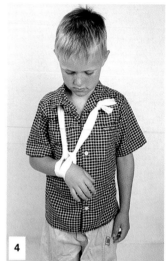

1. Grab a 1m (3ft) length of flannel or linen away from the centre so that you have one long end and one shorter end.
2. Fold two loops as shown.

3. Superimpose the two loops to form a clove hitch.
4. Place the superimposed loops carefully around the wrist of the injured arm and tie the ends securely together.

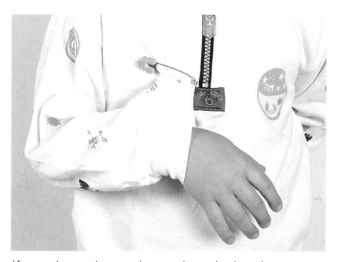

If you do not have a large triangular bandage, you can attach a long sleeve to the front of the child's shirt with a large safety pin. Do not bend the elbow beyond 90 degrees.

SPLINTING A FINGER

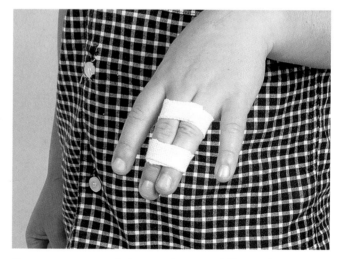

Do not try to straighten a fractured finger, but immobilize the injured finger by strapping it securely to the next finger.

SPLINTING FRACTURES BELOW THE KNEE

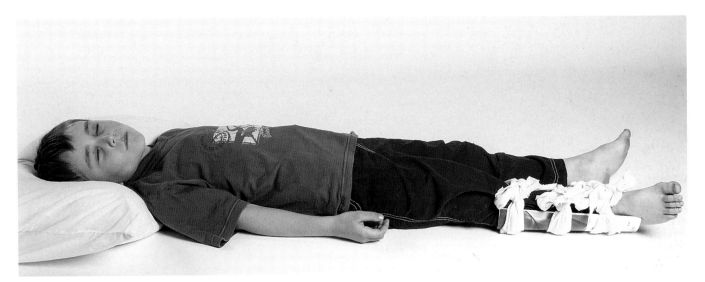

If you have called the ambulance, simply support the calf with a pillow, a rolled-up towel or blanket. If you must transport the child yourself, splint the lower leg with a rolled magazine, newspaper or any sturdy object that extends a few inches above the knee and below the ankle. Foot injuries do not need splinting, particularly if the child is small enough to be carried.

SPLINTING FRACTURES ABOVE THE KNEE

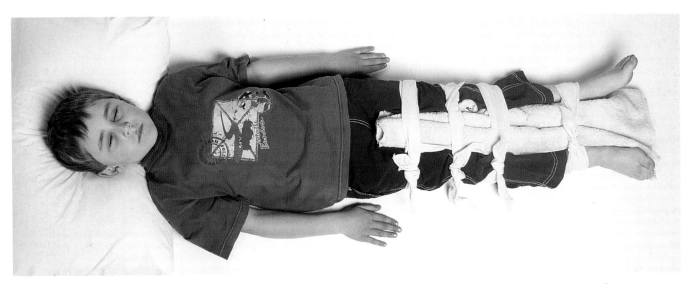

Splint the injured leg to the opposite limb using four 1m (3ft) lengths of linen or adhesive plaster. Do not move the child; wait for the ambulance and allow ambulance staff to move him.

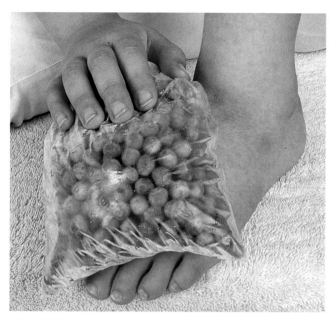

If a child's toes have been crushed, apply a cold compress (or frozen peas) to help reduce bruising and swelling, and take him to the doctor.

Pain relief – Pain at the fracture site is mostly due to the broken bone ends rubbing against each other. This can be minimized by splinting the limb and moving the child as little as possible.

Waiting for the doctor

Do not give a child with a fracture anything to eat or drink before a full medical examination has been done. Until X-rays have been taken, it is seldom possible to know which injuries require resetting under general anaesthetic. Food or drink in the child's stomach may delay treatment.

Aftercare

Most uncomplicated fractures and dislocations that are treated quickly and appropriately should heal completely. Although fracture treatment always attempts the best possible realignment of a broken bone, getting

it perfect is not always possible, or necessary. Slight angles or overlap at the fracture site will often be remoulded as the bone grows in the months after injury. Sometimes metal implants may be necessary to keep the healing bone in an acceptable position.

If the child's fracture is treated with a plaster of Paris cast or splint, ensure that before you leave the hospital you are given precise instructions about looking after the cast. The orthopaedic surgeon will also advise you about how long to restrict the child from sport or other physical activities.

A painful plaster cast

A fracture which has been properly reset and immobilized in a plaster cast may throb a bit, but mild painkillers such as ibuprofen – Brufen™ or Advil™ – or paracetamol (acetaminophen) – Panado™, Calpol™ or Tylenol™ – should suffice. Persistent or increasing pain inside a cast requires immediate medical attention to ensure that the blood supply to the limb is not obstructed.

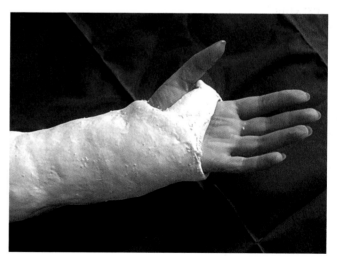

Ensure the plaster cast is not too tight. Any swelling may indicate constriction of the blood flow, so consult your doctor.

HEAD AND NECK INJURIES

Because the brain grows so rapidly in early childhood, a child's head is bigger and heavier in proportion to the rest of the body than that of an adult. By the age of five, the child's brain is almost as heavy as an adult's, although the rest of the body obviously is not. As you would expect, big heads perched on little bodies often get bumped – particularly at the stage when infants are taking their first shaky steps and toddlers are discovering the joys of running, jumping, climbing, and doing everything with more energy than judgement!

KINDS OF HEAD INJURY

Most childhood head injury is 'closed', that is, caused by blunt impact, so that the brain is 'shaken up' inside the skull to a greater or lesser degree, depending on the force of the impact. Penetrating (or 'open') injuries from bullets, knives, stones, and other projectiles are generally far more serious as they can cause severe brain damage.

The brain is well protected by the watery cerebrospinal fluid (CSF), membranes known as the meninges and the skull, which together absorb most of the impact in an injury. Closed head injuries that commonly occur around the home thus seldom damage the structure or substance of the child's brain. However, sudden movement or impact may temporarily disrupt the brain's electrical activity, causing the symptoms that are commonly referred to as concussion.

Cross-section of a skull

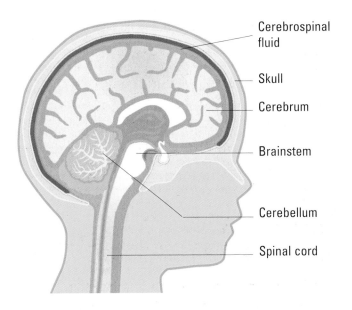

Cerebrospinal fluid

Skull

Cerebrum

Brainstem

Cerebellum

Spinal cord

More severe injury, for example, intentional blows to the head, or falls from a height of several metres, may cause bleeding inside or around the brain, even if the skull is not fractured. Severe, high-velocity impact may also cause the brain to swell so that pressure rises inside the skull. This may interfere with the blood supply to the brain. Brain swelling is an extremely serious complication of severe head injury, but can be minimized by quick and appropriate first aid and basic life-support measures.

The neck can absorb a fair amount of impact without being damaged, as it is protected by the elastic ligaments and discs between the vertebrae. However, the spinal cord may be stretched or damaged even when the spine is not fractured or dislocated.

Spinal cord damage

Neck vertebra

Fractures of the skull are mostly minor, and will heal without long-term effects. If the X-ray shows a fracture, this is a good indicator of moderate or severe impact to the brain. Most doctors will want to observe a child with a fractured skull in hospital, however well or unwell the child may be.

A fracture that causes an indentation (a depressed fracture) in the skull may press on the brain and need to be corrected surgically. Some fractures, known as compound skull fractures, may allow CSF to leak out from inside the skull. With these there is a risk of infection (meningitis) and the child may require hospital observation until the leak stops.

Most common skull fracture sites

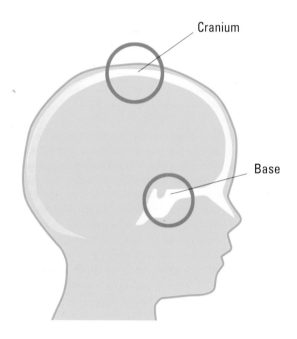

Cranium

Base

Cranial (crown) fractures are usually caused by a direct blow or falling on the head. Fractures of the base of the skull are the result of significant force, such as a road traffic accident or a fall. Raccoon eyes or bruising behind the ear suggest skull base fractures.

Signs and symptoms of head injury

Not all head injury is serious. The vast majority of children who bump their heads will cry lustily, and recover completely within half an hour.

- **The scalp** – You may notice a bruise or small cut at the site of impact.
- **The skull** – Fractures will cause a fairly large accumulation of blood under the scalp soon after injury and the child will inevitably have a headache. Clear or blood-stained fluid leaking out of the nose or ear may be CSF, indicating a compound skull fracture.
- **The neck** – The child may complain of pain or stiffness in the neck. Injury to the spinal cord may cause pins and needles or weakness in the arms or legs. Severe neck injury may cause breathing difficulty owing to paralysis of the diaphragm and chest muscles.
- **The brain** – Mild concussion may cause headache, irritability, nausea and vomiting. The child usually remains fully conscious. If the concussion is severe, however, temporary loss of consciousness and convulsions (fits) are possible, as is nausea. There may be injuries involving the neck and other parts of the body.

Delayed symptoms after head injury

A child may recover quickly after head injury, and then become drowsy or unwell over a period of minutes or hours. This may indicate brain swelling or bleeding around the brain and requires immediate medical attention.

Delayed symptoms – for example, headache, irritability, drowsiness or fever – that only present days after head injury may be due to an unrelated medical condition such as meningitis (*see* Meningitis, page 121). In such cases, consult your doctor as soon as possible.

✚ FIRST AID Treat the head and neck as one structure. The child's head is big and heavy, and the neck supporting it is fragile. Imagine an open sunflower on its narrow stem and you will have an idea of what a delicate piece of engineering this is. In response to impact, the momentum of the head inevitably pulls or stretches the neck forward, backward or sideways. This may injure the spine, the spinal cord or both. The more severe the head injury, the more likely the chance of associated neck injury. If your child has suffered a head injury, particularly if he is unconscious, protect his neck carefully until a medical examination and X-rays have shown there has been no damage to the spine or spinal cord.

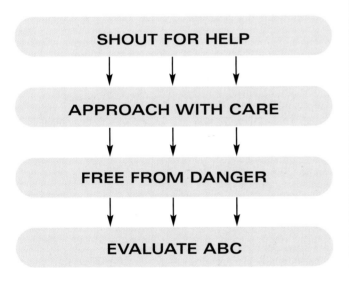

SHOUT FOR HELP

↓ ↓ ↓

APPROACH WITH CARE

↓ ↓ ↓

FREE FROM DANGER

↓ ↓ ↓

EVALUATE ABC

If the child is unconscious or not breathing
- Use the S-A-F-E approach (above).
- Ask someone to call for an ambulance.
- Steady the neck, avoiding any unnecessary movement of the spine.
- Begin basic life support, starting with establishing a clear airway, and continue until help arrives (*see* The ABC of Life Support, pages 22–31).

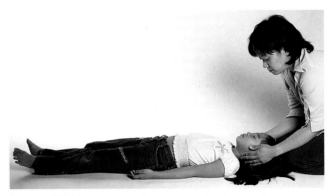

If the child is unconscious, steady the neck to prevent any movement of the spine.

If the child is conscious
- Press a clean dressing against scalp wounds to stop bleeding (*see* Open Wounds, pages 44–46).
- Treat bruises with a cold compress (ice blocks wrapped in a cloth, or a bag of frozen peas).
- Use a mild painkiller if the child complains of headache.
- Cover the ear with gauze dressing if you see fluid leaking out.
- If the neck is stiffly held in one position, leave it as it is. Support the neck by placing a heavy object on either side until the child is fully awake. Do not force him to straighten a stiff neck, as this may aggravate an underlying injury.
- Keep the child lying down quietly for a few hours. • Watch carefully for any signs of severe injury or deterioration which require medical attention.
- Do not force the child to take anything by mouth. Most children will remain nauseous for at least 30 minutes after head injury and vomit up anything given by mouth.
- Do not plug the ear or nose if you see fluid or blood leaking out.

Seek immediate medical help if:

- the child is not fully awake just after injury;
- he suffers a convulsion after injury, remains irritable or nauseous for more than an hour after injury;
- at first appears well, but becomes drowsy or unresponsive minutes or hours after injury;
- he complains of weakness or numbness affecting the hands, arms or legs;
- he complains of a painful or stiff neck;
- he has a pre-existing nervous system disorder which may make it difficult to assess the effects of injury;
- he has a large scalp swelling suggesting a skull fracture;
- he has clear or blood-stained fluid or blood leaking from the ear or nose;
- pupils are unequal in size;
- he has bruising behind the ear or around the eyes, suggesting a compound skull fracture.

If you suspect the injury or impact to have been severe, whatever the condition of the child, or if you are simply worried, consult the doctor anyway – for your own peace of mind.

Recovery after head injury

Most injuries that do not cause loss of consciousness or structural damage to the brain are followed by full recovery, with no permanent effect on the child's growth or development. He can resume normal activity at his own pace after minor head injury or mild concussion. With more severe injuries that have required hospitalization or surgery, consult the doctor about possible short- and long-term complications. She can advise how soon the child can return to school and resume normal activities. Children who have sustained any degree of injury to the neck may be at risk of re-injury for up to three months afterward. Consult the orthopaedic or neurosurgical specialist who treated the child about when it will be safe for the child to resume sport and other outdoor activities.

Although most children recover quite quickly and completely after head injury, some may be less lucky. Nerve tissue, particularly in the brain, is highly specialized, and once damaged is gone forever, leaving only scar tissue. Ensure your home is safe for children and do your best to prevent head injuries from happening in the first place.

Dealing with suspected skull base fractures

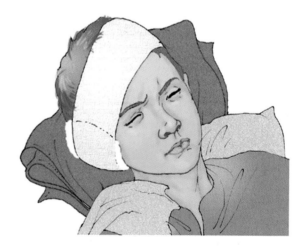

If fluid is leaking out of the ear, use a sterile pad and loose bandage but do not plug the ear.

EYE INJURIES

Of all the special senses, sight is not only the most precious – it is also the most vulnerable. Protect children from severe eye injuries by separating them from potential hazards by as wide a margin as possible – all the time.

- Do not let children of any age play with fireworks.
- Do not let pre-teen children have access to power tools.
- Keep toxic or concentrated chemicals locked up and out of reach.
- Keep firearms locked up in gun safes.

Cross-section of the eye

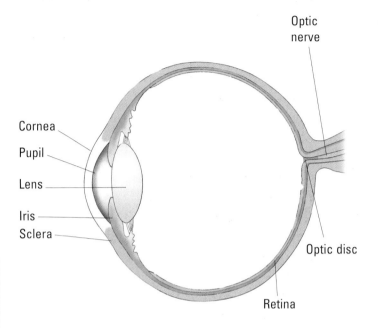

The eye is a highly specialized and delicate organ.

ANATOMY OF THE EYE

The eye is protected by a bony socket, and by the quick shutter-movement of the eyelids, but it is still more exposed than any other special sensory organ.

The eye can easily be damaged by:

- blunt trauma – for example, a punch or a sporting injury;
- sharp objects – for example, a pencil, a pellet from a pellet gun, or a stone thrown up by a lawnmower, foreign bodies, such as dust or sand, or even an eyelash;
- contact with corrosive or toxic chemicals;
- infection, which can complicate any injury that is not quickly or properly treated.

SIGNS OF EYE INJURY

All parts of the eyeball and surrounding tissues are extremely sensitive to any irritation and will show signs of inflammation immediately after any injury. Some of these signs are:

- redness (bloodshot eye) and watering;
- persistent blinking;
- not being able to see clearly;
- a gritty sensation in the eye;
- a bleeding or obviously abnormal-looking eyeball;
- pain (injuries to the cornea are extremely painful).

If both eyes show signs of inflammation, the cause may be an allergy or infection rather than injury. Consult a doctor urgently if you are unsure.

Preventing eye injuries

Although you cannot protect a child from every situation where a piece of grit might get into his eye, you can protect him from severe injuries caused by careless handling of domestic power tools or firearms. These accidents are as unnecessary as they are tragic.

➕ **FIRST AID** Since rapid diagnosis and treatment are essential to ensure the best possible recovery from eye injuries, the majority of eye injuries require emergency medical attention from an eye specialist. However, you can usefully apply the following first-aid procedures for foreign bodies in the eye and chemical burns or splashes.

With the exception of these injuries, where first aid can be useful before you seek medical help, all eye injuries should be seen by a doctor immediately.

Foreign bodies in the eye

- Do not let the child rub the eye. This will aggravate inflammation and increase the risk of infection.
- Wait for a minute or two before doing anything. Most foreign objects will be expelled by a combination of blinking and watering. Encourage the child to blink rapidly. If the gritty sensation persists, the object has not been expelled.
- Wash your hands before doing anything further.
- Moisten one end of a clean cotton bud with tap water and have this ready. (A piece of cotton wool moistened and teased into a point will do as well.)
- Gently grip the upper eyelashes and ask the child to look downward as you lift the upper lid forward and upward to get a better view of the eyeball. If you don't spot the foreign object, do the same with the lower lid as the child looks upward.
- If you spot the foreign object lying on the sclera (white part of the eye), dab it very lightly with the moist cotton bud until it comes away.

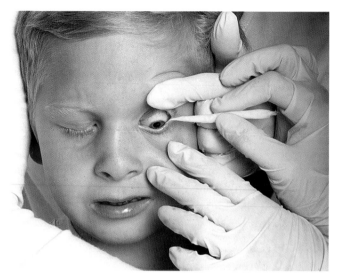

To remove a foreign body, moisten a clean cotton bud or piece of cotton wool. Lift the lid up and get the child to look down.

- Do not persist with trying to remove any foreign matter which seems stuck to the eyeball. What appears to be only a speck may in fact be the tip of a much larger object which has penetrated deep into the eyeball.
- Successful removal will usually bring immediate relief. If the discomfort persists, and you have been unable to spot the foreign object, it may be stuck to the inside of the eyelid. Seek immediate medical attention.
- Do not try to remove foreign objects from the iris (coloured portion of the eye). Cover the eye (as shown opposite) and take the child to a doctor.
- Do not try to remove foreign bodies if the eye already appears inflamed or infected.
- Do not use rigid or sharp implements to remove foreign bodies.
- Do not struggle with a child who is unable to sit still and co-operate with you.
- Do not put ointments or medications of any sort into the eye unless prescribed by a doctor.

Chemical burns and splashes

Rapidly diluting the chemical with tap water will stop the damage in its tracks. Hold the child's face under a cold running tap and let the water run over the eyeball while you hold the lid open. Continue washing for no less than 20 minutes. You must persist even if the child is uncooperative.

Do not splash water in the eye. This will just make the child blink and prevent water from reaching the eye. Blinking also aggravates corneal damage.

Cover the eye with an eye cup and seek medical attention immediately after washing. Take with you any packaging listing details of the chemical.

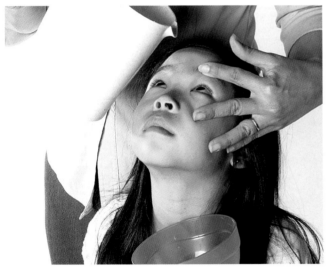

Carefully pour water into the eye to dilute and wash out dangerous chemicals, but do not splash.

Covering the injured eye

The irritated or injured eye is extremely sensitive to light and the child will usually blink continuously. This can aggravate damage that has already been caused to the iris – that is, the coloured portion of the eye. You can reduce blinking by blocking light from the eye, using the bottom half of a polystyrene cup secured over the eye with a crepe or gauze bandage (*see* First-aid Kits, pages 14–17). Use this method whenever there is even a slight possibility of corneal injury. (For black eye, or peri-orbital haematoma, *see* page 43.)

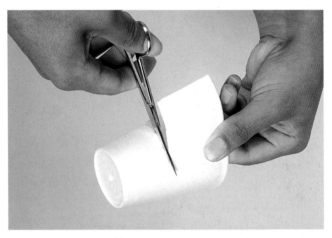

Cut the bottom off a polystyrene cup (above) and attach it with a bandage to protect the eye (below).

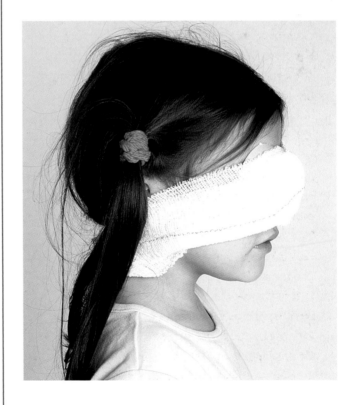

MOUTH, JAW, NOSE AND EAR INJURIES

The tissues of the face, mouth and upper airway are extremely delicate and easily damaged. Impacted foreign objects and lacerations are often self-inflicted, especially in infants and toddlers, who love to stick everything in everywhere. Although most facial injuries tend to be minor, they bleed lustily because of the rich blood supply to this area of the body.

MOUTH INJURIES

Injuries around and inside the mouth are most commonly seen in preschool children, and also in older children who play sport. Sharp objects such as pencils or lollipop sticks carried in the mouth while running may be pushed through any soft part of the mouth if the child falls. A front tooth may be chipped, loosened, or even forced out of its socket if the child falls against a solid surface, or is hit in the mouth with a fist or flying object.

Injuries to the inside of the mouth are dramatic because they are extremely painful and usually bleed a lot. Nevertheless, bleeding usually stops as quickly as it starts, and many of these injuries can be managed at home with a bit of first aid and a lot of reassurance. You can diagnose most injuries with a quick inspection of the open mouth. Use a pocket flashlight to see injuries behind the line of the teeth.

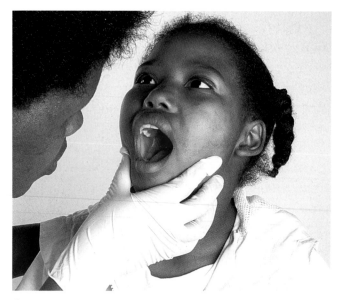

Check inside the mouth to assess the injury.

✚ FIRST AID   For any soft-tissue injury, get the child to lean forward and spit out blood rather than swallow it. You can control bleeding and relieve the pain quickly with a cold compress. Alternatively, get the child to suck an ice cube or rinse out her mouth once with iced water. When the bleeding slows or stops, assess the injury. Small cuts and bites which stop bleeding within minutes will heal quickly, and do not need stitches.

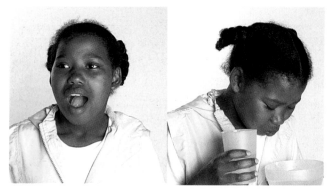

Suck an ice cube to reduce pain, swelling and bleeding or rinse out the mouth with iced water.

Avoid giving the child salty, spicy or acidic foods for five days after injury. Prevent infection with twice-daily tooth-brushing, and rinsing the mouth with water after meals. If gums or teeth have been injured, twice-daily gargling with a mild antiseptic mouthwash can substitute for tooth-brushing for the first few days. Mild bacterial infection sometimes causes injuries to begin bleeding again after two or three days, but good mouth hygiene should prevent this.

Seek medical help if the injury:

- causes difficulty with swallowing or breathing;
- involves the full thickness of the lip, cheek or tongue;
- involves the line where the lip meets the skin or the corner of the mouth;
- creates a large, loose flap of tissue anywhere inside or around the mouth;
- results in bruising or loss of gum tissue around the teeth;
- continues to bleed heavily after a few minutes;
- is at the back of the mouth or throat and difficult to see properly;
- shows signs of infection (bad breath or recurrent bleeding or swelling).

> If your child has orthodontic appliances (braces), the orthodontist or a dental surgeon should assess mouth or dental injuries as soon as possible.

Milk and permanent teeth

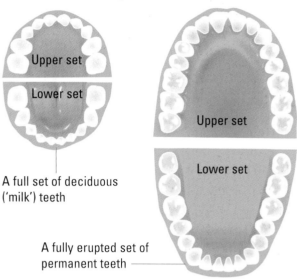

Upper set

Lower set

A full set of deciduous ('milk') teeth

Upper set

Lower set

A fully erupted set of permanent teeth

Tooth injuries

Just as their first set of teeth is established, children learn to run. Most dentists would probably prefer the sequence to be reversed! Tooth injuries are most common in children aged two to five years, although permanent teeth may also be damaged in older children during contact sports or fights. Front teeth (incisors and canines) are most at risk of injury, and damage to these may be associated with injury to the surrounding gum tissue or the jaw.

FIRST AID All tooth injuries should be assessed by a dental surgeon after you have provided first aid as recommended here. This applies equally to milk teeth and permanent teeth.

Chipped, cracked or broken teeth

- There should be little or no bleeding around the tooth.
- Try not to let the child swallow the loose fragment.
- Larger fragments should be soaked in milk or salt solution and taken along to the dentist.

Loose or displaced teeth

Control bleeding by having the child suck some ice or gargle with cold water. Consult a dentist as soon as possible. Do not try to correct the position of a displaced tooth yourself. This may aggravate bleeding or damage the root.

Lost teeth

Try not to let the child swallow the tooth. Handle the tooth carefully and avoid touching the root. Soak the tooth in milk or salt-water solution. This will prevent the delicate ligaments around the tooth from drying out for up to 30 minutes.

Control bleeding by pressing a gauze swab soaked in cold water against the tooth socket and then take the child and the tooth to a dentist as quickly as possible.

DENTAL INJURY

The speed with which you respond when your child's teeth are damaged can make all the difference. A dentist may be able to reimplant a permanent tooth which has been knocked out if the root and socket are undamaged. Broken or chipped permanent teeth can be repaired. If a milk tooth is lost, the dentist may use a spacing device to ensure the underlying permanent tooth comes through in the right place at the right time. Even after severe injuries involving several teeth, modern cosmetic dentistry can usually restore normal appearance and function.

Teeth jammed into the jawbone

Control any bleeding as recommended above and take the child to a dentist as soon as possible.

FRACTURES OF THE JAW

It takes a lot of force to fracture the upper or lower jaw. However, suspect this injury if:

- you notice marked swelling or bruising of the gums, in the floor of the mouth or around the lower half of the face;
- he cannot open or close the mouth normally;
- the upper and lower sets of teeth do not meet each other normally;
- two or more teeth appear to be displaced from their normal position.

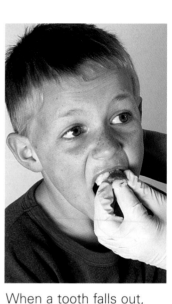

When a tooth falls out, saturate a piece of gauze in cold water and press it into the tooth socket to control the bleeding.

Common jaw fracture sites

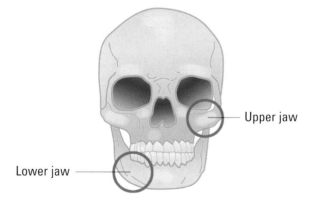

Upper jaw

Lower jaw

Seek urgent medical attention.

Fractures of the jaw require urgent medical attention. Get the child to lean forward and spit out any blood that may be collecting in the mouth. Do not give the child anything to eat or drink, as a general anaesthetic may be needed to reset the jaw, and this may be delayed if she has recently eaten.

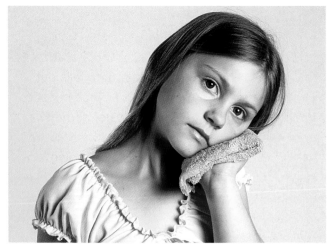

Place a cold compress on the painful side of the jaw and get the child to hospital.

NOSE INJURIES

Although it is a prominent feature on the child's face, the nose seldom lands up in big trouble. The 'bones' of a child's nose are mostly soft, pliable cartilage until they begin to harden with calcium in the early teens, so true fractures of the nose are uncommon in young children. A blow to the nose often causes swelling and some bleeding from one or both nostrils, but it will get better by itself, with little harm done beyond the temporary discomfort and distress at the sight of blood.

FIRST AID • Control bleeding with direct pressure (*see* The ABC of Life Support, pages 22–31).
- Reduce swelling with a cold compress (ice blocks wrapped in a cloth or frozen peas).
- Use a mild painkiller (acetaminophen or paediatric ibuprofen) for persistent pain.

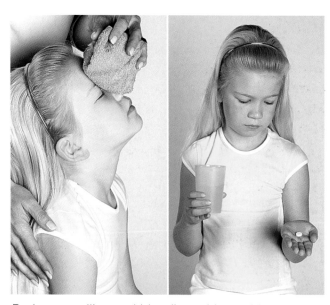

Reduce swelling and bleeding with a cold compress. Give a mild painkiller for persistent pain.

 Seek a medical opinion when:

- the nose appears crooked after swelling subsides;
- there is persistent or recurrent bleeding from the nose despite first-aid measures;
- the child cannot breathe through either nostril;
- the outer edge of the nostril has been lacerated;
- there is a foreign body stuck in the nostril (*see* Foreign Bodies in the Nostril, page 74).

INJURIES TO THE EAR

Like the nose, the outer part of the child's ear is mostly soft, flexible cartilage and is therefore fairly resistant to injury. (*See also* Foreign Bodies in the Ear, page 75.)

Bruising of the ear

Blunt impact can cause anything from mild redness and swelling to severe bruising under the skin. The main concern with severe bruising is the pressure that builds up under the skin, which may damage the delicate cartilage. Although rugby players shrug off such injuries, you would probably prefer your child not to develop 'cauliflower ears'!

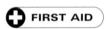 **FIRST AID**

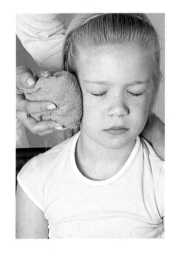

Reduce swelling and bruising by applying a cold compress immediately. Give the child a mild painkiller if needed.

Hold a cold compress against a bruised ear to reduce swelling.

 Seek medical attention if:

- the child complains of severe pain despite having taken medication;
- the skin covering the ear feels tense from built-up pressure;
- there is bleeding from inside the ear;
- the ear appears infected (red, hot and painful);
- the child develops a fever in the days following the injury.

Cross-section of the ear

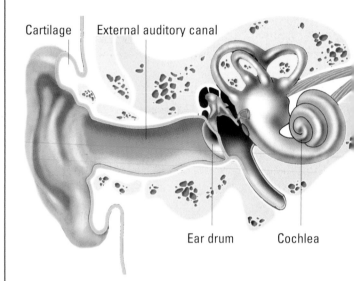

Cartilage   External auditory canal

Ear drum   Cochlea

Lacerations of the ear

Any cut involving the edge of the ear should be treated by a doctor after you have washed and cleaned it. Small nicks and scrapes can be managed at home (*see* Scrapes and Abrasions, page 47).

Bleeding from inside the ear

The eardrum and lining of the ear canal can be damaged by the transmitted force of a firm blow, or the impact of a loud noise or explosion close to the child. She will complain of temporary hearing loss, and there may be bleeding from inside the ear canal.

FIRST AID   Bleeding from inside the ear is usually minimal and stops quickly. If it persists, cover the ear with a few gauze pads kept in place with gauze or crepe bandage. Do not rinse the ear with anything, plug it, or stick anything inside it. A doctor will need to examine the inside of the ear, and may prescribe antibiotics if the eardrum is ruptured.

CHEST AND TRUNK INJURIES

The vital contents of the chest are protected by bone, and severe chest injuries are rare in the home environment. Most injuries sustained by children are cuts, scrapes and bruises of the chest wall, which require nothing more than first-aid attention (*see* Skin and Soft-tissue Injuries, pages 42–47). Where the injury is more serious, however, it is your job to notice the signs and symptoms and ensure the child gets medical attention.

Although a child's ribs are pliable and not as easily broken as an adult's are, a fall from a height or while riding a bicycle may fracture one or more ribs. These injuries are extremely painful, causing agony each time the child breathes deeply or tries to cough. It is usually necessary to admit the child to hospital for a few days.

What you should be most concerned about when your are dealing with a chest injury is the possibility that soft-tissue damage may have gone right through the chest wall – as when a child falls onto a sharp object. This may cause the lung to collapse, or blood may collect around the lung, causing severe breathing problems.

Your role as a first aid provider is to notice the signs that something is wrong with the child's chest, to provide basic life support where necessary (*see* The ABC of Life Support, pages 22–31), and to get the child to hospital as soon as possible.

Anatomy of the upper torso

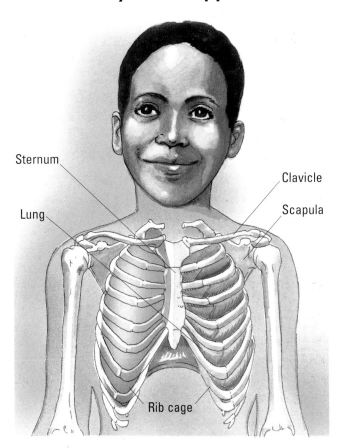

Sternum

Lung

Clavicle

Scapula

Rib cage

 Always seek medical attention if:

- the child complains of severe pain when breathing in;
- the child's respiratory rate and heart rate are above the normal range (*see* table on page 24);
- the child's complexion becomes pale or dusky (owing to lack of sufficient oxygen);
- one or other side of the chest wall moves abnormally or does not move at all;
- the windpipe just above the breastbone is pushed to one side or the other instead of being central;
- the blood in an open chest wound bubbles each time the child breathes in.

FIRST AID Provide basic life support if the child is unconscious or not breathing. Cover any open chest wound immediately with a clean, thick gauze dressing (two layers at least) fixed in place with short strips of adhesive plaster. Do not worry about cleaning the wound first.

Try to keep the child calm to minimize the body's oxygen requirements. Keep the legs raised above the level of the head if he appears pale or shocked.

Do not bind or strap fractured ribs with bandages; it only makes it harder for him to breathe normally.

Do not probe wounds with your fingers or instruments; this may cause bleeding or introduce infection.

Do not try to remove a sharp object stuck in the chest wall. This should only be done in hospital after X-rays of the chest are taken.

Seek medical attention for sharp objects in the chest wall.

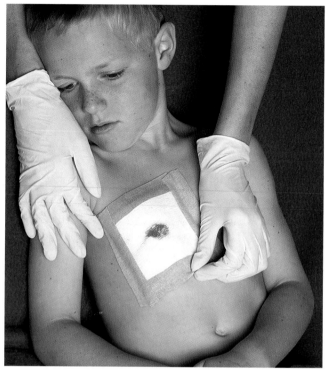

Reassure the child after covering the wound with a clean dressing (above). Keep his feet raised if he is suffering from shock (below).

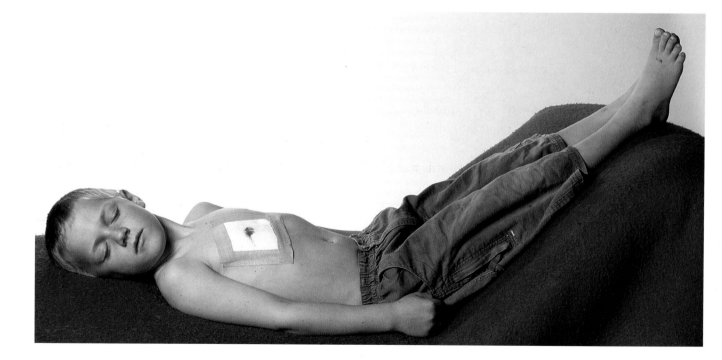

INJURIES TO THE ABDOMEN, PELVIS AND LUMBAR SPINE

The digestive tract and bony structures surrounding it are seldom injured by the activities typically enjoyed by children around the house and garden. However, injuries can be caused by blows or falls from a height, or while riding bicycles. Falls from a height onto an outstretched leg may cause pelvic fractures as well as injury to the leg itself. Smaller children should never be allowed to play in driveways, where they are difficult to see and at risk of being crushed by reversing vehicles. Crush injuries to the chest and abdomen are life-threatening. Your role as a first aid provider is to distinguish as early as possible between minor scrapes and bruises of the body wall, which you can treat yourself, and the possibility of internal injury or fractures, which must be dealt with by the doctor.

 Always seek medical attention for:

- deep penetrating injury of the skin and muscle, with or without protrusion of abdominal contents;
- abdominal pain that does not get better or disappear within 30 minutes of injury;
- nausea, vomiting or loss of appetite that does not get better within 30 minutes of injury;
- a child you have witnessed receiving a crush injury to the trunk – for example, the child was driven over by a car;
- pain in the lower abdomen, with difficulty in standing or walking (possible pelvic fracture?);
- a child who complains of numbness or weakness in one or both legs (possible spinal injury?);
- a child who passes blood in the urine minutes or hours after injury;
- a child who appears pale or shocked after injury to the trunk;
- a child whose abdomen becomes swollen.

✚ FIRST AID

- For trunk injuries, if the child is unconscious, appears shocked or has trouble breathing, use the S-A-F-E approach (below).
- Ask someone to call an ambulance immediately. Establish an airway and begin basic life support if necessary. Continue basic life support until help arrives (*see* The ABC of Life Support, pages 22–31).

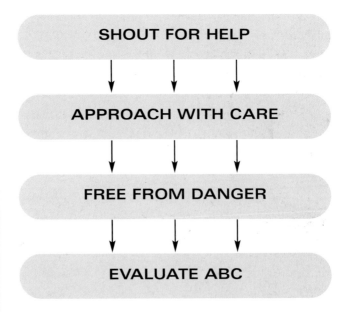

SHOUT FOR HELP

APPROACH WITH CARE

FREE FROM DANGER

EVALUATE ABC

- Do not move a child who is unable to stand or walk.
- Call for help.
- Cover the child with a blanket and raise the legs above the level of the head to improve circulation.
- Cover any penetrating wounds with a clean gauze dressing.
- Seek urgent medical attention for any child with signs of severe trunk injury.
- Do not give a severely injured child anything to eat or drink, because a general anaesthetic may be needed in hospital.

FOREIGN BODIES

The term foreign body refers to any object or material lodged in a part of the body where it does not belong. For example, an item of food that is normally welcome in the child's stomach becomes a foreign body when it is stuck in the ear or inhaled into the lung.

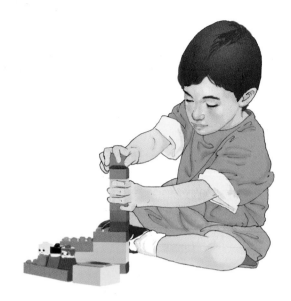

Beware of small toys or toy parts that can easily be swallowed or inhaled by young children.

Foreign bodies are a particular problem in small children, who stick objects into various parts of their anatomy out of curiosity or boredom. They do this with whatever they can lay their hands on, so the list of potential foreign bodies is limitless. Pencils, crayons and sticks may be used to scratch an itchy nose or ear, and then get stuck or break off. The mouth is a favourite place for storing coins or small toy parts when little hands are full, and peanuts and other small food items can go down the airway (the 'wrong way'), particularly when an entire handful is swallowed all at once, or the child is distracted by some other activity.

Objects stuck in the nose or ear may cause discomfort, but they are not a great danger to your child if spotted and removed as soon as possible. However, objects placed in the mouth may be dangerous. A small object such as a peanut or piece of popcorn inhaled into the lung and stuck there can cause chronic infection until the diagnosis is made and the object removed under anaesthetic. And any object stuck in the throat or upper airway may cause breathing difficulty or choking.

Choking on foreign bodies causes approximately 10% of injury-related deaths in small children. Almost all such deaths occur in the home. A combination of home safety measures and adult supervision can significantly reduce the risk of injuries of this kind. (*See* Safety in the Home, pages 35–41. For foreign bodies in the eye, *see* Eye Injuries, page 62.)

SWALLOWED FOREIGN BODIES

You will usually be aware of this problem after seeing it happen or the child is able to tell you about it. Otherwise, suspect a swallowed foreign body if:

- a contented, healthy child suddenly begins to drool or retch;
- the child refuses to eat, or vomits everything taken by mouth;
- any small object with which the child was playing suddenly disappears.

⊕ FIRST AID If the child is choking or has any breathing difficulty, follow these basic guidelines.

- Shout for help.
- Start basic life support.
- Use the 'choking' technique appropriate for the child's age (*see* The Choking Child, pages 32–34).
- Get a medical opinion as soon as possible. The doctor may take X-rays to see if there is a foreign object and if so, where it is, to decide whether an operation is needed to remove it. Objects that have passed into the stomach will usually be left to find their own way out in the stool. Do not use laxatives to speed up the passage of foreign bodies. This only increases the risk of damage to the digestive tract.
- Do not give the child anything to eat or drink, because a general anaesthetic may be necessary to remove the foreign body.

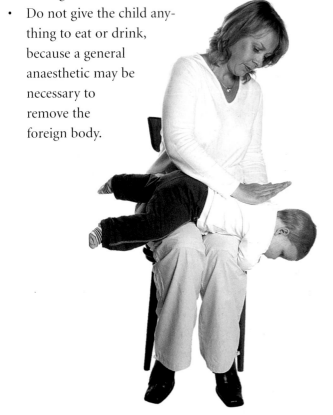

Deliver five firm blows with the heel of your hand between the shoulder blades to dislodge objects.

Foreign bodies in the upper airway

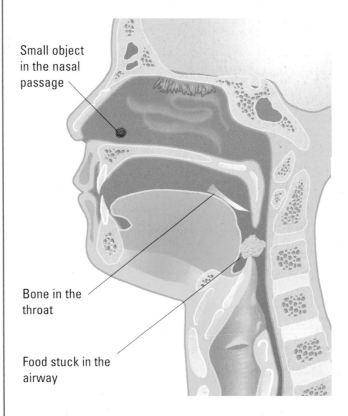

Small object in the nasal passage

Bone in the throat

Food stuck in the airway

Bones in the throat

Small bones from fish or chicken may become stuck at the back of the throat or in the gullet (oesophagus), causing a scratching or burning sensation when the child swallows. These bones often work their way loose if left alone. The discomfort may persist for a short while afterward. If the pain remains severe for more than an hour, get a medical opinion as soon as possible.

Do not try to push the bone out by forcing the child to drink fluids or to eat lumps of bread. The discomfort caused by the bone may make it difficult for the child to swallow normally and he may be liable to choke.

Never stick your finger blindly into the child's throat to try to feel for an obstruction.

FOREIGN BODIES IN THE AIRWAY

Choking may be caused by foreign objects that are too large for the child to swallow and become lodged in the back of the throat. In infants and small children the swallowing reflex is not fully developed, and choking may occur with foreign objects of any size. You should suspect a foreign body in the airway if a child:

- is choking;
- begins to cough, wheeze or struggle to breathe while eating;
- is well but suddenly begins to cough, wheeze, or struggle to breathe;
- develops a persistent cough with fever, which does not get better with antibiotics or other medication.

✚ FIRST AID If a child is choking or has any breathing difficulty, shout for help and start basic life support, using the 'choking' technique appropriate for the child's age (*see* The Choking Child, pages 32–34).

Even if after first aid the child is able to breathe without too much difficulty, obtain a medical opinion as soon as possible. All foreign objects stuck in the respiratory tract have to be removed.

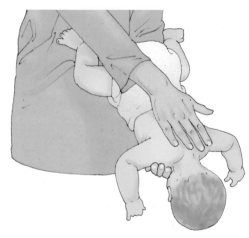

Foreign body obstruction of the airway is a life-threatening emergency.

FOREIGN BODIES IN THE NOSTRIL

You may see the child inserting something up her nose, or the child may tell you about it. Otherwise, you should suspect this problem if:

- she complains of a blocked nose affecting one nostril only;
- she has a foul-smelling discharge or blood coming out of one nostril;
- the skin around one nostril becomes inflamed.

Anything the child can fit into a nostril will be drawn upward with each intake of breath and, because the entrance to the nostril is wider than the deeper part of the nasal passage, it is likely to get stuck at a narrower point higher up. Most foreign bodies impacted in the nose are difficult to see without special lighting or instruments.

✚ FIRST AID Almost all foreign bodies impacted in the nose must be removed by a doctor. Attempt to remove the object yourself only if it is protruding outside the nostril and can be easily gripped with your fingers. If it does not come away easily, seek medical attention. Do not probe inside the child's nostril with tweezers (or anything else) nor encourage the child to blow his nose. With both manoeuvres there is a major risk of the object dislodging and going into the lung instead.

Successful removal of foreign bodies stuck in the nose or ear requires the child to keep very still. For this reason, many doctors will choose to perform the removal under general anaesthetic. Do not give the child anything to eat or drink before the doctor has decided how best to proceed.

 Seek medical attention for foreign bodies in the nostril.

FOREIGN BODIES IN THE EAR

A small child may try to copy an adult he sees cleaning an ear with a cotton bud or matchstick. Apart from the risk of damaging the delicate eardrum or the skin lining the outer ear canal, this is dangerous as an end may break off and become stuck in the ear. A child with a chronic ear infection or skin irritation inside the ear may use anything long and thin to scratch an itch his fingers cannot reach. Suspect a foreign body in the ear if:

- he keeps complaining of discomfort in one ear;
- he appears to be hard of hearing on one side;
- you notice a smelly discharge or bleeding from one ear;
- the skin of the outer ear has become red and painful from an infected discharge.

➕ **FIRST AID**　Almost all impacted foreign bodies in the ear need to be removed by a doctor. As with foreign bodies in the nose, do not give the child anything to eat or drink before seeing the doctor.

Attempt to remove the object yourself only if it is protruding outside the ear and can be easily gripped with your fingers. If it does not come away easily, seek medical attention instead. Do not probe inside the child's ear with tweezers (or anything else) as this will cause damage to the lining or the eardrum, and risk pushing the object in deeper.

Unwelcome insects

A small insect that flies into a child's ear can cause a lot of distress by buzzing and crawling close to the eardrum.

➕ **FIRST AID**　Warm a small quantity of cooking oil to just above room temperature and pour two drops into the ear canal with an ear dropper. Plug the

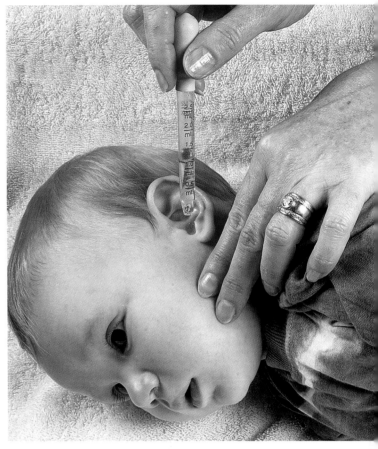

Put two or three drops of tepid cooking oil into the ear to suffocate an insect.

ear loosely with a small wad of cotton wool. The oil will provide immediate relief by suffocating the insect. With the plug still in place, take the child to a doctor to have the dead insect removed.

Foreign bodies in the vagina

This is a problem seldom seen in young children apart from those with mental disability. Foreign bodies in the vaginal opening or canal usually cause irritation and infection within a day or two, and should be suspected in any little girl with groin discomfort, or a vaginal discharge. Only a doctor should attempt to remove a foreign body from the vagina.

INJURIES CAUSED BY HEAT AND COLD

Two kinds of injuries can be caused by extremes of temperature:

- injuries from sunburn, burns and frostbite, which cause local tissue damage;
- injuries from environmental exposure, which cause the body temperature to become excessively high (heatstroke) or low (hypothermia).

Burns are among the most distressing injuries anyone can experience. Even the most minor burns are painful, but severe burns may leave a permanent scar on the child's memory well as on his skin. Children aged two to four years are most vulnerable to burn injuries, but entire families may fall victim to fire caused by faulty electrical circuits, burning cigarettes or leaking gas cylinders.

Only luck determines whether a burn wound will be small or large, superficial or deep. Unlike cuts, scrapes and bruises, which are part and parcel of growing up, burns should simply not happen, and are probably the best reason for taking safety in the home seriously (*see* Safety in the Home, pages 35–41.)

BURN INJURIES

No child should ever have to suffer the agony of a burn injury, and no parent should have to live with the regret of having let it happen. Where burns are concerned, PREVENTION IS EVERYTHING.

Children may be burned by:

- **Hot fluids** – tea, coffee and other hot drinks, boiling water spilled from pots and kettles, bath water that is too hot all cause scalds (*see* Safety in the Home, pages 35–41).
- **Hot oil**, which sticks to the skin, causing a contact injury rather than a scald. Tissue damage is more extensive than that caused by hot water.
- **Exposure to ultraviolet light (sunburn).**
- Contact with **heated surfaces** – pots and pans, stove plates, domestic heaters, even car engines.
- **Chemicals, dry or dissolved in a solution** – swimming-pool chemicals, bleaches and a range of domestic cleaners contain high concentrations of acid, alkali and other corrosive substances that burn on contact.
- **Flame and fire** – apart from burns, there are additional risks of suffocation and lung damage from inhaling hot smoke and poisonous fumes given off by burning chemicals or materials, particularly where children are exposed to fires in confined spaces.

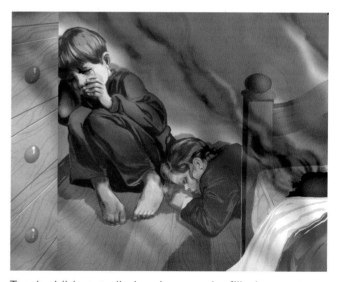

Teach children to lie low in a smoke-filled room to avoid smoke inhalation.

- **Electricity** – skin is a poor conductor of electricity, so it burns at the point of contact with electric current. There may also be a second 'exit' burn at the point where the current leaves the body (*see* Electric Shock, pages 87–88).

Damage from burn injuries is extensive. Heat from any source 'cooks' or 'fries' the skin, and underlying tissues, and the blood in small vessels under the skin may clot, making the damage worse. Serum may leak from the damaged skin and blood vessels, and the larger or deeper the injury the greater will be the risk of shock from loss of fluid.

Remember that any burn injury carries a high risk of infection, and particularly of tetanus (*see* Tetanus, page 50). This is largely because it destroys the skin, which is a natural barrier to harmful bacteria. The amount of tissue damage varies according to heat intensity and duration of exposure. For this reason the first-aid measures described below stress the importance of removing the cause and of cooling the site of injury.

Assessing the severity of a burn

To decide which burns and scalds can be managed at home and which require medical attention, assess the depth of the burn and the size of the surface area affected, using the following guidelines.

The depth

First-degree (*superficial*)	The skin is red, dry and very painful. The most typical cause is sunburn. Most first-degree burns heal within seven days without scarring.
Second-degree (*partial thickness*)	The skin is typically blistered and moist, and very painful. These burns may be caused by scalds or fire. They may require skin-grafting. There will be some scarring.
Third-degree (*full thickness*)	These burns are mostly caused by fire. They involve the deep layers of the skin, which may be pale or charred, and firm and leathery to the touch. Because the nerve endings are usually destroyed, these burns are often painless. All third-degree burns require surgical removal of dead tissue, and skin-grafting. Severe, permanent scarring is inevitable.

The surface area

This may be estimated using the child's hand as a measure. The palm of the child's hand is equivalent to 1% of her Total Body Surface Area (TBSA). As a rule, any burn involving more than 1% TBSA requires medical attention.

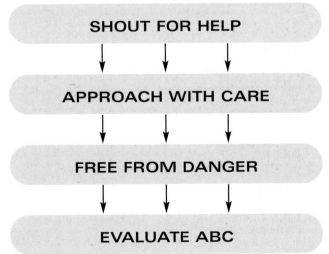

✚ **FIRST AID**   Follow these steps, regardless of what has caused the burn or whether the injury requires medical attention.

1. Follow the S-A-F-E approach

SHOUT FOR HELP

↓   ↓   ↓

APPROACH WITH CARE

↓   ↓   ↓

FREE FROM DANGER

↓   ↓   ↓

EVALUATE ABC

Shout for help

For anything more than the most minor burn, ask someone to call an ambulance.

Approach with care

As far as possible, avoid contact with whatever has burned the child. Wear gloves for protection against chemicals.

Free from danger

Remove the child from the source of the injury as quickly as possible. If his clothing is burning, douse the flames with water or smother with a blanket or by rolling him on the ground. Remove outer layers of clothing that are hot or burnt. Take care not to burn yourself in the process.

Evaluate ABC

Open the airway, and check the inside of the mouth for signs of smoke inhalation – redness, swelling, charring, soot particles. Smoke inhalation is life-threatening and requires immediate medical attention. Check breathing and pulse. Begin basic life support if necessary (*see* The ABC of Life Support, pages 18–27).

2. Limit the tissue damage

- Remove tight watches, belts, jewellery or shoes from anywhere close to the burnt skin before swelling or blistering occurs.
- Gently brush dry or powdered chemicals off the skin with a soft cloth before taking the next step.
- Take the container or packaging to hospital with the child, so the doctor can identify the chemical correctly.
- Cool burnt skin under a cool running tap for 20 minutes. Do not use ice or iced water, which will make the skin damage – and the pain – worse. Wash chemical burns for as long as possible but do not delay getting the child to hospital. Wash only the burned area. Do not submerge babies or small children in cold water – this may cause overcooling and hypothermia.

- Gently remove burnt or contaminated clothing that comes away easily, but do not pull at burnt clothing stuck to the skin. Rather use a large pair of scissors to cut around the stuck fabric.

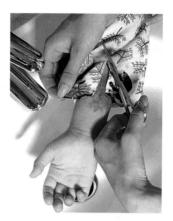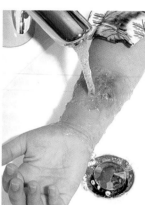

Cut fabric away from the burn site (left) and cool the skin under a running tap for 20 minutes (right).

3. Give pain relief

- The quickest and best relief you can give is to cool the burn. For small burns, acetaminophen (paracetamol) syrup or tablets may be helpful. Burns that are deep or cover large areas of skin will require stronger painkillers which can only be administered in hospital.

Heat remains in a burn wound long after the accident, and goes on destroying tissues until you cool it down. The quicker you can remove the heat source and cool the burnt area, the less tissue destruction and scarring there will be.

- Calamine lotion is soothing for moderate sunburn, but do not use it on blisters, second- or third-degree burns, or on dry peeling skin.

4. Dress and care for the wound

- Cool and cover burn wounds that require medical attention (*see* box on page 80) before taking the child to hospital.
- Use a single layer of kitchen cling film (Glad Wrap™) but remember not to wrap it tightly around a limb; this could cut off the blood supply.

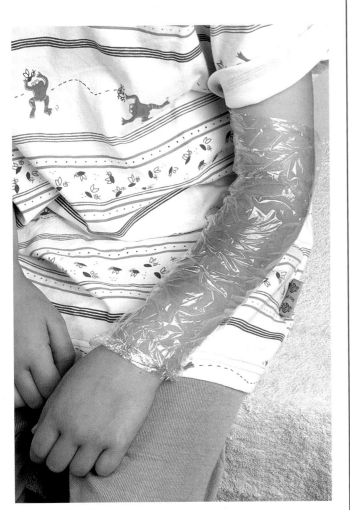

Wrap cling film loosely around a burn wound to seal it from oxygen and stop it from stinging.

- Protect a hand or a foot with a clean plastic bag tied loosely above the wrist or ankle.
- Do not cover the face with anything.
- Large burns may be covered with a clean, dry pillowslip or sheet.
- Do not pop blisters – they may become infected.
- Clean and dress small superficial burns in the same way as abrasions (*see* Scrapes and Abrasions, page 47). Paraffin-impregnated gauze squares are ideal dressings for small burns, and can be kept in place with a gauze bandage.
- Avoid fluffy or sticky dressings, which are very painful to remove.
- Do not put oil, butter, fat or other foodstuffs on a burn wound.
- Do not cover large areas of burnt skin with wet dressings. This may cause a dangerous drop in body temperature, particularly in infants.

5. Promote healing and prevent infection

- Ensure the child gets a tetanus shot (*see* Tetanus, page 50) – even for small burns you treat at home.
- Keep the wound covered with a clean dressing until completely dry. Most minor burns heal within seven days. Change the dressing only if it becomes damp or dirty. The easiest way to remove dressings is to let the child soak in a warm bath.
- Gently discourage your child from picking or scratching at dead skin. This may damage normal skin and delay healing. Reduce the itch by applying plain aqueous cream to the dry or peeling skin. If this does not help, ask your doctor to prescribe a mild antihistamine.

Consider the possibility of infection if:

- there is increasing redness, swelling or discomfort around the wound;
- you notice a nasty smell coming from the dressing;
- you see pus coming out of the burn wound;
- the child develops a fever.

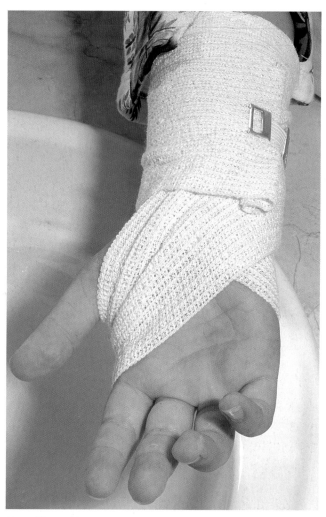

Paraffin-soaked gauze dressings are best for burn wounds. Cover with a clean, dry bandage.

 Take all infected burns to a doctor.

6. Be aware of some special cases

- Burns to the eye require immediate, prolonged (at least 30 minutes) washing with tap water. If you find this difficult to manage, seek medical assistance immediately. (*See* Chemical Burns and Splashes, page 63.)
- Electrical burns to the skin may be the tip of the iceberg, with much greater damage to the underlying muscle and nerves. Even if the visible burn mark is less than 1% Total Body Surface Area (TBSA), take the child to hospital immediately.
- If the child is caught in a house or room on fire, he may breathe in smoke which burns the airway and lungs, and poisonous fumes from burning materials. Even if there is no sign of external burns, anticipate breathing problems and get the child to hospital immediately.

BURNS REQUIRING URGENT MEDICAL ATTENTION:

- more than 1% TBSA affected;
- all second- and third-degree burns;
- burns affecting the eyes, face, hands, feet or groin area;
- all burn wounds that go all the way around the arm or leg, or a finger or toe;
- all burns caused by chemicals, electricity, fire or explosions;
- all infected burns.

NB: Check whether your child needs a tetanus booster.

FROSTNIP AND FROSTBITE

If a child is exposed to freezing or below-freezing temperatures without adequate protection, ice crystals can form inside the cells of the skin and deeper tissues. Blood may freeze inside small vessels so that the tissues are starved of oxygen, causing permanent tissue damage.

Infants and small children are most susceptible to cold injury, as they cannot control or conserve their body temperature as well as adults, and lose heat quickly. Although these injuries can be extremely painful, children having fun in the snow may be slow to notice what is happening to them.

Cold injury can vary from minor, reversible tissue damage (frostnip) to possible gangrene, with loss of fingertips or toes (frostbite). Damp skin or clothing, wind and prolonged exposure make things worse. Frostnip can usually be treated at home, but frostbite requires urgent medical attention.

✚ FIRST AID for frostnip

Take the child indoors immediately. Remove any wet clothing – gloves, stockings, and so on – and wrap her in a thick, dry blanket. Hold the frostnipped hand or foot in warm water until normal sensation returns. If the water cools, top it up with hot water. Use a cloth dipped in warm water for the face and ears. Give her a hot drink such as tea or cocoa.

✚ FIRST AID for frostbite

Get the child out of the cold immediately. Carry a child whose feet are frostbitten. Call for an ambulance or medical assistance. Remove wet clothes and replace them with warm, dry ones; wrap the child in a thick blanket. Hold the frostbitten hand or foot in warm (not hot) water. Keep it there until help arrives. Use a cloth dipped in warm water for the face. Give a warm drink such as tea or cocoa to restore normal body temperature.

SYMPTOMS OF COLD INJURY

FROSTNIP

- Mostly affects the fingertips, toes, cheeks, ears and nose.
- The child complains of tingling or experiences numbness.
- The affected skin appears red.
- Blistering is uncommon.
- Usually heals completely within six weeks.

FROSTBITE

- Commonly affects hands, feet and face, but can affect any part of the body that is not properly insulated against the cold.
- Affected parts are numb.
- Affected skin may initially appear red, but then becomes cold, white and hard to the touch.
- After a while, blisters may form on the skin of the frostbitten area.
- Even when treated, frostbite may progress to gangrene, with the affected skin turning black.

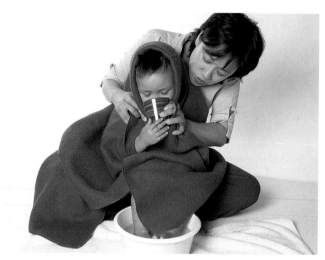

To rewarm a child, put his feet in warm water, wrap him in a blanket and give him a warm drink.

Watch carefully for signs of hypothermia (*see* pages 84–85), which may require vigorous rewarming of the entire body. Do not massage the affected skin or rub it with snow. This will only make the damage worse.

Do not use fires, heaters or hairdryers to rewarm the injured tissue, as this may cause burns. Avoid popping blisters, as this encourages infection.

Preventing cold injury

Before travelling to cold-climate destinations, ask your travel agent or travel clinic for advice on likely weather conditions and recommended clothing. This is particularly important if you plan to take children hiking, or anticipate spending a lot of time outdoors.

Dress children warmly in at least two thick layers of dry clothing before allowing them out into freezing weather. The outermost layer of clothing should be tightly woven and wind-resistant to reduce loss of body heat. Protect the face and hands with scarves, mufflers and mittens or gloves. Protect against dampness with water-resistant shoes and coats.

Clothes or accessories such as scarves should be removed if wet. Replace immediately with dry ones.

If you let children play outside in very cold weather, bring them indoors regularly. Check that all clothing is dry. Give them warm food and drinks, and inspect face and fingers for signs of frostnip. A shivering child should be kept indoors until properly rewarmed.

INJURY FROM EXPOSURE TO HEAT AND COLD

The human body can only function normally within a certain temperature range, and its internal 'thermostat' will maintain that range during brief exposure to excessive heat or cold. With prolonged exposure our ability to regulate body temperature may become exhausted, so that the entire body heats up or cools down too much for organs to function normally. Children are particularly at risk, and they need you to supervise and protect them when they are exposed to extreme heat or cold.

Heat exposure

When it is hot, sweating and changes in blood flow keep the body's temperature constant, and thirst reminds us to replace lost fluid. But although cold water and sports drinks may help to keep the body cool, some children are particularly at risk of overheating. For example:

- infants and small children may overheat after even 20 minutes of exposure to direct sunlight or hot, confined spaces such as a car;
- any child engaging in vigorous exercise;
- a child recovering from recent illness, particularly if he has had fever or diarrhoea.

Symptoms of heat exposure

Illness from heat exposure begins with mild symptoms, and progresses through the four stages shown below. The best thing you can do is protect the child from exposure; your next priority is to notice the problem early, cool her down, and replace fluid in good time.

✚ FIRST AID for heat exposure

Dehydration

The symptoms are thirst, flushed skin and dry mouth, tiredness, headaches, and dizziness. Move the child out of the sun and provide cool drinks. Only allow her back into the sun when all symptoms have completely disappeared.

Heat cramps

Symptoms are muscle pain or cramps during exercise under hot conditions, and possible signs of dehydration. Give the child water or, preferably, a sports drink to replace fluid and essential salts. Gentle stretching or massaging the affected limb may also help. Wait until the pain has completely gone before allowing the child to resume activity.

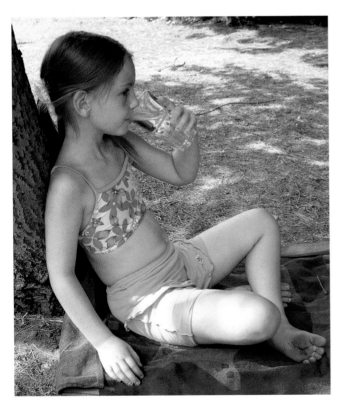

Get the child out of the hot sun, into the shade before doing anything else.

FLUID REPLACEMENT

Whether you are preventing or treating dehydration, cooled sports drinks that contain the correct balance of salt and sugar – and even plain water – are the best options. Avoid sweet, fizzy cold drinks or sodas, which have a high sugar content. The sugar acts like a sponge, drawing water out of the body via the kidneys, aggravating dehydration.

Heat exhaustion

In addition to the symptoms listed above, the child looks pale, sweaty and unwell, and may complain of stomach cramps, nausea, or feeling faint.

Move him to the coolest place available. Remove hot clothing and sponge the body with cool water. Encourage him to drink as much as possible. Obtain medical assistance if he does not recover rapidly, or shows signs of heatstroke.

Heatstroke

The symptoms are as for heat exhaustion, but the child's skin is very hot and dry and he may be drowsy and confused. His heart rate and breathing are rapid. He may vomit or have a convulsion.

Heatstroke requires urgent medical attention. While you wait for the doctor, remove all hot clothing and begin cooling the child down in a tub of cool – but not cold – water.

Alternatively, use wet towels, or a fan, even water from a hose if one is handy.

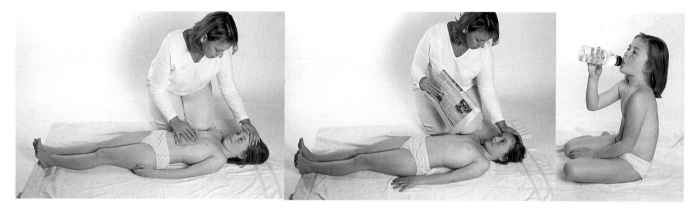

Sponge the child with a damp cloth and fan her skin to cool her down. Make sure she gets plenty fluids.

Preventing sunburn and heat exposure

During hot weather, schedule outdoor activities, outings to the beach, and outdoor games for the morning or late afternoon. Children should stay out of the midday sun (11:00–14:00).

Keep infants out of the direct sun entirely, as they can become dehydrated and sunburnt within minutes.

Following fever or any acute illness, children easily become dehydrated in hot weather and should return to normal outdoor activity gradually.

Protect children against UV light with lightweight clothing and hats. Apply sunblock or high factor sunscreen on all exposed skin. Always reapply after swimming. Consult your pharmacist or family doctor about which sun protection factor (SPF) preparation your child needs. Remember, swimming pools and seawater may keep a child cool, but skin under the water is still exposed to sunlight and must be protected with water-resistant sunscreen. Pack sunblock and sunscreen for holidays in the snow. As long as the sun is shining, sunburn can occur – even in icy conditions.

Encourage children to drink plenty fluids (ideally plain water) during hot weather, especially if exposed to direct sunlight, or playing outdoor sports. Do not wait for them to complain of thirst.

Remember, sunburn may occur together with heat dehydration, heat cramps, heat exhaustion or heatstroke if the child has been exposed to direct sunlight.

Hypothermia

In freezing or near-freezing temperatures, children may lose body heat more quickly than they can generate it. When this happens, their body temperature drops below the normal range. Hypothermia is a very serious condition that occurs when body temperature drops below 35.5°C or 96°F. As the body cools, the brain, heart and kidneys begin to malfunction, and the body will literally freeze unless rewarming occurs in good time.

Babies and small children are as ill-equipped to deal with extreme cold as with extreme heat. In cold climates, babies and infants can become hypothermic while sleeping in an unheated room. The process will be hastened if their clothing or bedding is damp.

The effects of hypothermia

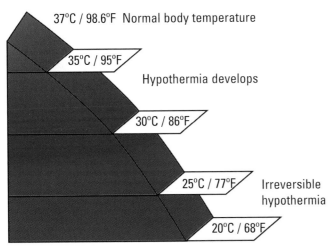

37°C / 98.6°F Normal body temperature

35°C / 95°F

Hypothermia develops

30°C / 86°F

25°C / 77°F — Irreversible hypothermia

20°C / 68°F

A child who accidentally falls into very cold or freezing water may have to be treated for hypothermia as well as near-drowning (*see* pages 100–103).

Signs of mild hypothermia

- The skin is cold to your touch, and has a pale or bluish appearance, particularly on lips and fingertips.
- The child is shivering (a reflex that generates body heat).
- An older child may be lethargic, with poor coordination, even for simple tasks.

+ FIRST AID • Move the child to the warmest possible place indoors. If necessary, raise the indoor temperature using a heater or fire.

- Remove and replace any wet clothing, or wrap the child in thick, woollen blankets. Placing the child in a warm (not hot) bath may also help to restore warmth.
- Give the child plenty hot, sweet fluids to drink.
- Check for signs of frostnip and frostbite, and treat as recommended on page 81.

Signs of severe hypothermia

- The body is very cold, almost freezing, to the touch.
- Shivering may be prolonged and impossible to control.

- The skin of the face and hands appears blue or purple.
- The arterial pulse may be irregular, and can be difficult to detect.
- Breathing may become shallow, irregular, or even stop completely.
- The muscles become rigid and feel hard when you touch them.
- The child becomes very drowsy and may be difficult to rouse.

+ FIRST AID • First, get yourself and the child out of the cold.

- Reduce heat loss as for mild hypothermia.
- Use your own body heat and skin contact to rewarm infants.
- Commence basic life support if necessary, and continue until normal circulation and breathing are restored, or until the child is rewarmed (*see* The ABC of Life Support, pages 22–31).
- Get the child to hospital or the closest medical help urgently, and continue to administer basic life support en route.

 Severe hypothermia is life threatening and requires emergency medical care.

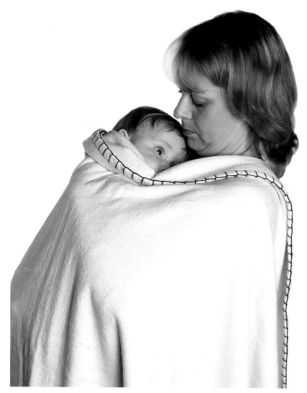

Use your own body heat and a warm blanket to rewarm an infant.

Should you check the child's temperature?

Accurate measurement of subnormal body temperature must be done via the rectum, for which you need a special low-reading thermometer. Leave this to the doctor. If your child shows any signs of hypothermia, taking her temperature is simply a waste of time. Do not delay first aid.

Preventing hypothermia (*see* Preventing Cold Injury, page 82)

Infants in cold climates

Where it is difficult to keep the indoor temperature warm during cold conditions, keep infants warm at night by letting them share the bed with you. Take precautions, however, to ensure that you do not roll over and suffocate the infant.

INFANTS AND THE COLD

Infants cannot tell you how cold they are. They do not even know they are freezing. They will cry for a while, as they do for all sorts of reasons. As they become exhausted from the combined effort of crying and trying to stay warm, they will go quiet and lie still. If left alone, without the necessary precautions during very cold conditions, they will freeze and die – quickly and quietly.

Ways of producing heat

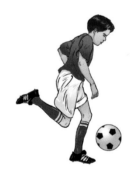

Physical activity

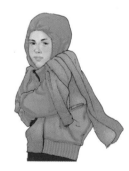

Warm clothing

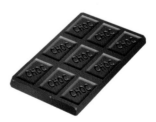

High-energy food

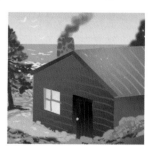

Heated shelter

ELECTRIC SHOCK

Most injuries caused by electricity occur in the home – from contact with electric appliances, power points, faulty wiring, or electricity conducted through water. Infants and toddlers are particularly at risk because they insist on exploring everything with fingers and mouths. Home electrical safety measures should focus on keeping any source of electrical current well insulated and preferably out of their reach (*see* Electrical Safety, page 37).

Because electricity supplied to your home is stepped down from high to low voltage, most domestic electric shocks are minor, causing only a brief, unpleasant 'buzz' and a scare before the child lets go. However, electrical current (particularly alternating current) can also cause muscles to contract involuntarily, so the child cannot let go of the source, which results in more sustained and extensive injury.

The electricity cables that supply our homes carry high-voltage current. Contact with these cables is almost always fatal. Do not let your children play on building sites or near road works where live cables may be exposed.

Depending on the kind of current and how long the contact lasts, electric shock may cause:

- interruption of normal heartbeat and cardiac arrest (heart failure);
- paralysis of breathing;

- damage to the brain and loss of consciousness;
- burn injury at the point of contact and where the current exits the body;
- 'cooking' of nerves and tendons, which conduct electricity better than other tissues; and
- muscle spasms, which may cause the body to jerk, resulting in fractures and dislocations of the spine and other parts of the skeleton, as well as internal injury.

SIGNS OF ELECTRICAL SHOCK

The diagnosis of electric shock is usually obvious when it happens in the home. However, if the injury occurs in your absence, the discovery of a distressed, immobile or unconscious child lying not far from an electrical appliance or power supply should make you suspect electrocution.

FIRST AID 1. The S-A-F-E approach

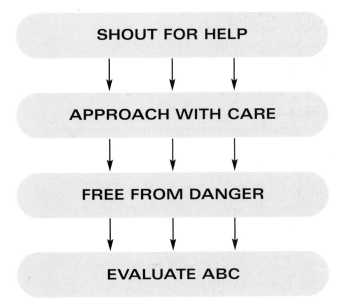

SHOUT FOR HELP

APPROACH WITH CARE

FREE FROM DANGER

EVALUATE ABC

- **Shout for help**
  If the child is unconscious or breathing abnormally, ask someone to call an ambulance immediately.

- **Approach with care**
  Protect yourself from the electricity. If there is water, electric wiring or any other electricity source near the child, you must regard the child as 'electrified', and a danger to yourself.
  Insulate yourself. Water may conduct electricity from the source or from the child to you. Do not approach the child across a wet floor if you are barefoot. Wear rubber gloves and shoes or stand on anything made from non-conducting material (clothing, paper, wood, plastic or rubber) before going near the child.
  Do not go near a child who is in contact with high-voltage electricity cables; call emergency services.

- **Free from danger**
  Unplug or switch off the electricity source only if you can do so without endangering yourself. If not, switch off the main supply at the switchboard.
  Push or pull the child away from the source of electricity, but do not allow your skin to touch his skin. Use a broomstick, chair or any dry, non-conducting object to move him, or simply pull on his clothes.
  No manner of insulation will protect you from high-voltage electrical cables. Stay away!

- **Evaluate ABC**
  If the child is unconscious, check the Airway, Breathing and Circulation. Begin basic life support if necessary (*see* The ABC of Life Support, pages 22–31). Continue until help arrives.

2. Consider other injuries
Keep the child lying still on his back or in the recovery position until help arrives. Unnecessary movement may make a neck fracture or other injuries worse.

3. Check for burns
Remember that there may be skin burns at the sites where current entered and exited the body (*see* Burn Injuries, pages 76–80).

 Call a doctor or take the child to hospital if he has:

- electrical burns involving the hand or mouth;
- infected burn wounds (red, weeping, painful);
- muscle pains or spasms;
- a cough or any difficulty breathing; or
- palpitations (irregular heartbeat).

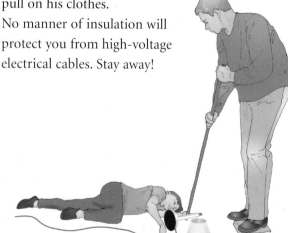
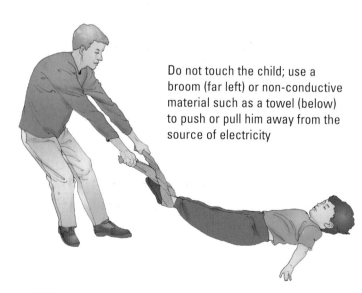

Do not touch the child; use a broom (far left) or non-conductive material such as a towel (below) to push or pull him away from the source of electricity

POISONING

Serious cases of childhood poisoning most commonly result when toxic substances are taken by mouth or inhaled in gaseous form. Volatile liquids such as paraffin (kerosene), solvents, household cleaning agents or aerosol sprays can cause poisoning by both of these routes. Poisons may also cause local damage through contact with the skin or the eyes.

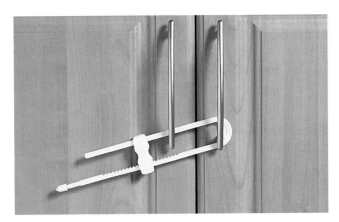

Keep harmful substances in a locked cupboard.

WHERE POISONS LURK

Since the substances responsible for most childhood poisoning are found in the bathroom, master bedroom, kitchen and tool shed or other DIY area, target these sites for poison safety (see Safety in the Home, pages 35–41).

As is the case in most childhood injuries, it is the two- to four-year-old age group that is most at risk of accidental poisoning. To a small child, paraffin (kerosene) stored in a lemonade bottle is lemonade, and sugar-coated prescription tablets or vitamins are sweets (candy). Although an older child will spit out anything that tastes revolting, the gagging reflex in infants and toddlers is not fully developed and they will inevitably swallow a certain amount of any poison they taste.

The combination of curiosity, perpetual craving for food and drink, and inability to read and tell one substance from another places toddlers at risk wherever and whenever they have half a chance to access toxic substances anywhere in the home. The key to protecting your child from poisons is to reduce that half a chance to zero. This is best achieved by a combination of adult supervision and blocking access through childproof packaging, and keeping poisonous substances well out of reach – preferably under lock and key.

The incidence of childhood poisoning from aspirin and other medications has dropped significantly in countries where the law requires them to be dispensed in child-resistant containers. However, even this does not guarantee safety: 20% of preschool children can open them. Constant adult supervision remains the most important child safety measure.

SWALLOWED POISONS

Poisons taken by mouth may make the child ill within minutes by being absorbed through the gut into the bloodstream, and may cause damage to the lining of the digestive tract itself. The toxic effects will depend on the nature of the poison, how much is swallowed, and how quickly it is passed out of the stomach.

Acid (used in swimming pools) and strong alkalis (such as domestic cleaners or bleach) are extremely corrosive; swallowing even small amounts can cause immediate, permanent damage to the delicate lining of the child's oesophagus.

Signs of swallowed poison

Consider the possibility of swallowed poison if your otherwise healthy child suddenly appears unwell, begins to gag or vomit repeatedly, complains of tummy-ache or moves or behaves abnormally.

Some poisonous substances, such as potassium permanganate, can be identified by their smell or a telltale stain on the child's lips and face.

Where the poison has affected the nervous system (for example, painkillers, sleeping tablets or alcohol), the child may be drowsy, difficult to rouse, or deeply unconscious. Finding an open or empty container near the child should help to clinch the diagnosis.

+ FIRST AID Call your local or national Poisons Control Centre or Helpline. (Ensure the Centre's phone number is clearly marked on the lid of your first-aid kit, and next to each telephone in your house. For good measure, ensure that the number is next to your neighbour's telephone as well.) If you do not have access to a Poisons Centre, get advice from your doctor or local hospital emergency unit.

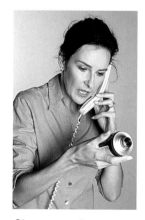

Give any package information to the poisons centre for speedy advice on what to do.

If the child is unconscious or having trouble breathing, use the S-A-F-E approach

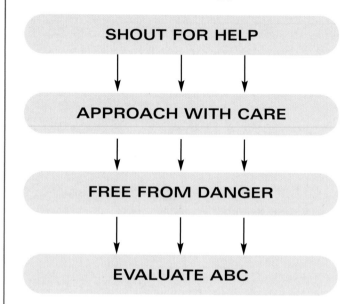

SHOUT FOR HELP

↓   ↓   ↓

APPROACH WITH CARE

↓   ↓   ↓

FREE FROM DANGER

↓   ↓   ↓

EVALUATE ABC

- **S**hout for help. Ask someone to call an ambulance, and then contact the local Poisons Control Centre or Helpline.
- **A**pproach with care. Beware of spilt liquid near the child that may be dangerous to yourself.
- **F**ree from danger. Get the child away from any toxic substance that may be a danger to either of you.
- **E**valuate ABC. Open the airway. Clear away any unswallowed tablets or other poison which you can see in the mouth. Begin basic life support and continue until help arrives.

If the child is conscious
- Get her to spit out any poison left in her mouth.
- Give her half a glass of milk or water to drink. This dilutes poison already in the stomach and limits corrosive damage from acids or alkalis.
- Nurse a drowsy child in the recovery position (*see also* page 27) to protect the airway if she vomits, which is likely.

- Call your Poisons Centre or doctor for advice. Have available the following information:
    - the age and approximate weight of the child;
    - the approximate length of time since the poison was taken;
    - the details of the poison (check the packaging), and how much was taken;
    - any abnormal physical signs you have noticed.
- Follow the advice you are given and take the child to hospital if necessary.
- Do not try to make the child vomit, either by giving a remedy to induce vomiting or sticking your finger down the throat. This is of no benefit whatsoever, and can do significant damage if the vomited poison is inhaled into the lungs.

INHALED POISONS

The common hazards found in the home are:

- leaking gas from a faulty gas supply pipe or canisters used for cooking and heating;
- carbon monoxide that accumulates when open fires are allowed to burn in poorly ventilated indoor spaces;

> ### IPECAC NOT RECOMMENDED
>
> Syrup of Ipecac induces vomiting, and was recommended for many years as a first-aid measure and an essential item in all home first-aid kits. In 2003, however, it was established that administering Ipecac or inducing vomiting by any means is of no benefit in most poisoning cases, as it eliminates very little of the poison already in the stomach. Some children will vomit repeatedly after being given Ipecac. As this may interfere with other treatments they need to be given in hospital, we do not recommend that Ipecac is used in the home.

- flammable materials that catch fire, releasing toxic gases which are breathed in together with smoke (*see* Burn Injuries, pages 76–80).

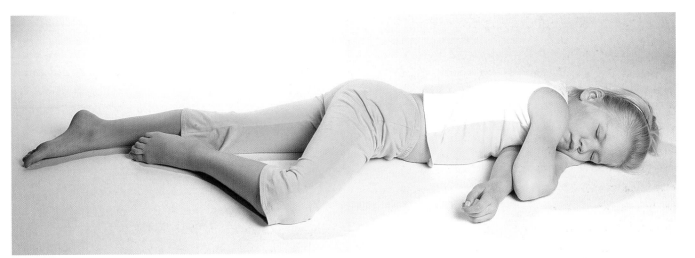

Place the child in the recovery position to ensure the airway remains open in case she vomits.

Intentional poisoning is rare before children reach their teens. Poisons most commonly taken intentionally by adolescents are alcohol, prescription medication and so-called recreational drugs. Teenagers requiring prescribed medication for behavioural or psychiatric disorders should be given only short-term supplies, to reduce the temptation to overdose intentionally. If an older child has harmed himself deliberately, seek medical advice for the underlying emotional or psychological disorder as soon as the effects of the poison itself have been dealt with.

The signs of toxic inhalation are usually obvious – particularly in the event of a fire. In fact, if you are alert, you may smell leaking gas even before you come across a child in distress.

If the child swallows a volatile liquid (for example, paint stripper, turpentine or paraffin, or the contents of an aerosol can), it can give off fumes that are inhaled into the lungs as well – two kinds of poisoning in one.

➕ FIRST AID

- Use the S-A-F-E approach.
- Ask someone to call an ambulance.
- Think twice before putting your own life at risk.
- Get the child out of an enclosed space containing toxic fumes.
- Begin basic life support if required. Continue until help arrives.

SHOUT FOR HELP

↓ ↓ ↓

APPROACH WITH CARE

↓ ↓ ↓

FREE FROM DANGER

↓ ↓ ↓

EVALUATE ABC

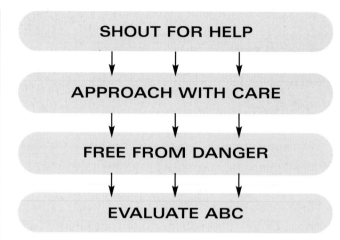

Sadly, the most common poison inhaled by children is cigarette smoke exhaled by their own family members and other adults. While passive smoking may not cause any sudden crisis, it has negative long-term effects on the health, growth and development of your child. Keep your home and your children smoke-free.

If the child is conscious and breathing normally, and there is no risk of fire or other danger to your family, it is still a good idea to call your local Poisons Centre or hospital emergency unit for advice. Have the necessary information about your child and the likely poison available when you call.

Contact poisons: Treat as for chemical burns – *see* Burn Injuries, pages 76–80.
Poison in the eye: *see* Eye Injuries – Chemical Burns and Splashes, page 63.

VENOMOUS BITES AND STINGS

With some animal-inflicted injuries the risk of poisoning is of more concern than the damage caused by the bite. Non-venomous insect bites are usually harmless, causing only local discomfort, itching and swelling, but the venom injected by insect stings and the bites of certain snakes and spiders may cause a systemic reaction (one affecting the whole body), sometimes requiring basic life support and a dose of anti-venom.

A poisonous bite or sting may cause an unusually severe reaction in some children who are allergic to the venom, and such children should be protected as far as possible from exposure to this type of injury. During warm weather and when camping or hiking in open countryside, you can avoid stings and bites by wearing protective clothing in neutral colours and closed shoes, and spraying with insect repellents (diethyl toluamide or DEET), particularly if you are out of doors at dawn and dusk – mealtimes for insects. Scented cosmetics and brightly coloured clothes both attract insects, and should be avoided.

(For treating bites by dogs, cats and other animals *see* Bites, pages 49–50.)

⊕ FIRST AID If your child has a severe allergic reaction to a bite or sting, such as an itchy rash with swelling, and difficulty in breathing:

1. Use the S-A-F-E approach (avoid getting bitten or stung yourself).

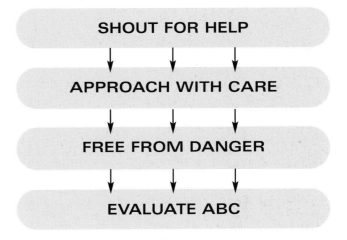

SHOUT FOR HELP

↓ ↓ ↓

APPROACH WITH CARE

↓ ↓ ↓

FREE FROM DANGER

↓ ↓ ↓

EVALUATE ABC

2. Start basic life support (ABC).
3. Open the child's airway.
4. Check for breathing and circulation. If absent or doubtful – continue until help arrives (*see* The ABC of Life Support, pages 22–31).

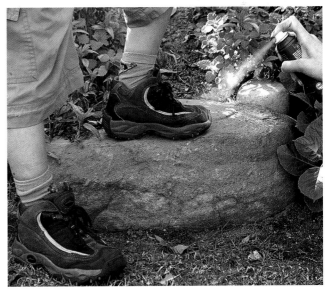

Before a hike in the bush, spray the child's shoes with insecticide to prevent tick bites.

Snake bite

- Never apply a tourniquet!
- Never cut the wound and try to suck venom out 'cowboy'-style.
- A bite or sting that becomes more red, swollen or painful three to five days after injury may be infected. Take the child to the doctor if she seems generally unwell following a bite or sting.

Anti-venom

Specific anti-venoms exist for a variety of venomous creatures. However, we do not advise that you carry these in your first-aid kit unless you have been trained in how and when to administer them. Even then, use them only when you can identify the creature beyond any doubt. Incorrect use of an anti-venom may do more harm than good.

Emergency drugs

If your child is known to be allergic to certain insect bites or stings, your doctor may advise you to keep a pre-packed adrenaline pen or syringe handy at home or in your first-aid kit. Given into the thigh muscle, this drug may be life-saving in the event of severe allergic or anaphylactic reaction (*see* page 111), but must be given correctly. Follow the manufacturer's instructions and – most importantly – your doctor's advice about using it.

FLYING INSECTS

Bees, wasps, hornets and yellow jackets

Flying insects sting anything or anyone who disturbs them or comes near their nests or hives. Honey bees die after stinging, but hornets and wasps can sting again and again.

Children should be warned that even dead insects can sting. In addition, beware of stinging insects floating in your swimming pool.

Symptoms

The sting of a flying insect usually causes a painful red swelling, which gets better within 24 hours. These are dangerous only if there are multiple stings and a large amount of venom is injected, which may cause toxic reactions such as fever, vomiting and malfunction of the kidneys – or if the child is allergic to the venom which can lead to severe allergic reaction.

➕ **FIRST AID** Honey bees leave a barb or 'stinger' in the skin. This looks like a small dark splinter in the centre of the sting site, and is attached to a poison sac. Scrape the stinger out gently, using your fingernail, a blunt knife or a credit card. Do not use tweezers – there is a chance you may squeeze additional poison into the child. Relieve pain by applying an ice block or cold compress to the sting area for about 10 minutes. Creams or gel containing the local anaesthetic benzocaine may soothe the sting. Alternatively, try gently rubbing meat tenderizer or baking soda onto the skin around the sting.

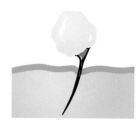

The barb of a bee sting

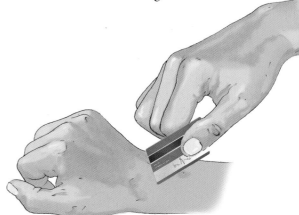

Use a credit card to scrape off the sting; tweezers can make extra poison enter the skin.

Seek urgent medical attention if:

- there is marked swelling, or if it persists for more than 24 hours;
- the child has an urticarial rash (*see* Urticaria, page 143) or facial swelling;
- the child has breathing or swallowing difficulties;
- there are more than 10 stings;
- there is a sting inside the mouth; or
- the child feels unwell after the sting.

CRAWLING INSECTS
Spiders
Only a small fraction of the huge number of spider species is poisonous and only the female bites. The most dangerous spiders are: the **brown spider** (also known as the brown recluse or violin spider), which is widely distributed in warmer countries; the **American black widow**; the **South African button spider**; and the **Australian funnel web spider**

Signs of spider bites
The bite of the brown spider can cause local pain, swelling and a large sore that heals slowly. The black widow, button and funnel web spiders inject venom that attacks the nervous system, causing severe muscle paralysis and breathing difficulty.

 FIRST AID   Apply ice or a cold compress to the bite area. Seek urgent medical help for a child who develops any symptoms after a spider bite, especially if you cannot identify the spider. Symptoms of severe poisoning may be mild at first, then become life-threatening within minutes or hours. The smaller the child, the greater the risk of fatal poisoning. If possible, take the dead spider to the hospital to be identified.

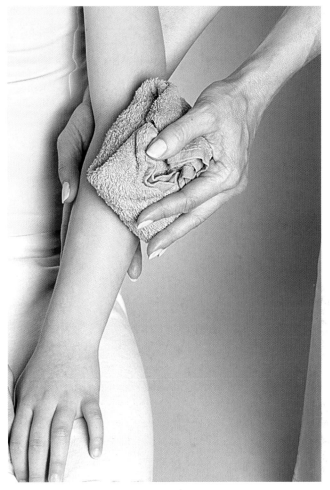
Hold a cold compress on the bite area.

 Seek urgent medical attention for spider bites that cause severe poisoning symptoms.

Scorpions
Scorpions lurk in cool, dark places. Children may be stung when playing near woodpiles or pulling bark off trees. Poisonous scorpions are recognizable by their small pincers and large tails. The venom is injected through a sting at the point of the tail. Most bites that appear 'out of nowhere' are caused by scorpions.

Signs of a scorpion sting

Although most stings cause only severe local pain, some may cause muscle pains, weakness, coma and convulsions.

➕ **FIRST AID** Apply ice or a cold compress to the sting. This will relieve pain and slow down the spread of venom. If the child does not develop any signs of systemic poisoning, wash the sting with soap and water, and watch for signs of infection. Seek urgent medical attention if the child develops a generalized rash or other symptoms after a scorpion bite. Most hospital emergency rooms carry a supply of anti-venom to neutralize the poison.

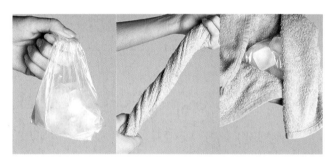

Wrap ice in a damp towel to make a cold compress.

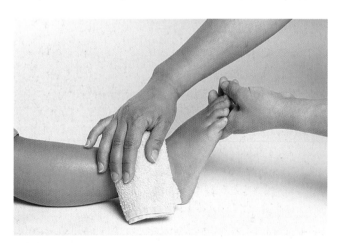

Apply the cold compress to a scorpion sting to relieve pain and inhibit the spread of the venom.

Ticks

These small brown insects are plentiful in wooded areas and farmland. They attach to the skin with hook-like mouthparts and suck blood. Most tick bites are harmless, but some (for example, the Australian scrub tick) contain venom that can cause a general paralysis which only clears up on removal of the tick. Other ticks contain bacteria and can transmit infections when they bite.

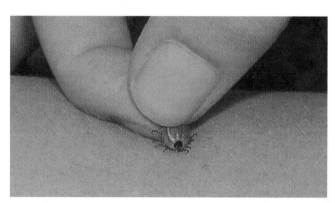

Remove ticks gently; do not leave parts behind.

Tick-bite fever

This is caused by the rickettsia micro-organism and is common in African countries. The bite is followed 10 to 14 days later by fever, a rash, headaches and painful swelling of lymph glands near the bite – usually the neck, armpit or groin. The area around the bite itself may become inflamed. A dark scab in the middle of the bite is characteristic of tick-bite fever.

Lyme disease

This infection is caused by bacteria carried and transmitted by the deer tick. Most infections occur in summer. Within days a red rash appears around the tick bite, with fever, headache, muscle and joint pains appearing weeks or even months later. If Lyme disease is not diagnosed and treated, the child may develop muscle paralysis and other severe complications.

⊕ FIRST AID Remove the tick by gripping it close to the skin, and pulling gently but firmly with your fingers or a pair of tweezers. Too much force can leave the mouth parts of the tick embedded, and this can result in a persistent sore. Carefully check the child's body for additional ticks.

Seek medical attention if:

- your child becomes unwell in any way in the weeks following a tick bite (both tick-bite fever and Lyme disease can be successfully treated with antibiotics).

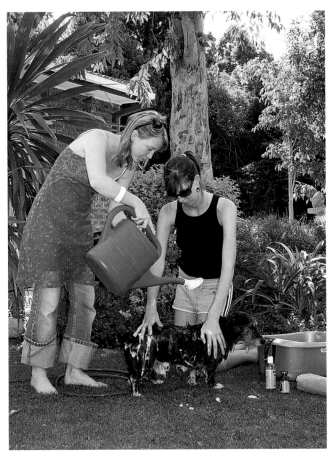

Check domestic animals for ticks and have them dipped or dosed regularly.

Fleas and bedbugs

Papular urticaria (*see* Urticaria, page 143) from insect bites is common in the hot months. Repeated bites from fleas or bedbugs may result in hypersensitivity and severe itching at the site of both fresh and old bites. The spots often become infected from scratching, frequently with streptococci.

⊕ FIRST AID

Crotamiton™ cream applied three times daily to the itchy spots is soothing and antiseptic.

A blitz on fleas within the house is essential. Spray mattresses, skirting boards and cracks in the floor with insecticide. Keep your house as dust-free as possible. Ask your veterinary surgeon to dip your domestic animals or use an effective flea-killer, particularly during the warmer months of the year.

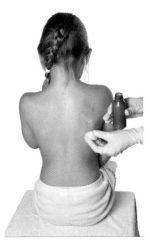

Calamine lotion helps to soothe itchy bites.

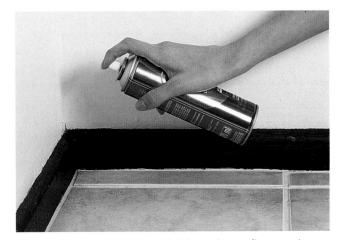

Spray skirting with insecticide to keep fleas at bay.

SNAKE BITES

Worldwide, there are nearly 3000 varieties of snake, but only about 300 are venomous, and even fewer are a danger to humans. Sea and land snakes are generally non-aggressive unless molested, and bites to children are uncommon. Adders and vipers (including the rattlesnake) may be trodden on accidentally and strike at the ankles and lower legs. The cobra rears up when cornered and will strike higher on the body; the spitting cobra is able to eject venom with force and accuracy at the eyes, causing severe pain and often permanent blindness.

Familiarize yourself with the types of snakes present in your area and find out whether anti-venom is available at your local hospital. (Species of dangerous snakes vary so much from region to region that this book cannot do justice to them. We advise the reader to obtain a good illustrated country-specific book on snakes and snake bite, as a companion to this book.)

Venomous snakes usually have fangs, large heads, and elliptical eyes.

There are three main types:
1. *Cytotoxic (adders and spitting cobras)* – these cause local tissue damage, resulting in large, painful or infected ulcers at the site of the bite.
2. *Neurotoxic (cobras, black and green mamba, rinkhals)* – these affect the nervous system, causing slurring of speech, drooling, muscle weakness and breathing difficulty.
3. *Haematoxic (boomslang, birdsnake)* – these cause generalized bleeding.

Non-venomous snakes usually have teeth instead of fangs, small heads and round eyes. Their bites can become infected, and some of these snakes even leave teeth behind in the wound. Others may leave tiny scratch marks or irregular lacerations on the skin, instead of the characteristic puncture marks of the venomous snakes.

Snake features

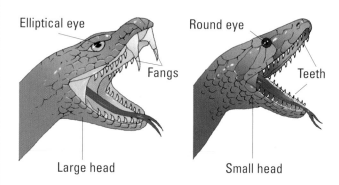

Poisonous snake   Non-poisonous snake

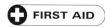 **FIRST AID**

- A snake bite is extremely frightening, so calm and reassure the child.
- Keep her still – movement increases the spread of venom to other parts of the body.
- Remove any jewellery or tight clothing from the bitten area in case swelling develops.
- Apply a firm overlapping bandage to the limb, starting over the bite site, and winding it as far up the limb as possible to the armpit or groin. This will reduce the spread of venom through the lymphatic system.

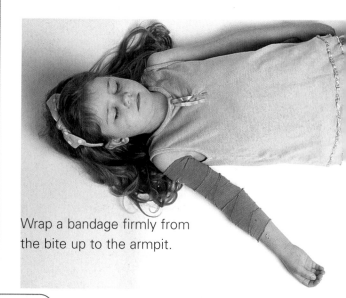

Wrap a bandage firmly from the bite up to the armpit.

- Do not clean the bite area. A venom sample may be taken to help identify which anti-venom should be used.
- Transport the child to hospital on a stretcher if possible to limit movement. Watch carefully for breathing difficulties on the way and commence basic life support if necessary.

Even a small amount of snake venom can be fatal in a child. so it is best to treat all snake bites as dangerous, and get the child to a hospital as soon as you have administered first aid.

MARINE CREATURES

Children can be stung by a variety of venomous fish, sea snakes and shellfish when exploring rock pools during beach vacations, or accompanying adults on fishing trips. Supervise children carefully during these outings, and teach them to inspect jellyfish, spiny fish, sea urchins and other sea creatures with their eyes only.

The large group of venomous sea creatures known as jellyfish includes the Portuguese man-of-war, blue-bottle, sea anemone, sea nettle and sea louse, found in warm coastal waters around the world and often washed ashore. They appear dead when washed up by the tide, but the sting remains alive and is dangerous for some time.

All varieties possess tentacles that fire off toxin to paralyze their prey. The box jellyfish commonly found on the northeast coast of Australia has a toxic sting which is extremely dangerous. Emergency services at coastal resorts where this species is commonly found will usually have a specific anti-venom for the box jellyfish.

Most popular beach resorts have signs that warn you about any dangerous marine life likely to be found in the area, so be observant.

Signs of jellyfish sting

- intense pain and burning at the sting site;
- a raised, red, whip-like swelling;
- an itchy rash that erupts one to two weeks after the sting;
- muscle pains, breathing difficulty and shock.

➕ **FIRST AID** Call for help and begin basic life support (*see* pages 22–31) if the child has any breathing difficulty. Wash the sting area with vinegar for at least one minute. This inhibits the firing of toxin from any tentacles still adhering to the skin. Carefully remove these tentacles. Apply cold compresses to the skin for pain relief.

Seek immediate medical attention if the child shows any signs of generalized toxic effects. When calling the ambulance, mention that jellyfish anti-venom may be required.

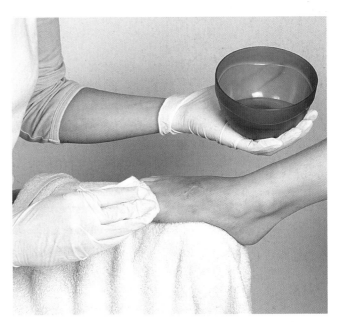

Wash a jellyfish sting with vinegar to restrict the poison from being fired from any leftover tentacles.

NEAR-DROWNING

Drowning is the second most common cause of injury-related death in children. Every child is vulnerable, but children under four years of age are especially so; they account for 80% of fatal drowning accidents.

PREVENTING DROWNING

A small child can drown in any liquid deep enough to cover the mouth and nose – as little as 2.5cm (1in) is a hazard. Bathtubs are the main water hazard to children under one year of age, while swimming pools and spas are a risk to toddlers and older children. In particular, any child with special needs or with a neurological disorder such as epilepsy should be introduced to water with the utmost care and always supervised one-on-one by an adult.

The most vital factor in preventing drowning in children is adult supervision – whether the child can swim or not. Many safety measures can substantially reduce the risk of accidental immersion in water but none can substitute for constant adult vigilance (*see* Water Safety, page 39).

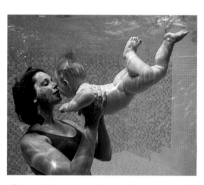

From five months of age, professional lessons can make less likely for your baby to drown.

How children drown
Within seconds

You may see a child drowning, but you will not hear him. This is because instead of kicking and screaming (as seen in the movies), he simply struggles to breathe.

Any water that passes through the mouth before the child sinks is more likely to enter the stomach than the lungs. As she sinks and water enters the throat, breathing stops, the windpipe is closed off, and the heart rate slows. These reactions are all part of a protective reflex called the diving reflex, which we share with other mammals.

Within two minutes

Lack of oxygen for two minutes or more will cause loss of consciousness. The child may start to breathe again, in which case water, and anything floating in the water, will enter the lungs. From this stage onward, the chance of survival rapidly deteriorates.

Breath holding, inhalation of water and suffocation all contribute to progressive oxygen starvation – the main cause of death from drowning.

Within four minutes

Lack of oxygen for four minutes or more will result in permanent brain damage. Tragically, this is the outcome for one child out of every five children who survive near-drowning.

Associated injuries

Hypothermia may complicate near-drowning in any child submerged in very cold water for even a short time (*see* Hypothermia, pages 84–85).

Head and neck injuries should always be suspected in a child who might have dived or fallen into shallow water (less than 3m, or 9ft), particularly if the child is unconscious when she is rescued (*see* Head and Neck Injuries, pages 57–60).

After rescue

Delayed complications may occur in children who are successfully rescued and resuscitated. These include lung infection, brain swelling and hypoglycaemia (a fall in the blood sugar level).

The effects and outcome of near-drowning are the same whether a child falls into salt water or fresh.

In cases of near-drowning, it is all about rescue, resuscitation and speed. If there is a single situation where the speed and skill with which you provide basic life support makes a difference, it is near-drowning. Rapid restoration of ABC can save a life that might otherwise be lost, and reduce the chance and degree of permanent brain damage in survivors.

Here is how you do it.

 FIRST AID   The S-A-F-E approach

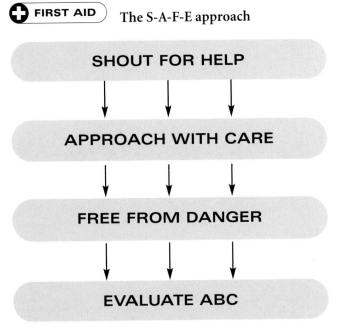

Call a doctor to attend to any near-drowning victims.

Shout for help

If you cannot swim, call for someone else to rescue the child from deep water. Only experienced lifeguards or competition-fit swimmers should attempt to rescue anyone from the open sea.

Approach with care

Never put your own life at risk. If you cannot swim, find someone who can. If the child has fallen through cracking ice, do not do so yourself. You are no use to a drowning child if you are drowning yourself!

Free from danger

Get the child out of the water as quickly as possible to reduce the risk of hypothermia and exhaustion. If you rescue a child in water far from land, keep him face-up and begin rescue breathing while you swim for shore.

Older, conscious children may be pulled from frozen water, streams or pools using a rope, towel or anything long enough and easy to grip.

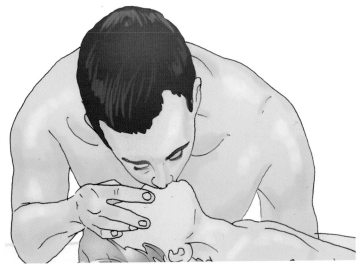

Get the child out of the water and begin rescue breathing (see page 28) as soon as possible.

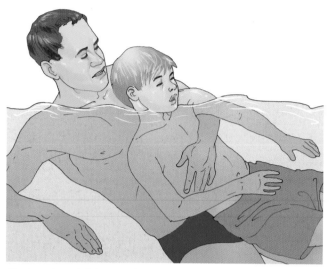

Swim the child to safety, making sure you keep his head above water.

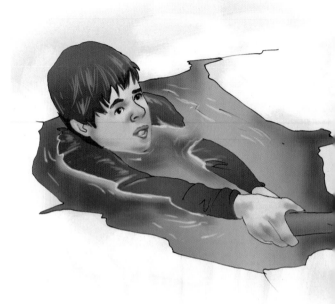

Evaluate the ABCs

Continue resuscitation until help arrives (*see* The ABC of Life Support, pages 22–31). Consider possible head or neck injury (*see* Head and Neck Injuries, pages 57–60) and avoid neck movement in an unconscious child.

Check for signs of hypothermia. Keep the child warm by removing wet clothing and wrapping her in a blanket or dry towels. Because of the risk of head or neck injury, as well as delayed complications, all near-drowning survivors should be examined by a doctor after being successfully resuscitated.

Do not give food or drink to a child who has been submerged in water. The stomach may be filled with air (because the child has been gasping) and swallowed water, so vomiting commonly occurs after rescue. If she is not fully conscious, vomited stomach contents may pass into the lungs, aggravating the injury and increasing the risk of pneumonia.

Do not try to pump water out of the lungs as often shown in the movies. The key to resuscitation is getting oxygen in – not water out.

But the most important thing of all is: do not let drowning happen in the first place!

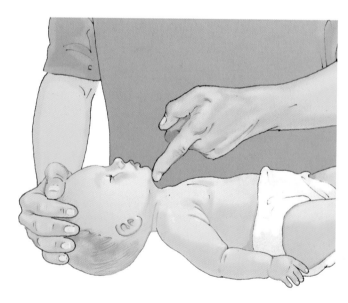

1. Open the airway using the chin lift.

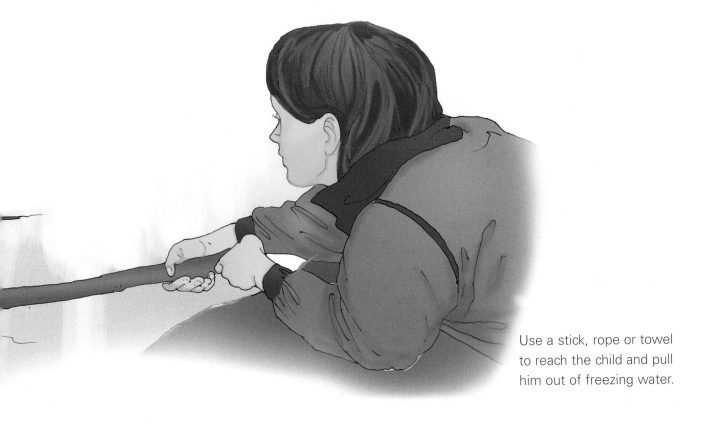

Use a stick, rope or towel to reach the child and pull him out of freezing water.

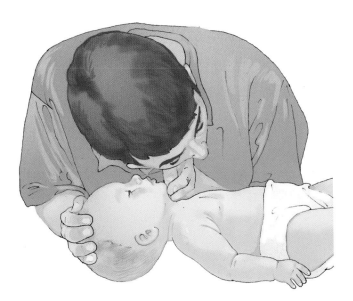

2. Look, listen and feel for breathing.

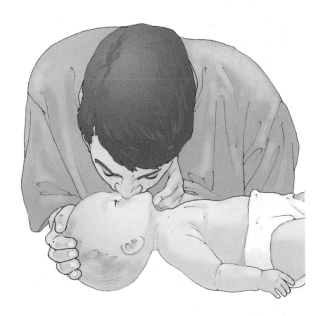

3. If he is not breathing, give up to five rescue breaths.

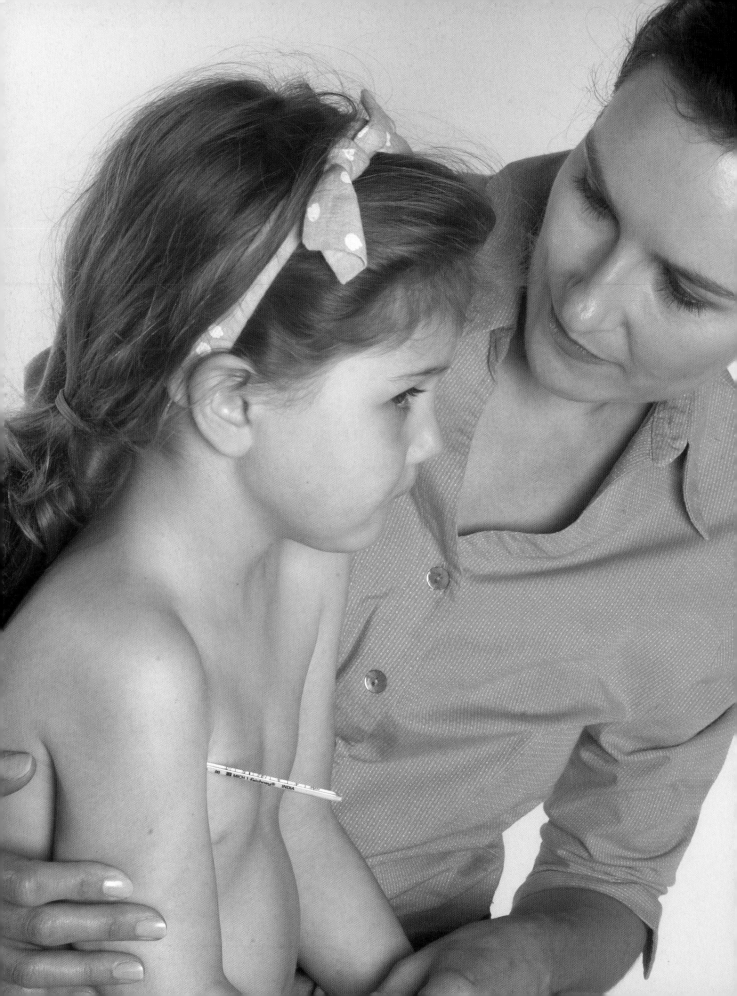

First Aid for Medical Conditions

MEDICAL EMERGENCIES

- Is your baby experiencing any illness in the first four weeks of life? Illness in the first month could be serious.
- Does your child have a temperature over 40°C (104°F)?
- Is he refusing all feeds, including breast milk?
- Is he tired, listless and drowsy, refusing to play, not smiling, just staring ahead? Does he cry when touched or moved? Is he unable to sleep? Crying constantly? These symptoms may indicate severe pain or illness.
- Does he cry or push your hand away when you press gently on his tummy?
- Is his scrotum tender or swollen? This may indicate a twisted testis (*see* Torsion of the Testis, page 134).
- Does he have any difficulty breathing? Is there a crowing sound on breathing in?
  Is there wheezing?
  Is there rapid breathing? (*see* Breathing, page 23).
- Is there a drawing in of the lower chest?
- Is there a blue or grey colour to the lips?
- Is there inability to swallow, or drooling?
- Is he not walking when previously able to? Or limping?
- Is he dehydrated? (*see* Signs of Dehydration, page 126).
- Is the neck sore or stiff?
- Are there small blood spots or bruises in the skin? (*see* Rashes and Spots, pages 135–145).

SYMPTOMS REQUIRING IMMEDIATE MEDICAL HELP

As with minor injuries, illnesses are part of growing up. Colds, sore throats and diarrhoea are in a sense necessary because they help children develop immunity against infections. Nevertheless, the minor problems of infancy and early childhood can cause parents considerable anxiety. This section will help you understand and cope with common childhood illnesses – and to know when to get professional help.

Severe symptoms such as bleeding, unconsciousness or convulsions are obvious to anyone, but milder symptoms may not initially seem important. In the box on the left is a list of some that could mean your child is seriously ill or in pain and needs medical attention as soon as possible.

Pain and discomfort in children

If your child can talk to you and describe her feelings, it is easy to tell something is wrong, but if she is very young it is less easy. Consider five aspects of her behaviour to decide whether she is not her usual self:

- **Sleep pattern.** Is she sleeping well? Or is she waking at frequent intervals, or constantly awake?
- **Crying.** Does she moan or whimper, or cry steadily, or scream?
- **Activity.** Is she peaceful and contented? Or is she fussy and restless, or thrashing about? Or is she irritable or lethargic?
- **Feeding.** Is she feeding normally or regularly refusing feeds?
- **Can you distract her?** If she is crying or unhappy, can you distract or console her easily? If not, she may be ill or in pain and not just being 'difficult'.

FEVER
What is a fever?

A fever is a temperature above 38°C (100.4°F). The normal body temperature ranges between 36°C (96.8°F) and 37°C (98.6°F).

A raised temperature is a likely sign of illness, and the cause is generally an infection due to a virus or bacterium. Fever is one of the body's ways of attacking infection. It is in itself only an emergency if:

- there is fever in a baby under three months;
- the fever is excessively high – over 40°C (104°F);
- the fever causes a convulsion.

The most common cause of fever in children is an infection of the upper respiratory tract (colds, flu and tonsillitis). Fever and generally 'feeling rotten' are often the only initial symptoms – runny nose, sore throat, earache or cough may only develop after a day or two.

Some other possible causes are:

- pneumonia;
- a rash caused by a virus;
- mumps;
- a bowel infection;
- a urinary tract infection;
- heatstroke (*see* page 83).

Fever in an infant may indicate a germ in the blood stream (bacteraemia) or early meningitis.

 FIRST AID To bring the child's temperature down you can give liquid paracetamol (acetaminophen) in the dosage recommended by a pharmacist. Do not give it more often than eight-hourly. Never give aspirin to children, except on a doctor's advice.

Remember fever is there for a purpose. It does not need to be brought down unless the child's temperature is very high – that is, above 39°C (102.2°F) – or if he is uncomfortable, or cannot sleep. Do not wake him to take his temperature or to dose him; sleep is a great healer!

Do not dress the child too warmly or cover him with too many blankets. Give him frequent drinks (for example, water or fruit juice) in small amounts. Finally, sponge him with lukewarm water if his temperature rises above 40°C (104°F).

Get medical help if:

- the infant is younger than four months;
- there is rapid breathing (*see* Pneumonia, page 110);
- the child loses consciousness or has a convulsion;
- there is any rash;
- there is persistent vomiting or a stiff neck;
- the fever lasts for more than three days.

TAKING THE TEMPERATURE

Measure your child's temperature with a mercury or digital thermometer in the armpit. Do not place it under the tongue if the child is younger than seven. Alternatively, use a temperature strip on the forehead, but remember when you take a skin temperature to add 0.6°C (1°F) to get the true body temperature.

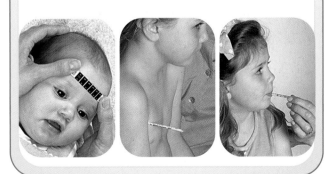

RESPIRATORY TRACT AND LUNG DISORDERS

The air we breathe passes through the nostrils, past the larynx, and down the trachea and bronchial tubes, which become progressively smaller until they reach the lungs. The most common causes of respiratory disorders are viral and bacterial infections that can affect any part of the respiratory tract. Young children are particularly prone to these infections as their immune systems are so immature. Allergic disorders such as asthma are also common in children.

COLDS AND FLU

All young children catch **colds** regularly, as often as five or six times a year. You will no doubt know the symptoms: a scratchy feeling in the throat, runny nose, sneezing, coughing and, in babies, a fever. A cold is particularly distressing for a baby, and the blocked nose makes it difficult for you to feed him. Colds are caused by viruses and usually clear up in three or four days.

Flu (or influenza) is an upper respiratory infection caused by the influenza virus. The symptoms are more severe than they are in the common cold – high fever, muscle aches, headache, tiredness and weakness – and they last longer.

Unfortunately, colds and flu are sometimes complicated by bacterial infection, which may lead to ear infection, sinusitis or pneumonia.

✚ FIRST AID for a cold

Where possible, keep infants out of close contact with anyone with a cold. Give more fluids than usual, in frequent small quantities. Paracetamol (acetaminophen) in liquid or tablet form will bring the temperature down and make the child feel better.

You can use a bulb aspirator to unblock your baby's nose. Saline nose drops are also helpful. Get a sterile saline (salt) solution from your pharmacist for this purpose.

The best decongestant is humidified air. Use a vaporizer, or place a wet towel near a heater. You can also boil a kettle in the room to create steam – but make sure it is safe! Alternatively, take the child to the bathroom and run the hot water tap. Stay with her to avoid accidental scalding.

A good home remedy is a teaspoon or two of honey or syrup and a little lemon juice in a cup of warm water, given three times a day. We do not recommend that you use nasal decongestants, whether in nose drop, spray or oral form. (They can have a rebound effect, making the problem worse.) Do not give the child cough suppressants. The cough helps get rid of mucus in the throat.

Colds generally clear up on their own and there is no need for antibiotics. However, see the doctor if there is prolonged fever or earache or if the symptoms do not clear up within a few days.

✚ FIRST AID for flu

Treat as for a cold, except in cases as listed on page 109.

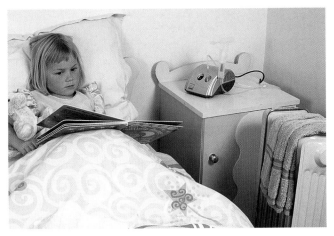

Use a vaporizer and a wet towel on a heater to humidify the air and ease breathing.

Seek medical attention if:

- the child's temperature is above 40°C (104°F);
- there is abnormally fast breathing (*see* Pneumonia, page 110);
- the child is drowsy or unwilling to feed.

Flu is dangerous in a child under two or with a chronic illness. After a dose of flu a child should not take part in vigorous games for two weeks.

For advice about flu vaccines, *see* Immunization, pages 146–148.

SINUSITIS

The sinuses are air spaces in the cheekbones and above and behind the nose, linked to the nasal passages. A cold may be followed by acute sinusitis, an infection that causes thick yellow nasal secretions, bad breath, a cough, fever, and pain and tenderness over the affected sinuses – usually the forehead or cheeks. A child may get sinusitis repeatedly over a long period, with recurrent fever and ill health. If untreated, infection can spread beyond the sinuses, causing serious complications.

FIRST AID Decongestant (vasoconstrictor) nasal drops help to open up the narrow openings into the inflamed sinuses. Do not use them for more than three or four days; they may make the congestion worse when the effect of the drops wears off.

If your doctor prescribes an antibiotic, ensure the child completes the full course so that the infection does not recur.

If you suspect sinusitis, consult your doctor.

Diagram of the sinuses

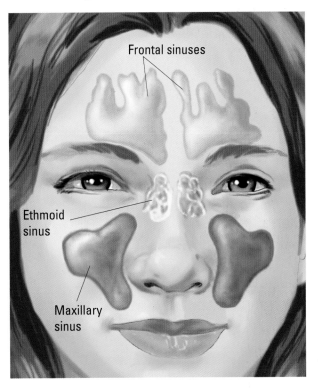

Frontal sinuses

Ethmoid sinus

Maxillary sinus

Make your own nose or eye drops by thoroughly dissolving half a teaspoon of clean salt in a cup of warm, previously boiled water.

PNEUMONIA

Pneumonia is an inflammation of one or both lungs due to bacteria, viruses or other organisms. It often develops after a cold, when germs in the nose and throat are carried into the lungs, or it may complicate another illness, such as whooping cough or measles.

In babies or infants it may also indicate an underlying problem in the lung, such as inhaled feed. In toddlers, it may be the first sign of obstruction by an inhaled foreign body (*see* Foreign Bodies, pages 72–74). Pneumonia is generally more severe in children who are malnourished or have a chronic illness.

Pneumonia may be complicated by painful inflammation of the membranes of the lung (pleurisy) or fluid collecting around the lung.

A child with pneumonia:

- is feverish and unwell;
- has a persistent, initially dry, cough;
- may cough up brownish or blood-stained sputum;
- breathes rapidly (*see* page 23);
- may or may not have pain on breathing.

 Take the child to hospital if there is:

- indrawing of the chest on breathing;
- blueness of the lips and tongue;
- marked drowsiness;
- inability to feed;
- convulsions.

After consulting a doctor, treat the child at home unless she is very ill. Give her food frequently in small amounts, and paracetamol (acetaminophen) syrup in the recommended dosage to relieve fever and headache.

The doctor may prescribe an antibiotic. In an uncomplicated case the child should be better in a few days. A chest X-ray must be done after recovery to check there is no residual disease or underlying abnormality.

WHOOPING COUGH (PERTUSSIS)

Whooping cough is an acute and highly infectious disease caused by a bacterium, *Bordetella pertussis*. The illness is usually prolonged – it has been called the 90-day cough.

It starts as a mild cold with a cough, especially at night. These symptoms worsen, and at the end of the second week spasms of severe coughing develop, during which the child becomes red in the face and saliva drools from the mouth. Each spasm ends with a crowing indrawing of breath – the whoop – and there may be vomiting. In very young infants the breathing may stop altogether at the end of the spasm.

During the convalescent phase the whooping gradually disappears. It may return over a number of months, whenever the child develops a fresh cold. The spasms are exhausting for the child and can cause haemorrhages in the eyes and other complications, including pneumonia, marked weight loss from poor appetite and vomiting, and even (rarely) brain damage.

FIRST AID If your child has been in contact with someone with whooping cough, or any prolonged cough, get medical help at the first sign of any illness. An antibiotic can stop whooping cough at this stage.

Once the whooping starts, only time will stop it. Get medical help as soon as possible.

Whooping cough is preventable. Make sure your baby is fully immunized at the correct times (*see* Immunization, pages 146–148). Immunization does not prevent all cases, but the illness is likely to be much less severe if it does occur.

BREATHING DIFFICULTIES

One of the most common breathing problems is the blocked nose associated with the common cold. This is very troublesome to infants, who cannot breathe through their mouths or blow their noses. Enlarged adenoids cause snoring at night and continuous mouth breathing, while croup is a difficulty with breathing in, resulting in a crowing sound and barking cough. Infection of the bronchial tubes causes wheezing, which is difficulty in breathing out. Lung infection shows itself by rapid and difficult breathing. Finally, complete obstruction to breathing results in asphyxiation – an extreme emergency.

ASPHYXIATION

Young infants are particularly vulnerable to asphyxiation – breathing being obstructed by food or a small object. Common offenders are such things as a peanut, a piece of sausage, or an uninflated balloon. A baby can also suffocate by getting a plastic bag over his nose and mouth, or his head stuck between the side of the cot and the mattress or between the cot slats. A baby who is choking will be red in the face, or blue, and he will be unable to cry because he is struggling to breathe.

(*See also* The Choking Child, pages 32–34, and Foreign Bodies, pages 72–74.)

Correct sleeping position for babies

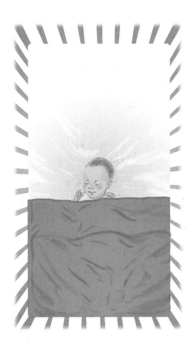

Put your baby to sleep on his back, with his feet near the bottom of the cot. This prevents him from slipping down under the blankets, where he may become overheated or even suffocate.

ANAPHYLACTIC SHOCK

This is a severe allergic reaction to a food, such as nuts or seafood, an insect sting, or a medication such as penicillin. Though uncommon in children, it is dangerous when it does occur.

The reaction comes on a few minutes after exposure. There is a sudden feeling of anxiety, followed by:
- a generalized itchy rash;
- burning of the lips and throat;
- swelling around the eyes;
- increasing difficulty with breathing;
- shock and collapse; and even
- loss of consciousness.

⊕ FIRST AID   Sometimes shock and collapse come on very suddenly without any of the other warning signs. Get medical help immediately. Call for help or ask someone to summon an ambulance.

Place the child in a semi-sitting position to ease the breathing. If she loses consciousness begin basic life support (*see* The ABC of Life Support, pages 22–31).

A doctor or nurse can give her an injection of adrenalin, which is usually rapidly effective. Other drugs may also be given.

When your child is better, consult a paediatrician or allergy expert to try to find out what she is allergic to. If you know she is allergic to something she should wear a wrist band (MedicAlert) indicating this. Keep an adrenalin injection (Epipen™) at hand in case of emergency.

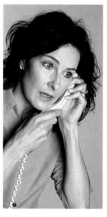

Call for medical help if the child collapses.

CROUP

Croup is an acute viral infection, most commonly affecting children aged six months to three years. It affects the upper airway, usually starting with cold symptoms and fever. This may be followed within a few days by inflammation of the upper windpipe just below the voice box, causing a hoarse barking cough and breathing difficulty. Typically, the child with croup makes a crowing sound, particularly on crying. In older children the croup virus simply causes hoarseness and cough (laryngitis).

Croup tends to come on at night and is always very frightening to both child and parents. The progress of this illness is unpredictable, and it is important to recognize the symptoms as soon as possible and take appropriate action.

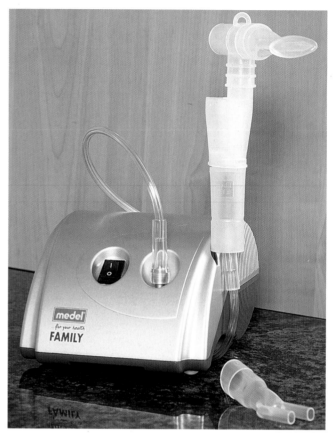

If your child has difficulty breathing, invest in a nebulizer to humidify the atmosphere.

⊕ FIRST AID   Be calm, and stay with the child – crying usually makes the symptoms worse. Give a dose of paracetamol (acetaminophen). Give him warm drinks, and humidify the air to ease breathing (*see* Respiratory Tract and Lung Disorders, pages 108–110).

 Get medical help if:

- the child does not improve, or cannot feed normally;
- there is indrawing of the lower chest on breathing in;
- the lips, tongue or skin look blue;
- the child appears exhausted, or breathing suddenly becomes shallow.

Croup can be greatly eased by an aerosol or injection of adrenalin, or other medication which a doctor may decide to use.

A very dangerous form of croup, acute epiglottitis, is caused by a bacterium, *Haemophilus influenzae*. It should be suspected if:

- there is high fever;
- there is complete loss of voice;
- there is drooling and inability to swallow;
- the child is only comfortable in a sitting position.

Fortunately epiglottitis has become rare since the introduction of immunization to prevent it. If your child shows these symptoms, get him to a hospital or clinic at once.

BRONCHITIS

Bronchitis is an inflammation of the larger airways (bronchi). It may follow a cold. Thick secretions and spasm of these airways make the child cough and wheeze (have difficulty in breathing out). There may or may not be fever. If a child develops bronchitis after every cold, it may be the first sign of asthma.

 FIRST AID Encourage the child to drink in order to help to prevent dehydration. Humidify the air to ease breathing (*see* Respiratory Tract and Lung Disorders, pages 108–110).

Place the child face down over your knees and gently tap the back of the chest on each side with a cupped hand for a few minutes to help bring up the mucus. Or tickle her to make her laugh – this usually causes coughing. If the secretions are yellow, your doctor may prescribe an antibiotic. Do not give cough suppressants. A bronchodilator such as salbutamol eases the spasm and releases mucus. It is available on prescription as syrup, tablets or aerosol. Ask your pharmacist for dosage instructions.

The bronchial system

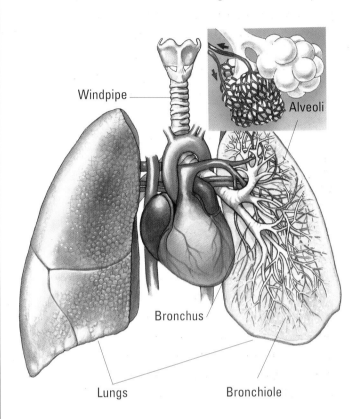

Windpipe

Alveoli

Bronchus

Lungs

Bronchiole

Get medical help if the child:

- has difficulty breathing;
- is breathing rapidly (*see* Pneumonia, page 110);
- is exhausted.

BRONCHIOLITIS

This is an acute viral infection affecting the smallest airways (bronchioles) inside the lungs. It occurs mostly in infants under 12 months and can be a dangerous condition in very young or weak babies.

At the start the illness may resemble a cold. The baby then becomes increasingly distressed and feverish and may refuse feeds. There is a cough and breathing difficulty. The chest is bloated with air trapped in the lungs. The baby may stop breathing for a few seconds at a time.

Because the course of bronchiolitis is unpredictable, get medical help immediately if your child shows these symptoms. She may need oxygen therapy in hospital.

✚ FIRST AID After the doctor has seen her, home treatment may include:
- giving plenty of fluids;
- humidifying the air to ease breathing (*see* Respiratory Tract and Lung Disorders, pages 108–110);
- giving paracetamol (acetaminophen) for the fever.

The child usually gets better within a week, but the cough can persist for much longer. There is no permanent damage to the lungs, but she may subsequently be prone to wheezing attacks.

See also Pneumonia and Whooping Cough, page 110.

ASTHMA

Asthma is a common condition affecting about one in 10 children, and is twice as common in boys. Only about half of the children who have asthma still have attacks after the age of 10 years.

The first symptom is usually a nagging cough, especially at night. Other symptoms are recurrent attacks of wheezing, tightness of the chest and shortness of breath, especially after exercise. Often the child has other allergies, such as hay fever or eczema, and other family members may be similarly affected.

Asthma is caused by a narrowing of the lung airways and accumulation of secretions. In a susceptible child, it may be brought on by excitement, infection, exercising in cold air, and allergy to house dust, pollens, pets, pollutants such as tobacco smoke, and some foods.

✚ FIRST AID If your child has repeated attacks of coughing or wheezing, ask your doctor for a full assessment. She will rule out other causes of cough and wheezing, as well as doing tests for asthma.

Various medications are available for a child with asthma. You can teach him how to use them in an attack. You will need to assist a younger child. Relieving medicines are now usually given in the form of an inhaled spray or an aerosol, or nebulizer. Preventive medicines are also available. When given every day, they will prevent most attacks.

Keep your asthmatic child well away from tobacco smoke and any other kind of smoke.

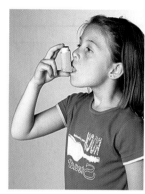

Asthma pumps must be kept handy.

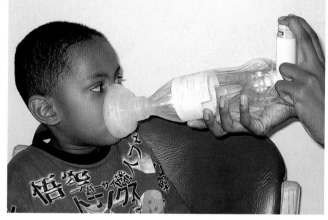

For young children use a spacer attached to the pump as they cannot synchronize breath intake with the puffs from the pump. A small plastic bottle makes an inexpensive spacer. Cut a hole in the bottom for the pump nozzle. The aerosol is pumped into the bottle at one end while the child breathes in at the other.

MOUTH, THROAT, NOSE AND EAR PROBLEMS

The nose and mouth are entry points for micro-organisms in the air we breathe and the fluids and food we ingest so, not surprisingly, nose and throat infections are the most common in children. The middle ear is an air-filled space closed to the outside by the eardrum. Its only exit is a narrow tube leading to the back of the nose. This tube is readily blocked by enlarged adenoids, when the child has a cold, or by abrupt changes in pressure caused by air travel – with resulting infection.

MOUTH ULCERS AND COLD SORES

The herpes simplex virus that causes these is widespread in the community. In fact, most of us carry it unnoticed. Children infected with it for the first time may develop a very sore mouth and throat. The child is feverish, the throat is inflamed and there are many ulcers (blisters that have burst) inside the mouth. The gums are usually inflamed and swollen. Sometimes there are also cold sores (fever blisters) on the lips or around the mouth, and even on one or two fingers the child has sucked. This is a significant illness in children under five. They take seven to 10 days to get better and during this time feeding is very painful.

✚ FIRST AID In mild cases, control discomfort with tannic acid and lignocaine gel, or Dequadin Mouth Paint™ applied to the mouth ulcers; give paracetamol (acetaminophen) for the fever eight-hourly; give milk and bland fluids (preferably chilled) in small amounts at regular intervals, but not acidic fruit juices; give 5ml (one teaspoon) of a multi-vitamin mixture daily.

 For severe cases consult a doctor.

THRUSH

Thrush (*oral candida* or *monilia*) is a common fungal infection of the mouth in infants. You will see white patches on the tongue, inside the cheeks and sometimes in the throat. If severe, the condition causes some discomfort, and feeding may be affected. It can also cause severe nappy rash (*see* Nappy Rash, page 140). In older children thrush may develop after the administration of antibiotics, or the use of a nebulizer for asthma.

✚ FIRST AID Thrush can be cured with oral anti-fungal drops such as nystatin or by putting one drop of 1% acqueous gentian violet inside each cheek three times a day. If thrush is persistent, seek medical advice as it may be an early sign of immune deficiency.

Some children get mouth ulcers from time to time without other symptoms. The cause is unknown. Rinsing the mouth with a mild salt solution may be soothing, or ask a pharmacist for a suitable medication.

Some also get recurrent cold sores on the lips – usually a minor complaint requiring no treatment. When they cause burning, discomfort or embarrassment, a doctor may prescribe a cream containing the anti-viral agent acyclovir to clear them more quickly.

HAND, FOOT AND MOUTH DISEASE

Other viruses can also cause sores in the mouth and throat. Hand, foot and mouth disease is a common viral infection that tends to occur in summer. It is generally a mild illness, starting with slight fever and a few ulcers in the mouth. After a day or two blisters appear on the hands and feet, and often on the knees. The blisters on the arms and legs usually disappear after three or four days.

✚ FIRST AID For treatment of mouth ulcers, *see* Mouth Ulcers and Cold Sores, page 115. Apply calamine lotion to blisters on hands and feet to relieve itching and dry out the sores.

MUMPS

Mumps is a common viral infection of the salivary glands, which lie in front of and below the ears, under the jaw and under the tongue. It starts with a day or two of fever, which may be so mild as to pass unnoticed in young children. The face becomes tender and swollen on one side or both, and there may be vomiting and headache. The swellings last for up to a week, after which the child rapidly gets better.

Feeding may be painful, especially anything acidic, so give him milk and bland foods.

✚ FIRST AID Mumps can be prevented by the MMR vaccine, so have your baby vaccinated (*see* Immunization, pages 146–148). Although it is generally a mild disease, consult a doctor.

Get medical attention urgently if the child has severe headache and vomiting, or abdominal or testicular pain. These symptoms may indicate a complication of the mumps virus.

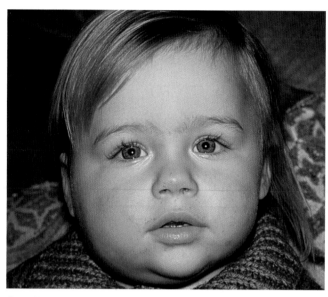
Swollen glands are characteristic of mumps.

TEETHING AND TOOTHACHE
Teething

This is a natural process and you should not attribute such symptoms as fever and diarrhoea to this cause. The appearance of the larger teeth (canines and molars) may be associated with some redness of the gums, discomfort and dribbling. Paracetamol (acetaminophen) syrup will relieve discomfort. Biting on a teething ring or a rusk may also help.

Toothache

Usually there are no symptoms until there is advanced tooth decay. Then there may be sensitivity to heat or cold and sometimes severe pain. Paracetamol (acetaminophen) syrup will help relieve the discomfort until you can see the dentist.

How to prevent tooth decay
- Encourage your child to brush twice a day with a fluoride toothpaste.
- Keep her diet low in sugar and do not allow sugary snacks between meals or last thing at night.

- Take her to the dentist for regular check-ups from age two and a half.
- If the water in your area is adequately fluorinated, no additional fluorine is needed. Ask your dentist about this.

(*See also* Tooth Injuries, pages 65–66.)

THROAT INFECTIONS
Pharyngitis and tonsillitis

The tonsils are situated on either side of the back of the throat. They serve two important functions: preventing harmful germs in the mouth and throat from entering the body, and making antibodies to fight infection. The adenoids, situated higher up in the back of the throat, do the same job.

In any throat infection in a child, whether due to viruses or bacteria, the tonsils will be enlarged and painful (tonsillitis), and the rest of the throat will usually be inflamed also (pharyngitis). A child with a very sore and red throat, high fever and enlarged tender glands at the angle of the jaw may have a bacterial infection ('strep throat', from streptococci), which requires antibiotics. But it is often impossible to tell a streptococcal throat infection from one caused by a virus, unless the doctor does a throat culture (to grow the germs so as to identify them). Consult a doctor, who will decide whether to prescribe an antibiotic.

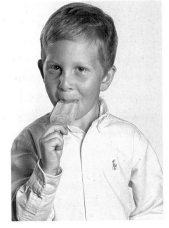

Sucking an ice lolly relieves a tender throat.

As a general rule, you can make the child more comfortable with:
- paracetamol (acetaminophen) syrup, given four times a day;
- throat lozenges;
- gargling with salt water;
- cool liquids, such as fruit juice or milk, or ice cream, to relieve pain on swallowing.

EARACHE

Earache commonly occurs in children between the ages of six months and two years. It is most often caused by an infection behind the eardrum and usually follows a cold, when the drainage tube from the middle ear to the back of the nose gets blocked. The fluid behind the drum raises the pressure and causes pain – and sometimes rupture – of the paper-thin eardrum. If this happens, the fluid or pus drains out, and pain is relieved. With proper treatment the eardrum reseals itself and full recovery should occur.

The tonsils

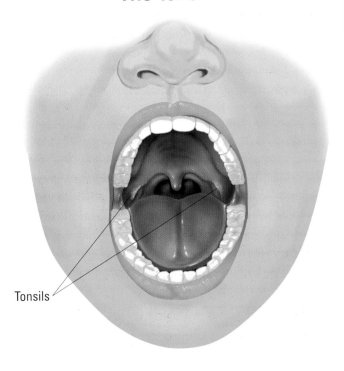

Tonsils

⊕ FIRST AID If you suspect earache consult a doctor. (Babies with ear infection may simply be irritable and sleepless, or frequently touch or rub the ear.)

Give prescribed medication exactly as directed and complete the full course. Give paracetamol (acetaminophen) for pain or if the fever is over 39°C (102.2°F). Do not put drops in the ear. (They obscure the eardrum and make it harder for the doctor to assess the infection.) Visit your doctor after two weeks to ensure the infection has cleared up and hearing is normal.

A child's middle ear cavities can become filled with thick, glue-like fluid, causing hearing loss. Drainage of the fluid may be required. A drainage tube (grommet) will be inserted through a small incision in the ear drum to allow fluid to escape and to equalize pressures in the middle ear. However, your doctor may want to wait three months as there is often spontaneous improvement.

NOSEBLEEDS

Nosebleeds are common throughout childhood. They are usually caused by picking the nose during colds, or vigorous sniffing or nose-blowing, and are frequent in children with hay fever (allergic rhinitis).

⊕ FIRST AID Get the child to sit, leaning forward, so that the blood can be spat out rather than swallowed. Have a basin handy for this. Swallowed blood is irritating to the stomach, so it is often vomited

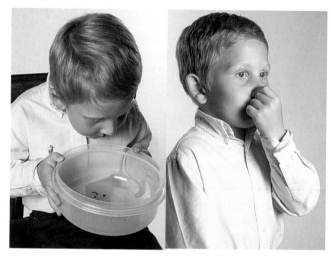

Lean forward over a bowl to spit out any blood. Pinch the nose shut and breathe through the mouth.

up. Let him blow his nose free of large clots. Then apply firm pressure by pinching the soft part of the nose against the central wall with your fingers, and maintain this pressure continuously for 10 minutes. Do not worry – he will breathe through his mouth. If bleeding continues, insert a piece of gauze soaked in vasoconstrictor nose drops (for example, phenylephrine) or coated with petroleum jelly, and continue pressure for a further 10 minutes. Leave the gauze in for a further 10 minutes before removing it.

A cold object placed on the back of the neck or elsewhere does not help to stop a nosebleed!

 Get a medical opinion if:

- bleeding continues;
- the child feels dizzy or faints;
- there are any signs of bleeding elsewhere, such as bleeding spots in the skin;
- he has recurrent nose bleeds – repeated bleeding from one side may mean that a small vein needs to be cauterized.

EYE INFECTIONS

Common eye infections in children are conjunctivitis (affecting the mucous lining of the eyelids and eye), styes and blepharitis (affecting the eyelids). Fortunately, involvement of the eye itself, which is much more serious, is also much rarer. Get a medical opinion immediately if there is pain in the eye, marked sensitivity to light, and/or haziness of vision. There may be a scratch or sore on the cornea (the transparent part of the eye), a foreign body in the sclera (the white of the eye), or a problem within the eye itself. (*See also* Eye Injuries, pages 61–63.)

CONJUNCTIVITIS

Conjunctivitis (also called 'pink eye') is an infection of the thin membrane that covers the whites of the eyes and the inside of the eyelids. It may be caused by a virus, bacterium or, in the newborn, by a microorganism called chlamydia.

Viral conjunctivitis results in red eyes, irritation and watery discharge. In bacterial conjunctivitis, on the other hand, the discharge is yellow and the eyelashes are matted together after sleeping. Both eyes are almost always affected.

Other causes of red inflamed eyes include allergy – in which case the eyes are usually itchy as well – and irritation resulting from smoke or chlorine in swimming pools.

Conjunctivitis

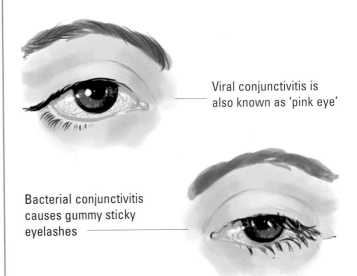

Viral conjunctivitis is also known as 'pink eye'

Bacterial conjunctivitis causes gummy sticky eyelashes

⊕ FIRST AID If the eyes are simply red without yellow discharge, bathe them frequently with mild salt solution (*see* box on page 109). Pour a few drops into each eye, wiping the excess away with cotton wool. Do this at least every hour while the child is awake. The conjunctivitis should clear in four to seven days.

If there is a sticky discharge, it is bacterial conjunctivitis, requiring antibiotic drops or ointment. Follow instructions from your doctor or pharmacist.

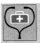 **Always seek medical advice if:**

- your baby (under six weeks) has inflamed eyes;
- only one eye is involved – this may mean the cornea has been scratched, or there is a foreign body in the eye (*see* Foreign Bodies in the Eye, pages 61–63);
- the eyelids become swollen;
- the child's vision is blurred.

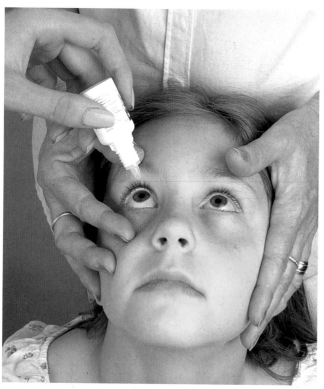

Putting eye drops into a young child's eyes may require two adults. One of you holds the child while the other puts them in.

APPLICATION TIPS

- If you cannot open the eyelids sufficiently, put drops in the inner corner of the eye with the child lying down and they will run into the eye itself.
- Put in drops every two hours.
- If you have difficulty applying ointment, apply it to the eyelid corners; it will reach the conjunctiva as it melts.
- Ointment is longer acting than drops; apply every four to six hours.

STYES

Styes are boils affecting the eyelashes. A stye will get better by itself, but you can help bring it to a head by applying heat.

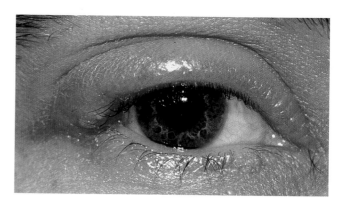

A stye is caused by inflammation of a hair follicle.

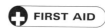 **FIRST AID**

Warm a teaspoon in warm water (not too hot!) and get the child to apply it to her eye. Repeat this frequently. Applying an antibiotic eye ointment three times a day for a few days is a good idea. Get this from your pharmacist or doctor.

BLOCKED TEAR DUCTS

In infants and young children, the tube carrying tears from the eyes into the nose may be blocked on one or both sides, resulting in constant watering of the eye. There may be a bead of pus at the corner of the eye – sometimes mistaken for conjunctivitis.

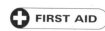 **FIRST AID**

Open a blocked duct by rolling your finger in the angle between nose and cheek bone, just below the eye. Though the problem usually resolves itself with time, see a specialist if it has not by the age of one year. Probing of the duct may be required.

HEADACHES

Headache is as common in children as in adults. It accompanies many childhood infections and is seldom the most troublesome symptom. But headache may also be the only, or earliest, indication of serious illness such as meningitis or other conditions that raise the pressure inside the head.

RECURRENT HEADACHES

Many children have recurring headaches with no apparent physical cause. Chronic non-progressive headaches occur at irregular intervals, become more severe during the day and are brought on by stress or tiredness. Eye strain is often blamed, and it is a good idea to have your child's eyes tested. Sinusitis or a tooth infection may also be responsible.

Migraine headaches occur at regular intervals and there is often a history of migraine in the family. In a young child the main symptoms may be vomiting and/or abdominal pain. The classic visual effects that can precede a migraine – wavy patterns or dots to one side of the line of vision – occur only in older children.

If your child regularly gets headaches, first look for possible stresses within the family, school or peer group and deal with them. Then get a full medical assessment. Once the more serious causes are excluded (which is most likely) your doctor may diagnose migraine. Effective treatment is available to stop, even prevent, these headaches.

PROGRESSIVE HEADACHES

Headaches that steadily increase in severity are a different matter. These may be caused by raised pressure in the head, or high blood pressure. They are the only headaches that will wake a child from sleep. Effortless vomiting without preceding nausea is a particular danger sign. Get medical advice urgently.

MENINGITIS

Meningitis is an infection of the membranes around the brain, and may be caused by a variety of micro-organisms. The symptoms of viral and bacterial meningitis are similar in the early stages, but bacterial meningitis tends to be much more severe. In infants the symptoms may be vague – crying, restlessness, refusing feeds, vomiting, fever, or abnormal drowsiness, and sometimes convulsions. Older children can tell you they have a severe headache, cannot stand bright light or loud noises and have a painful stiff neck.

In one common and dangerous form (meningococcal meningitis) there may be bleeding spots in the skin – tiny red spots that do not blanch on pressure, or larger bruises (*see* Meningococcal Infection, page 139).

 Get medical advice urgently if:

- a child complains of severe headache;
- she vomits persistently;
- she has a stiff neck;
- she is drowsy or lethargic;
- she has a convulsion;
- she has small bleeding spots in the skin.

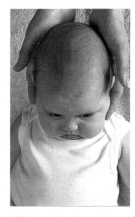

Tilting the head forward onto the chest will be painful if the child has meningitis.

CONVULSIONS AND SEIZURES

Convulsions and seizures are brief passing attacks of disturbed consciousness, sometimes accompanied by abnormal movements of limbs or body. There are many causes – sudden rise of temperature, low blood sugar or poisoning – so always consult your doctor if your child experiences a 'funny turn'.

FEBRILE CONVULSIONS

A convulsion (or fit) happens because of an abnormal electrical discharge in the brain, most commonly caused by a sudden rise in temperature brought on by an infection (a febrile convulsion).

These attacks are most frequent between the ages of six months and four years, when the brain is especially sensitive to rises in temperature. They are generally quite harmless, though frightening to parents and onlookers. The child will suddenly pass out, stiffen or develop twitching of the limbs, and the eyes will squint or roll upwards. She may feel hot, but sometimes the temperature rises so quickly you cannot immediately feel it in the skin. Most attacks last only a few minutes.

STAY CALM AND ASK FOR HELP

- Make sure the child's airway is clear and that she cannot injure herself against hard objects.
- Do not shake or slap her.
- Do not put anything in her mouth to prevent her biting her tongue.
- Take off her clothes and sponge her all over with lukewarm water, starting at the head.
- If her temperature is very high – above 40°C (104°F) – apply an ice pack or cool her with a fan.
- When the attack is over, put her in the recovery position (*see* page 27), with a light covering.

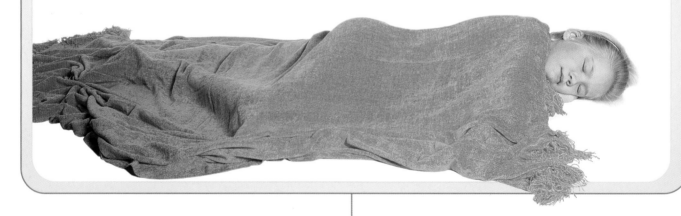

FIRST AID In most children this is a one-off event, but some may experience further convulsions with fever. In these cases, prevent attacks by giving a sedative (diazepam) rectally at the first sign of fever. Febrile convulsions generally have no ill-effects, and few children who have them later develop epilepsy.

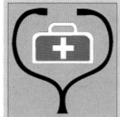 **Call the doctor if an attack lasts more than 10–15 minutes. Medication is needed.**

EPILEPSY

Epilepsy is a tendency (sometimes inherited) to have recurrent convulsions. It takes many forms and the diagnosis is not often made before the age of five. You should always get a specialist opinion to establish the cause and nature of recurrent fits. There are a number of effective medications to prevent convulsions or lessen their frequency and severity. An epileptic attack usually lasts only a few minutes.

 FIRST AID Follow the instructions for convulsions above. Do not try to stop the convulsion. Once it begins it cannot be stopped. If it lasts longer than a few minutes, or if the child is blue in the face or choking, get medical help immediately

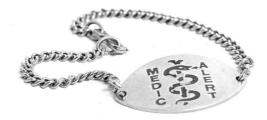

Every child with epilepsy should wear a MedicAlert wristband indicating the nature of the problem.

BREATH-HOLDING SEIZURES

When some young children start to cry, they hold their breath on breathing out and cannot breathe in. Their faces become red or purple and they may pass out for a few seconds. They then relax and normal breathing is restored. Loss of consciousness is due to slowing of the heart, in other words, to a temporary shortage of oxygen in the brain and not to an electrical discharge as in a convulsion.

These attacks are harmless and not related to epilepsy. They disappear as the child matures, usually by four years. Never allow fear of an attack to interfere with normal discipline. Ignore the attack, not the child!

If you are concerned, call the doctor. She may want to check the child's blood count, as the attacks may be worsened by anaemia.

FAINTING

This is sudden loss of consciousness with extreme pallor of the face, brought on by such things as an empty tummy combined with a stuffy room, standing in the heat, or a sudden fright. It is caused by a brief shortage of oxygen in the brain when the heart slows down or there is a drop in blood pressure. A child who faints regularly must be investigated by an expert.

STOMACH AILMENTS AND ABDOMINAL PAIN

Digestive system problems are frequent in children, second only to colds and sore throats. Although the common symptoms of vomiting and diarrhoea are upsetting, they are rarely persistent enough to be a serious threat to health. Other digestive disorders are less common but may cause chronic illness that can affect growth if left untreated.

VOMITING IN INFANTS

Vomiting is the forceful ejection of stomach contents. It should not be confused with regurgitation (posseting), which is an effortless spitting up after feeds, often with a wind. This is a normal feature in babies. The infant who possets and is otherwise well and gaining weight requires no special treatment.

 Consult a doctor if:

- regurgitation is frequent and copious;
- there is no gain in weight;
- there are any other symptoms, such as excessive crying or a cough.

A single vomiting episode is seldom cause for concern, but there are many possible reasons for vomiting in infants – if your baby keeps doing it you would be well advised to check with the doctor.

 FIRST AID After a single episode of vomiting, give no feeds for one hour, then offer sips of clear fluids (such as water or fruit juice) every 15 minutes for one hour. Do not give any medications to stop the vomiting. Once there is no further vomiting, begin to introduce regular feeds in half quantities, then work up to the usual quantity.

 Get medical advice if:

- your baby has a fever above 38°C (100.4°F);
- he has a cough or diarrhoea;
- he vomits persistently;
- he is drowsy;
- your baby is dehydrated (*see* Signs of Dehydration, page 126);
- there is pain or the baby's abdomen is tender when you press it.

Get urgent help if:

- the vomit is greenish or blood-stained;
- the vomiting is forceful and happens after every feed.

VOMITING IN CHILDREN

Some children are more prone to vomiting than others. Common, harmless causes of a single bout of vomiting are overeating, overexcitement or travel sickness.

In other cases vomiting may be the first sign of an infection. The commonest is a bowel infection (gastroenteritis), when vomiting is soon followed by the passing of loose, frequent stools. Sometimes contaminated food can cause an outbreak of vomiting in a number of people at the same time (known as food poisoning).

Other possible causes of vomiting

- ingestion of a toxic substance (*see* Poisoning, pages 89–92);
- acute appendicitis;
- an obstruction of the bowel;
- an infection of any kind (*see* in particular Meningitis, page 121);
- injury.

+ FIRST AID Reassure the child and let her rest quietly. Do not give her any food or drink for an hour, and then offer her sips of water – or any non-fizzy clear drink – every 15 minutes. Never give any medications to stop vomiting. If there is no further vomiting, increase fluids steadily, and introduce solid food after six hours.

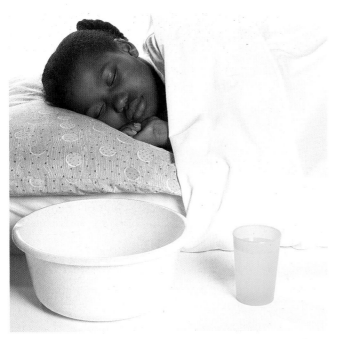

Place a basin near the child's bed for her to vomit into. Keep fluids nearby to prevent dehydration.

 Take the child to the hospital if:

- she vomits persistently or for more than three hours;
- you suspect a head injury;
- she shows any symptoms of meningitis (*see* Meningitis, page 121);
- you suspect she has ingested a drug or poison;
- the urine is dark in colour;
- the vomit is greenish or blood-stained;
- there is any abdominal pain or tenderness (*see also* Hernia, page 129).

DIARRHOEA

Diarrhoea – abnormally frequent or liquid bowel movements – is a common symptom in children, most often due to gastroenteritis, an infection of the bowel caused by viruses or other organisms. The first signs may be tummy rumbling and vomiting and there may be cramping abdominal pain and tenderness. Gastroenteritis caused by bacteria is more severe, and the stools may contain blood and mucus. When blood is present the term dysentery is used.

Diarrhoea may also be caused by infection elsewhere in the body, drugs or poisons accidentally swallowed, anxiety, or many other causes. The main danger is that if diarrhoea is severe, your child can become dehydrated.

+ FIRST AID Simply replace the fluid lost from the body. Do not use medications to make the stools firmer or less frequent – the body will take care of this in its own time.

If the diarrhoea is mild, the child can continue taking the usual feeds. Replace lost fluid by giving additional water, sugar and salts (*see* box on page 126). A toddler or young child who is still breast-fed can continue nursing. Continue normal feeds in frequent small amounts and give extra fluids.

For a child under two years give 50ml to100ml (a quarter to half a cup) of liquid after each loose stool. For an older child give 100ml to 200 ml (half to one cup) after each loose stool. If the child vomits, wait 10 minutes, then give the solution more slowly (for example, a teaspoonful every two to three minutes). If the child is very thirsty, give more fluid.

Do not give any medication to stop vomiting. Check the child's weight after recovery, and give her an extra feed a day for at least a week after she has recovered.

What fluids to give

Oral rehydrating solution (ORS) can be bought ready-mixed in a packet or as a prepared drink (Pedialyte™ or Resol™). These contain just the right amounts of salts and sugar and are the best way to replace fluid.

Get medical help if:

- the diarrhoea lasts for five days or longer;
- the child is feverish;
- vomiting is continuous;
- the child is unable to drink;
- the child is lethargic or becomes drowsy;
- there is blood in the stools;
- breathing is rapid and deep;
- signs of dehydration increase (*see* below).

Recognizing severe diarrhoea
Signs of dehydration

You can recognize dehydration by the following signs:

- a dry mouth and tongue;
- sunken eyes;
- absence of tears when crying;
- decreased urination;
- lethargy and drowsiness;
- skin that goes back slowly when pinched.

REHYDRATING SOLUTION

If you do not have an oral rehydrating solution, make your own sugar and salt solution by mixing eight level teaspoonsful of sugar and half a teaspoonful of table salt in one litre (two pints) of water (preferably boiled first and allowed to cool). A child older than two can be given non-fizzy fruit drinks instead, or add a little fruit juice to the salt solution for flavour.

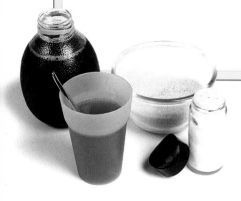

DEHYDRATION CHECK

The pinch test is a very simple way to check for dehydration. Gently pinch the skin on the side of the abdomen and then let go. If the child is not dehydrated the skin will flatten immediately. If there is some dehydration, the fold will take a second or two to disappear. In cases of severe dehydration the fold of skin will stay raised for several seconds.

In the absence of these symptoms, a few days of diarrhoea are generally not cause for concern. But diarrhoea caused by a virus or bacterial infection may be contagious, so wash your hands well to avoid spreading germs, especially to those particularly at risk, such as other young children, the elderly, or people with weakened immune systems.

Preventing diarrhoea

Make sure you wash your hands well, particularly after nappy changes, before and after handling food (especially poultry) and after touching pets and cleaning aquariums or cat litter trays. Lessen the risk of food poisoning by thoroughly washing all kitchen and eating utensils, cleaning surfaces where you prepare or cook food, and cooking meat until it is cooked through and no longer pink.

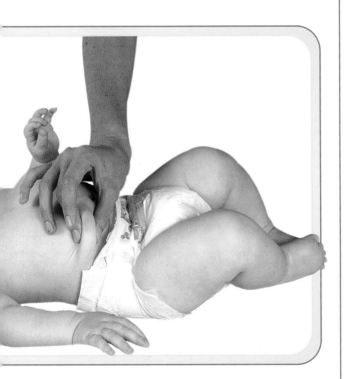

PAIN IN THE ABDOMEN

Occasional abdominal pains are common in children, but although there are some serious causes – and the pain is a symptom you should not disregard – most are minor upsets.

Abdominal pain in infants
Infantile colic

Colic in the first three months of life is probably just an extreme variety of the behaviour normal for this age, but can cause distress. It is characterized by regular vigorous crying, usually in the late afternoon or early evening. During these spells the infant cries, cannot be soothed, and draws up her legs or arches backward as though in pain. In all other respects she is well: she is not vomiting, she is gaining weight, and bowels, feeding and weight gain are normal. These spells have no lasting effect on the baby's health.

If the baby has a fever, or any symptoms other than the crying, the diagnosis is not infantile colic. If you are worried, consult a doctor or nurse.

➕ **FIRST AID** Ensure you are using the right techniques for feeding the baby and bringing up wind (burping). Avoid overfeeding; do not feed her every time she cries.

Allow her to suck a pacifier (dummy) – but remember to keep it clean – or, better still, to suck her fingers or thumb. This is a harmless practice. Carry her in a harness or sling at your front or back.

Do not stop breast feeding or change the feed formula. Milk allergy is seldom the cause of colic in infants under three months.

Do not use medications or sedatives.

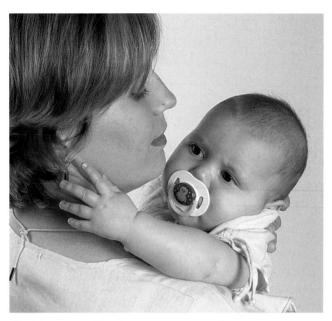

Sucking a pacifier helps to ease colic.

Hernia

A hernia, or rupture, is a weak spot in the abdominal wall that allows a segment of bowel to come through. The usual place for a hernia is the groin, in both boys and girls. The bowel can normally be pushed back with gentle pressure, but if it twists, or strangulates, it causes serious intestinal obstruction.

When a hernia strangulates, the baby shows sudden great discomfort:
- he refuses feeds;
- he vomits, and often the vomit is green in colour;
- the abdomen may become distended;
- there may be a firm tender lump in the groin, which cannot be pushed back with gentle pressure.
If your baby shows any of these symptoms, call an ambulance immediately.

The bulging of the navel (an umbilical hernia) is quite common in infants and usually disappears with time. These hernias very seldom strangulate. See a doctor if you are concerned.

These three conditions require urgent medical attention:

1. Intestinal obstruction

Babies may develop a bowel obstruction because of some defect they were born with. Symptoms will be:
- sudden abdominal discomfort;
- refusing feeds;
- vomiting;
- abdominal distension.

2. Appendicitis

Very rarely a baby may develop appendicitis, and the symptoms may not be as apparent as in older children. You should suspect this if the baby has a fever and the stomach is swollen and tender.

3. Torsion of the testis

This can be the cause of abdominal pain in young male infants (*see* Torsion of the Testis, page 134).

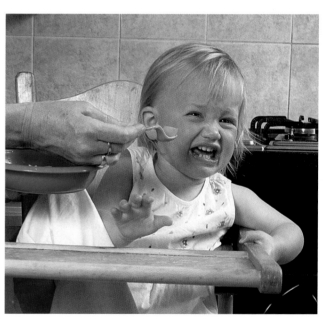

Refusing feeds is common in children but may also be an indicator of an intestinal obstruction.

Abdominal pain in older children
Intestinal obstruction

This may have various causes. One is intussusception, which occurs usually between the ages of three and nine months. This is an infolding of a segment of bowel, causing obstruction that may need surgical repair. It affects previously healthy, well-nourished infants, coming on so suddenly that she may wake with a surprised shriek of pain. There are then intermittent attacks of severe cramps, sweating and disturbed sleep. Other symptoms are:

* vomiting of greenish-yellow material;
* failure to pass stools;
* later, passage of blood-stained mucus;
* fever and swelling of the abdomen if treatment is delayed.

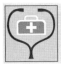 **The above symptoms require urgent attention. Call an ambulance.**

Appendicitis

This is fairly common in children. The appendix, a worm-like structure attached to the large bowel in the right lower abdomen, easily becomes obstructed or infected. Symptoms appear fairly suddenly, with pain in the centre of the abdomen which steadily worsens, and later becomes localized in the right lower abdomen. Slight pressure on the tummy increases the pain. There is some nausea or vomiting, and fever. If neglected, the appendix can burst, resulting in an abscess or infection of the abdominal cavity – a very serious condition called acute peritonitis.

Acute abdominal pain in children may also be caused by inflamed glands in the abdomen (mesenteric adenitis), secondary to a throat infection. This can be difficult to distinguish from appendicitis.

Position of the appendix

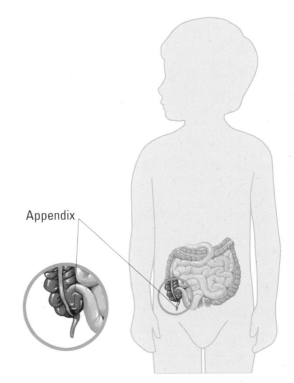

Appendix

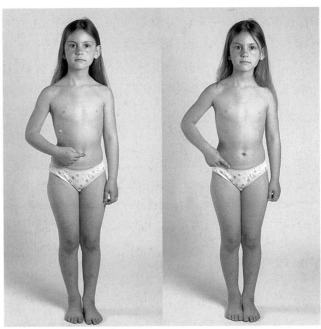

Appendicitis pain usually begins at the navel and moves down toward the right lower abdomen.

Another cause of acute abdominal pain is an infection of the bladder, tubes or kidneys (*see* Urinary Tract and Genital Problems, pages 133–134).

➕ **FIRST AID**   If your child has sudden abdominal pain, it is difficult to tell whether this is a temporary upset or something more serious. Do not give him painkillers or other remedies that may mask a serious condition. Do not give him anything to eat or drink. A hot water bottle held against the tummy may provide some relief. If symptoms are severe, or continue for more than three hours, get medical help.

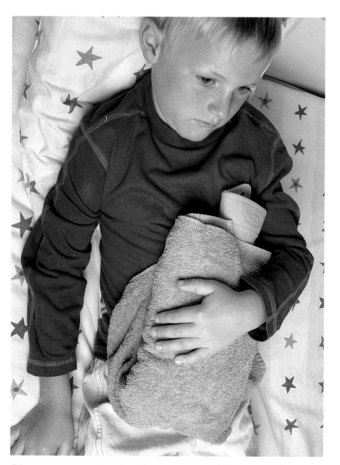

Place a hot water bottle – wrapped in a towel to prevent scalding – on the abdomen to relieve pain.

Functional abdominal pain

About 10–15% of children will experience recurrent abdominal pain, particularly if they are highly strung and anxious. It is rare before five years of age and is most frequent between 10 and 12. No cause for the pain can be found, so we term this 'functional' abdominal pain. The pain is generally vague and in the centre of the abdomen. It seldom wakes a child from sleep. If it does, you should suspect a more serious cause, particularly if the pain is not in the centre of the abdomen but to one side.

If your child has this kind of pain without any other symptoms, get him checked by a doctor to make sure there are no other possible causes. Your doctor will assure you that, although there is no serious illness, the pain is real and not in the child's head – which will help relieve your anxiety and the child's. The next step is to discover what is troubling him and deal with any stresses within the home, school or peer group. Abdominal pains of this kind should then become fewer and less frequent. It is not a good idea to give medicines to such children.

Some young children (one to five years) who experience attacks of abdominal pain at intervals of weeks or months, with or without vomiting, will later display the classic symptoms of migraine, especially if there is a family history of migraine (*see* Recurrent Headaches, page 121).

Constipation

Children differ in the frequency with which they pass stools. As long as the stools are soft and normal in consistency and are passed painlessly, do not worry about regularity. Constipation is the infrequent passage of hard stools with straining and discomfort. Although it may seem a minor problem, it can become a major one for an older child as a result of over-forceful toilet training as an infant, a painful anal fissure, or even reluctance to use unsanitary toilets at school.

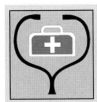 **FIRST AID** Constipation is rare in breast-fed babies, although stools may be passed only every five to seven days, but a baby fed on cow's milk formulae may pass hard stools. To relieve constipation in babies:
- add 2.5ml (half a teaspoon) of brown sugar to each feed;
- increase fluids by giving the baby more water or fruit juice during the day;
- give 5ml (one teaspoon) of prune juice as a laxative if the problem persists.

To relieve constipation in older children:
- see that they drink plenty of fluids;
- ensure they get roughage in their diet (cereal, brown bread, vegetables and fruit);
- get them into the habit of regular, unhurried toilet visits each morning.

Consult your doctor if your child's constipation does not improve, or the abdomen is painful or swollen.

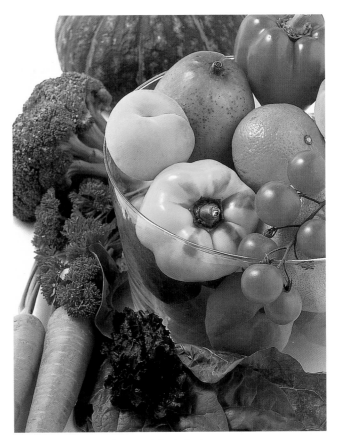

Fibre in vegetables and fruit helps to prevent constipation naturally.

Anal fissure

Sometimes a small tear in the lining of the anus may result when the child passes a large, hard stool. This causes pain on defaecation and the stool may show a streak of fresh blood. Treat this promptly.

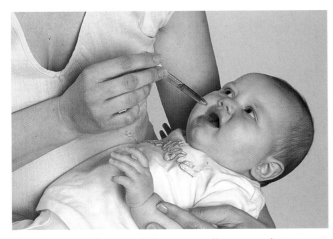

A teaspoon of prune juice can relieve persistent constipation problems in babies.

FIRST AID Buy a mild anaesthetic cream from your pharmacist (for example, Remicaine™) and apply it with your little finger, gently inserted into the anus. Repeat three times a day, and before a stool is passed.

Give the child a stool softener such as Dufalac™ for a week, or give a vegetable laxative (Senokot™) every night for one week.

Worms

Two common types of worms in the bowel are round-worms and thread (or pin) worms.

Roundworm

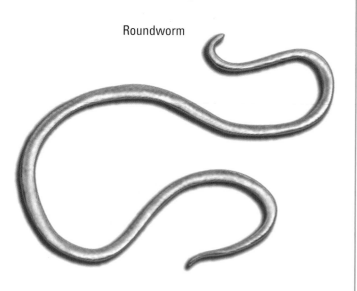

Roundworms

Roundworms are much larger than threadworms – up to 15cm (6in). One or two may be found in the child's stool, or may even be vomited up. When there are large numbers of worms in the bowel they can become knotted up and cause an obstruction. Occasionally worms get stuck in odd places – resulting, for example, in an obstructed appendix or bile duct. If the child has been infested with roundworms for a long time, larval worms passing through the lungs may cause persistent wheezing or pneumonia.

Other worms, such as hookworm, whipworm and tapeworm, are less common in temperate climates but can cause more severe symptoms.

Threadworms

Threadworms are tiny white worms that live in the lower bowel. The only symptoms are itching around the anus caused by the sticky eggs they deposit. There may be infection from the child's scratching. The worms may be seen wriggling in the stool. In girls the vulva may also be itchy.

Threadworms are easily spread from one child to another by eggs transferred on the fingers, so ensure you teach your children to wash their hands regularly, especially in daycare centres and wherever they use an outdoor play area. Also remember to make sure that you wash vegetables thoroughly.

✚ FIRST AID   All worms are easily eliminated by modern medications (abendazole or mebendazole), which are safe and effective. Consult your pharmacist.

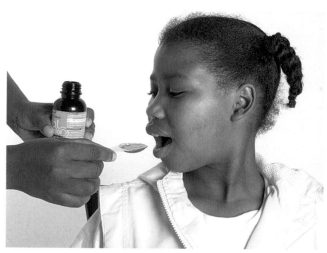

Intestinal worms can easily be eliminated with the appropriate medication.

URINARY TRACT AND GENITAL PROBLEMS

Urinary tract infections (UTIs) are infections of the bladder and the tubes carrying urine from the kidneys – the ureters and urethra. They are more common in girls, as the urethra is much shorter than in boys, so bacteria can more easily enter the bladder from the bowel.

URINARY TRACT INFECTIONS

Learn to recognize UTI symptoms, such as:

- burning on passing water;
- unusual frequency of passing water;
- bed-wetting in a previously dry child;
- in children under two, diarrhoea;
- urine that is smoky or pink in colour and may be odd-smelling;
- fever, irritability and vomiting;
- pains in the back or abdomen (*see* Stomach Ailments and Abdominal Pain, pages 124–131).

Have a specimen of urine tested. Your doctor will explain how to collect it. If the doctor prescribes an antibiotic, make sure your child completes the course as prescribed.

 See a doctor within 24 hours if you suspect a urinary tract infection.

The urinary tract

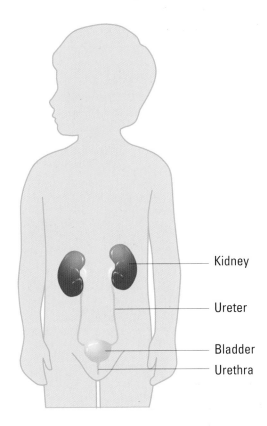

Kidney

Ureter

Bladder
Urethra

How can UTIs be prevented?

Children should be encouraged to pass urine every four hours or before each meal and especially before going to bed. It is a good idea to encourage 'double urination' in a child who has had a UTI – going back a second time and trying to produce a drop or two more. Both girls and boys should be encouraged to wipe their bottoms from front to back after using the toilet.

Girls' problems
Vulvovaginitis

Burning or itching of the vulval area, vaginal discharge and discomfort on passing water may be caused by:

- infrequent changing of nappies and poor hygiene;
- wearing tight pantyhose (tights);

- bubble baths;
- threadworm infestation;
- in older girls, thrush.

A smelly discharge may indicate a foreign body in the vagina (*see* Foreign Bodies in the Vagina, page 75).

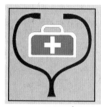 **FIRST AID** Sit her in a warm bath twice a day for a week, and wash her (or encourage her to wash herself) with a mild baby soap. Dry well and apply barrier cream, such as Siopel™ (see Nappy Rash, pages 139–140). Ensure she wears panties made of cotton rather than synthetic fabric, and she wipes herself from front to back after using the toilet.

If the problem persists, or symptoms are severe, consult your doctor.

Boys' problems
Balanitis
This is swelling and itching of the head of the penis and foreskin, with redness and a white discharge. As in vulvovaginitis, this usually results from poor hygiene.

FIRST AID Wash the child (or encourage him to wash himself) regularly with a mild baby soap. Dry the area well and apply a barrier cream, such as Siopel™. Try to make sure he wears light cotton under-wear rather than synthetic fabrics.

If the problem persists, or symptoms are severe, consult your doctor. Circumcision may be needed in severe cases.

Phimosis
This means an unretractable foreskin, which is normal in infancy. In some boys the foreskin is not retractable till the age of four.

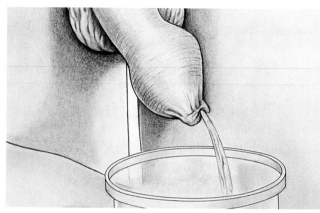

The opening in the foreskin is abnormally small in phimosis, which may make passing urine difficult.

Paraphimosis
This term means a retracted foreskin, which is stuck behind the glans, causing severe pain and swelling.

 Seek medical help urgently.

Torsion of the testis
The testis can become twisted on its appendages, caus-ing severe pain. The scrotum on the affected side is swollen and red and the testis hard and extremely ten-der to touch. In an infant, the cause of the screaming may not be apparent until the genitalia are examined.

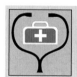 **Seek medical help urgently. This condition requires immediate surgery.**

RASHES AND SPOTS

Your child has a rash...

This chapter describes some common childhood rashes. There are a number of other less common ones, some of them serious, some not. If your child develops a rash that does not fit any of these descriptions, see a doctor as soon as possible.

Many childhood infections cause rashes. They can be:

- spotty rashes (multiple pink spots, either flat or slightly raised);
- patchy rashes (irregularly shaped patches or generalized redness);
- blistery rashes;
- blood spots in the skin.

Most rashes are not serious, but some are outward signs of an infection needing urgent medical attention. Consult a doctor about any rash occurring with fever, in case it is measles, which is a serious illness. Any blistery rash in a very young infant requires urgent attention.

(For advice on general management of rashes with fever, *see* Fever, page 107, and Respiratory Tract and Lung Disorders, pages 108–110.)

SPOTTY RASHES

Probably the commonest rash in children under two is a virus infection called 'rose rash' (*roseola infantum*). It usually starts with three days of high fever and irritability, after which light pink spots appear on the body. The temperature then settles and the child feels better. There are no other symptoms, although there may occasionally be a febrile convulsion at the start, as the temperature rises very suddenly (*see* Convulsions and Seizures, pages 122–123). The condition is mostly harmless.

✚ FIRST AID You do not need to do anything other than bring the child's temperature down if he feels uncomfortable (*see* Fever, page 107). Give lots of fluids. Once the rash appears, the temperature will go down and the child will be well again.

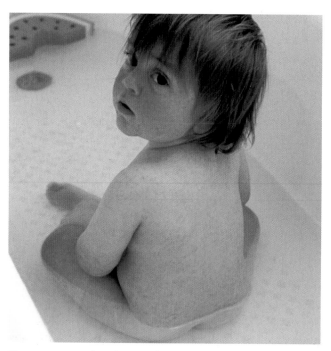

German measles is not dangerous to children.

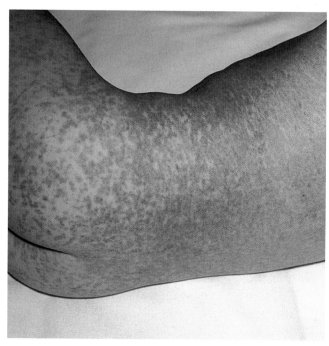

Measles can be prevented by vaccination.

German measles (rubella)

German measles is caused by the rubella virus and usually occurs in children over two who have not been vaccinated against it. There is very little fever. The child simply feels unwell and has a rash lasting for two or three days. At first the rash is separate pink spots, mostly on the trunk. On the second day it runs together into a generalized redness and then fades. The glands at the back of the head and in the neck are usually enlarged. Older children may have sore joints for some weeks after an attack of rubella.

➕ **FIRST AID** Unless the rash causes discomfort, you do not have to do anything. However, it is advisable to have a doctor confirm the diagnosis, because rubella is dangerous to a woman in the first three months of pregnancy. Her growing embryo can develop serious eye, ear, brain and heart problems.

Measles

This is the most serious of the common childhood rashes. It is extremely contagious, and is most severe in infants and in children who are weak or chronically ill. It is a notifiable disease. Thanks to an effective vaccine it is now uncommon but still accounts for 50% of deaths from common vaccine-preventable illnesses in poorer countries.

Measles starts with fever, cold symptoms and red eyes, all of which get steadily worse for four or five days before the rash appears. The child is sickest as the rash is coming out, which can take as long as three days. It starts as spots and blotches deep in the skin of the face, neck and chest. These spread to the rest of the body and the limbs. Because the virus also affects the lining of the respiratory and digestive tracts, cough and diarrhoea are common additional symptoms, and the illness may be complicated by ear infection, severe croup or pneumonia.

FIRST AID If your child is feverish, give paracetamol (acetaminophen) syrup eight-hourly as needed. Give plenty of fluids, and small, regular meals. A multivitamin mixture (especially with Vitamin A) will protect against secondary infections.

Ensure your baby is vaccinated against measles.

Glandular fever (infectious mononucleosis)

This is a common viral infection in older children. The symptoms usually include a sore throat and enlarged tonsils, as well as enlarged glands in the neck, armpits or groin. If it is incorrectly diagnosed as 'strep throat' and treated with an antibiotic, the child may develop a spotty rash.

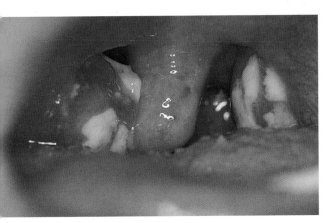

Enlarged tonsils covered with white membranes (resembling strep throat) are characteristic of glandular fever.

FIRST AID There is no specific treatment for glandular fever, but the child is likely to be tired and listless for some weeks. See your doctor if you are worried. She can check him for possible complications, such as disorders of the blood or nervous system.

PATCHY RASHES
Scarlet fever

Now uncommon, scarlet fever is caused by a strepto-coccus, which produces a toxin that causes a red rash. It starts suddenly, with high fever, sore throat, headache and vomiting. Within 12 hours the rash appears, first on the neck and chest, then the rest of the body. The face is flushed, with a pale area around the mouth. Tonsils and throat are inflamed and the tongue is white-coated. After a few days the coating peels off, leaving a red tongue with redder taste buds (a 'strawberry tongue'). Skin affected by the rash feels rough. After a week there is peeling, especially of the palms and soles.

FIRST AID Consult a doctor to confirm the diagnosis. She will prescribe an antibiotic to shorten the course of the illness and prevent complications, such as rheumatic fever and kidney disease. Make sure your child takes the full course.

Give paracetamol (acetaminophen) liquid to reduce high fever and make the child more comfortable. Keep him away from other children for a week.

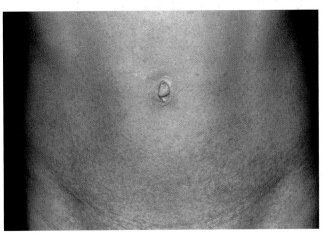

Scarlet fever – also known as scarlatina – produces a sore throat with widespread rash.

Slapped cheek disease

This common mild illness seldom has complications. It is caused by a virus that is widespread in the community, so young children are often infected without any symptoms. Typically, the child comes home from school with very red cheeks, as though he has been slapped. There are no other symptoms and no fever of note. A pink spotty rash then comes out on the trunk and spreads to the limbs, forming an irregular lacy or spotty appearance. The rash can persist on the limbs for as long as six weeks but the child remains quite well.

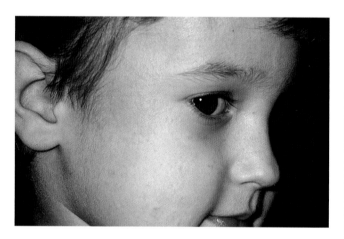

Slapped cheek disease is not accompanied by fever.

➕ **FIRST AID** No specific treatment is required, but keep the child away from any pregnant woman, because if she is not immune the foetus may be severely affected. The virus may also badly affect children with chronic illnesses.

BLISTERY RASHES
Chicken pox

This infection, caused by a virus, is generally a mild illness in children but more severe in older people. Typically there are only a few hours of fever and feeling unwell, then small red spots appear, usually on the trunk. These rapidly become small round blisters containing clear fluid. Soon more appear elsewhere and the process continues for a day or two. The severity of the rash varies, from only a few spots to involvement of the whole body. The blisters are itchy and easily popped on scratching. The resulting little ulcers turn into scabs and often become secondarily infected. Sometimes there are a few blisters inside the mouth and in the genital area. The scalp almost always has a blister or two – a good way of telling that the rash is chicken pox.

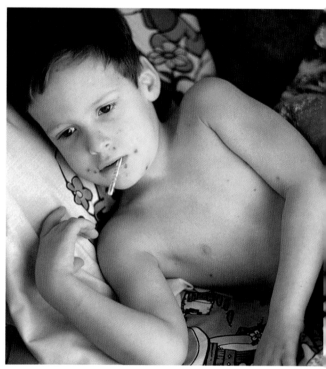

Small, round, red blisters containing clear fluid are characteristic of chicken pox.

➕ **FIRST AID** Apply calamine lotion to relieve itching and dry the sores. Consult a doctor, who may prescribe antibiotics for secondary infection of the blisters, and watch for any unusual complications.

Hand, foot and mouth disease

This viral infection causes blisters on the arms and legs, as well as mouth ulcers (*see* Hand, Foot and Mouth Disease, page 116).

Blood spots under the skin

You can tell a rash is caused by bleeding under the skin if the spots do not fade when you press them. These can be tiny bleeding spots or larger ones (bruises).

Bruises are usually caused by the mishaps that are a fact of life for all children. Sometimes small blood spots under the skin may be caused by the pressure of a garment, such as sleeping in clothing with a raised pattern, when the spots take on its pattern on the chest or abdomen. However, bleeding into and under the skin is a symptom of a number of significant, though generally rare, conditions so get a doctor's advice unless the cause is obvious.

Meningococcal infection

Meningococcus is a bacterium that causes a dangerous blood infection, sometimes also meningitis (*see* page 121).

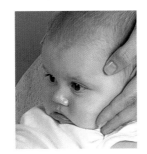

A stiff neck is a sign of meningitis.

The illness usually starts with fever and a few small blood spots that appear anywhere on the body, including the eyes and mouth. There are often early signs of meningitis (headache, vomiting and stiffness of the neck). In the most severe cases there is widespread progressive bruising, shock and collapse.

See your doctor immediately if you see blood spots or bruises in your child's skin, unless you know they were caused by a bump or a fall.

Bleeding into the skin and elsewhere may follow viral illnesses such as rubella or chicken pox.

Seborrhoeic dermatitis

This is common in babies between one and six months. It generally gets better by itself. The baby may have thick greasy crusts (cradle cap) on the scalp, neck, nose and ears and red scaly patches on the body. The neck, groin and armpits may become reddened and weepy, which can lead to secondary infection by yeasts or bacteria. The rash does not itch, and causes little discomfort.

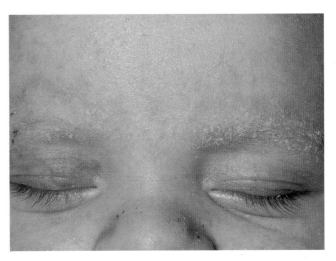

Greasy scales on eyebrows and forehead indicate that the baby has seborrhoeic dermatitis.

➕ FIRST AID Remove the scales and crusts by massaging olive oil into the scalp and leaving it on overnight. Then shampoo and gently remove the scales with a comb. Regular bathing and short periods of exposure to sunlight are often beneficial.

Get medical advice if the rash is infected.

Nappy rash

A baby's skin easily becomes irritated or infected if he wears a soiled nappy for too long. There are many kinds of nappy (diaper) rash. At first all you may see is redness over the buttocks or thighs, around the anus,

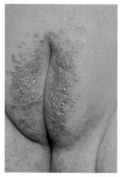

Raw skin and blisters make nappy rash a source of great discomfort.

or in the skin folds of the groin. Later the area becomes inflamed and weepy, and there may even be blisters or raw open areas. When there is a yeast (candida) infection you will see roundish red patches that spread and are scaly around the edges.

The main causes of nappy rash are heat, damp, friction and diarrhoea. Less commonly, it may be an allergy to elastic, soap powder or fabric softener.

FIRST AID Change the nappy more often, cleaning the skin thoroughly each time with warm water and mild baby soap. Dry thoroughly and apply a protective cream such as zinc oxide ointment, Fissan Paste™, Nivea™, or a barrier cream such as Siopel™.

Good hygiene and short periods of exposure to sunlight will help prevent more severe rashes. For severe rash ask your pharmacist for an effective anti-bacterial, anti-fungal and anti-inflammatory cream. See your doctor if the rash does not clear up or if the baby is also unwell or not thriving.

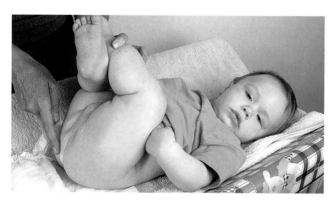

Careful washing, drying and application of a protective cream helps prevent nappy rash.

Impetigo

This is an infection caused by skin bacteria (staphylo-coccus or streptococcus). It appears as golden crusted sores or pus-filled blisters anywhere on the body. Staph infection is more likely if there are sores on the face, and if it started by itself, not with scratching. Strep impetigo tends to occur with scabies and insect bites, which the child scratches. It is found more often on the child's legs and produces more severe skin damage. If the lymph glands in the groin, armpits or elsewhere are enlarged, strep is more likely.

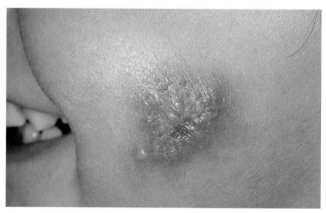

Impetigo sores are often covered by golden crusts.

FIRST AID Consult your doctor for a prescription for the appropriate oral antibiotic treatment. Treat the rash with Vioform™ emulsion or povidine-iodine cream, but never with anti-histamine or antibiotic creams.

Boils

Boils are caused by the same germs as impetigo, but the infection starts off in a hair follicle rather than in the surface skin, producing a painful red swelling. The boil gradually comes to a head and discharges pus, bringing relief. It can occur anywhere on the body. A splinter or small wound may be the entry point for infection.

FIRST AID If the boil is small and not causing much pain, apply a poultice – a paste made of Epsom salts (magnesium sulphate) and a little warm water. Cover with gauze to encourage the boil to come to a head. When it bursts, gently wipe the pus away with cotton wool soaked in antiseptic. Cover it with a dressing, kept in place with pieces of plaster placed well away from the boil. Do not apply sticking plaster to the boil itself and never squeeze or poke the boil.

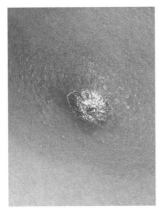

A boil is a round sore with a yellow head surrounded by tender redness.

A large boil that is very painful, or one that is getting bigger or not coming to a head after two days, must be opened by a doctor as soon as possible.

Get medical help if:

- the child has a fever or is unwell;
- the child has recurrent boils;
- you see red lines extending from the boil – this indicates a more serious condition (cellulitis) that requires urgent attention.

Recurrent boils

When boils occur recurrently on the head and neck, or on the buttocks and lower half of the body, your child may be harbouring a staphylococcus germ in the nose or anogenital region.

Sometimes recurrent boils are a sign of a more serious condition, so get a medical check-up to obtain the correct treatment.

Fingernail infections (whitlows)

A finger (less often, a toe) may become infected at the side of or under the nail. The side of the finger is red, tender and swollen, and a yellow head of pus may form.

FIRST AID Soak the finger for 15 minutes three times a day in warm water containing a little antiseptic. You can apply a poultice as for boils. If the whitlow comes to a head, you may be able to release the pus by gently pushing the skin aside at the edge of the nail.

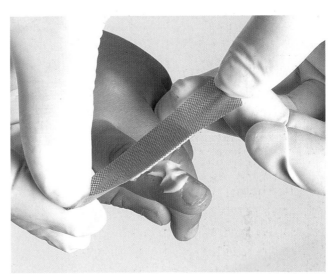

Apply a poultice to a whitlow to clear the infection.

See your doctor if:

- the finger is swollen and tender;
- the finger has not improved in 48 hours;
- the infection has not completely cleared within seven days.

Styes

These are boils that affect the eyelashes (*see* Styes, page 120).

Eczema

Eczema – like hay fever and asthma – commonly runs in families. Children with eczema are generally allergic to several things, though seldom to foodstuffs. The rash is intensely itchy, red and often weepy.

In young children the cheeks, forearms, front of the legs and trunk are most often affected. In older children the front of the elbows and back of the knees are more commonly involved, and the itchy skin is dry, cracked and often thickened.

⊕ FIRST AID A child with eczema must see the doctor. The condition is treated by applying plenty of moisturizing creams, using topical cortico-steroids where necessary, and using wet wraps.

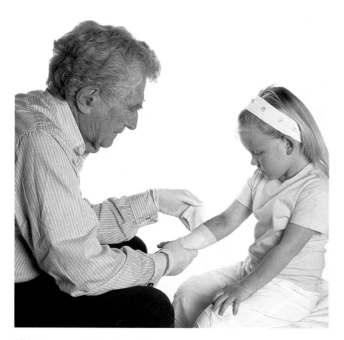

Wet wraps help to relieve eczema.

Wet wraps are cotton bandages moistened with hot water, applied to the affected areas and kept in place for up to 24 hours at a time. Apply them daily at first, and then less often as the skin heals. Stop when the itch-scratch-itch habit is controlled, but continue if the child starts to scratch again. This extremely effective treatment is recommended by dermatologists.

Some children develop chronic, non-itchy, pale patches, with a fine scale that looks like bran on the face or neck (*pityriasis sicca alba*). The cause is unknown, but it may be a mild form of eczema. Consult your doctor for appropriate medication.

A rash around a child's mouth may be due to the habit of lip-licking or lip-sucking ('lick eczema'). Moisturizing creams can help, or consult your doctor.

Psoriasis

This is a common chronic skin complaint that runs in families and is marked by sudden flare-ups with long remissions inbetween. It consists of red, scaly, thickened patches, which are not particularly itchy but may be uncomfortable, mostly on the scalp, elbows, knees and lower back.

⊕ FIRST AID Control mild cases by keeping the skin well moisturized with aqueous cream and exposing affected areas to the sun for short periods.

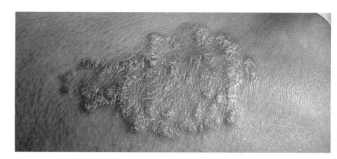

Raised, red, scaly patches are typical of psoriasis.

In more severe and distressing cases, consult a doctor, preferably a dermatologist, as there is a range of effective remedies she can recommend.

Urticaria (hives or nettle rash)

Urticaria may be caused by a virus infection or an allergic reaction to a foodstuff, drug or insect sting. It is an intensely itchy rash consisting of irregularly shaped, slightly raised pale blotches surrounded by a red border (weals). It may cover a small area or be very widespread. The weals shift their position – each one rarely lasts longer than 12 to 24 hours.

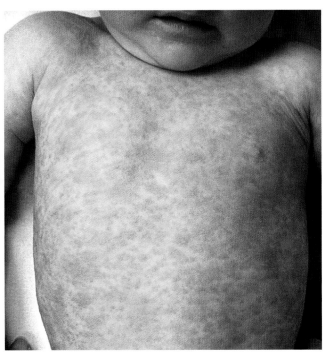

Raised, itchy, irregularly shaped patches are indications of urticaria.

➕ FIRST AID Antihistamine syrup or tablets from your pharmacy may relieve the symptoms. If your child has chronic urticaria (recurring frequently or lasting longer than six weeks) see the doctor so the cause can be identified and eliminated. In severe cases there may be facial swelling, even anaphylactic shock. An adrenaline injection under the skin is often effective (*see* Anaphylactic Shock, pages 111–112).

Pityriasis rosea

This starts as a ring-worm-like patch on the trunk, followed five days later by a rash on the trunk, but not the face. It consists of fawn-coloured or dark pink, slightly scaly spots that follow the lines of the ribs, so that they have a 'Christmas tree' distribu-tion. Sometimes there is

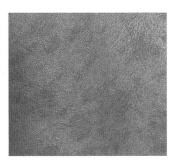

The trunk is covered by slightly scaly patches that do not itch.

mild itching, but no other symptoms. It is a harmless condition of unknown cause that tends to occur sea-sonally and gets better by itself. Exposure to sunshine or ultraviolet lamp treatment helps it get better faster.

Warts

These are caused by a virus infection which may spread from one child to another. Common warts are raised, have a rough surface and usually affect the hands and feet. Plane warts are flatter, with a smooth surface, and affect the face, neck or hands. Warts are harmless

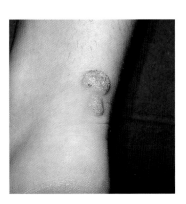

Warts are best left alone unless they are in an awk-ward spot.

growths which are best left alone as they generally disappear in six to 12 months. However, a wart on the sole of the foot (plantar wart) can be very painful and requires treatment. Otherwise, treat a wart if it is in an awkward place or if it looks ugly and your child is embarrassed about it.

 FIRST AID Cover the wart with a wart plaster, and change it daily. For a plantar wart, first remove the layer of hard skin with a pumice stone before applying a plaster. Where a plaster cannot be applied, use a wart paint daily until the wart disappears, first protecting surrounding skin with petroleum jelly. Get plasters and paint from a pharmacy. If the child has many warts, a doctor can remove them with liquid nitrogen.

See a doctor for warts on the face.

Another common childhood skin condition is *molluscum contagiosum* – pearly white or pink nodules, often with a dent in the centre, appearing on the trunk, face or hands. These are contagious and caused by a virus. They are best left alone, as they disappear in time, but see the doctor if the child has a large number of them.

FUNGAL INFECTIONS

Fungi are yeast-like organisms that are widespread in the environment. Some may cause skin problems. Children may get infected by touching animals, from contact with other children, their clothing, or the soil.

Ringworm of the body

This is a fungal infection of the non-hairy skin, the face being particularly affected in children. The circular or oval patches have a well-defined raised border and they gradually enlarge as they clear in the centre.

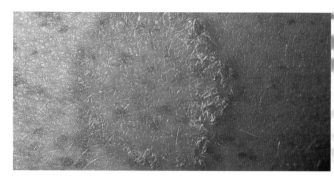

Note the raised border of ringworm infection.

 FIRST AID Ringworm can be cured by applying anti-fungal skin cream daily for two to three weeks. Ask your pharmacist about suitable medication.

Ringworm of the scalp

Here the fungus establishes itself deep in the hair roots, making hairs break off close to the skin and leaving a large scaly bald patch or several smaller patches over the scalp. In the early stages it may resemble severe dandruff. If the child develops an allergy to the fungus, the patches become inflamed, weepy and crusted, and the glands at the back of the head and neck become enlarged.

Ringworm of the scalp can be confused with other conditions such as impetigo, so consult your doctor for diagnosis and treatment.

Pityriasis versicolor

This is a fungal disorder that causes multiple small patches with clearly defined borders. They may be lighter or darker than the surrounding skin. The upper portion of the trunk, neck and lower half of the face are most often affected.

 FIRST AID Consult your doctor for a diagnosis and a prescription for a suitable anti-fungal treatment that you can apply at home.

Athlete's foot

This fungal infection cause itchiness and cracked tender skin between the toes. Toenails sometimes become thickened, discoloured and cracked. It is usually acquired from the floors of communal changing rooms and swimming baths. It is not common before puberty.

✚ FIRST AID   Effective remedies are available; ask your pharmacist to recommend one.

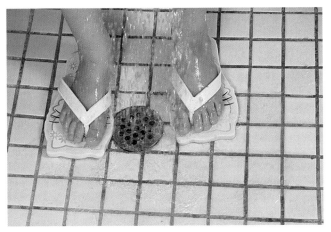

Use slip-on rubber sandals in public showers.

SCABIES

Extremely itchy, this is caused by sensitization to scabies mites, or their eggs and excreta. Mites burrow into the skin, preferring the chest, abdomen, genitalia and extremities, particularly wrists and hands. In hot climates they remain in the top skin layers, producing only small raised spots. In cold climates the burrows go deeper to form little lines. Children usually catch scabies from skin-to-skin contact, not from clothing and bed linen.

Suspect scabies if a rash is extremely itchy and friends or family members have it too. It is highly contagious so it is essential to treat the whole family. Consult your pharmacist.

✚ FIRST AID   An effective, safe, and cosmetically acceptable treatment is Permethrin™ (synthetic pyrethrin). Benzyl benzoate can also be used but is less pleasant. Other remedies are crotamiton, sulphur cream, and Tetmosol™ soap, but none will cure severe cases.

HEAD LICE

Lice are a common infestation of the scalp in children. The eggs (nits) can be seen as little white specks glued to the scalp hairs. The adult louse feeds on blood by biting into the scalp, producing itchy raised spots which often become infected from scratching, resulting in impetigo of the scalp. The lymph glands in the child's neck are frequently enlarged. As with scabies, treat the whole family, as the condition is highly contagious. Consult your pharmacist.

✚ FIRST AID   Permethrin™ scalp lotion is a safe and effective treatment. This kills nits as well as lice, so that the hair need not be cut or shaved. Malathion™ (0.5% in alcohol) or benzyl benzoate can also be used.

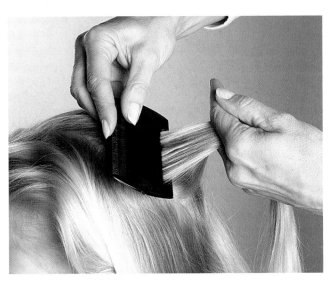

After shampooing, comb out nits with a lice comb.

IMMUNIZATION

Immunization is a simple, effective way of protecting children against dangerous illnesses. There are some infections the human body cannot make itself immune to without help. Give your child this help by seeing that she gets the right vaccines so her body will develop immunity. This also helps others, because if the level of immunity in the community is high enough, then the infection cannot spread so easily from one person to another.

IMMUNIZATION SCHEDULE

At birth	Polio and BCG
6 weeks	DPT, Polio, Hep B and HiB
10 weeks	DPT, Polio, Hep B and HiB
14 weeks	DPT, Polio, Hep B and HiB
9 months	Measles
18 months	Booster DPT, Polio, Measles or MMR
5 years	Booster DT, Polio, Measles or MMR

FREQUENTLY ASKED QUESTIONS
What do these abbreviations mean?

BCG is the Bacillus Calmette-Guérin vaccine, for protection against tuberculosis (TB).

DPT is the combined Diphtheria, Pertussis (whooping cough) and Tetanus vaccine.

DT is the Diphtheria and Tetanus vaccine, without Pertussis.

Hep B is the Hepatitis B vaccine.

HiB is the Haemophilus influenzae B vaccine.

Measles is the anti-measles vaccine.

MMR is the combined Measles-Mumps-Rubella vaccine.

Polio is the Poliomyelitis immunization – the injected Salk vaccine or the oral Sabin one.

Can I expect a reaction after immunization?

Mild fever and irritability are common, particularly after DPT, Measles and MMR immunizations. With DPT this occurs six to 12 hours after the injection. The site of the injection may also be red or sore for a day or two. With Measles and MMR, mild fever can be expected about seven days after vaccination. Some 10–20% of infants will develop a slight rash or other measles-like symptoms. There are virtually no reactions after the Hepatitis B and HiB vaccines.

Side-effects can be alleviated by giving three doses of paracetamol (acetaminophen) in the recommended dosage at four-hourly intervals. If a child has shown more severe reactions to a particular vaccine it should not be given again. Consult your doctor.

Does immunization cause cot deaths or autism?

Extensive research has shown that immunization does not cause either of these conditions.

Can the Polio vaccine cause paralysis?

Most Western countries are using the Salk vaccine in which the virus is inactivated. With this vaccine there are virtually no reactions.

With the oral Sabin Polio vaccine there is a genuine, though extremely small, risk. This vaccine contains live altered viral particles which spread the immunity to polio around the community. As a result – although rarely – the child himself, or one of his contacts, is paralyzed by the virus, just as happens with real ('wild') polio.

In Africa and some other countries, the oral Sabin vaccine is still widely used because it is effective and cheap and spreads immunity through the community. As a result of its use polio has virtually been eliminated throughout the world.

My baby was premature. Is she too delicate to be immunized?

Premature infants respond to immunization just as well as mature babies and should be immunized at the same time intervals after delivery.

What about the child who is HIV positive?

These children are especially in need of protection. A child who is HIV positive should receive the regular schedule of immunizations.

Does my child really need the Hepatitis B vaccine?

Hepatitis B is endemic in less advantaged communities in many parts of the world. In these communities mothers can transmit the infection to their infants during or after pregnancy, or the children can acquire

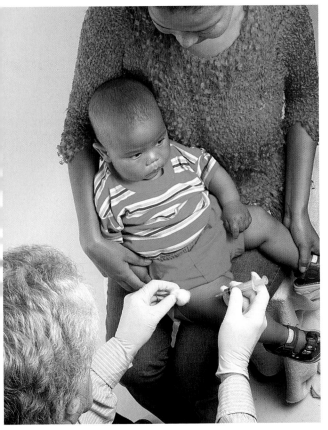

Immunization injections are not nice – but it is better to be safe than sorry.

My baby is allergic. Could immunizing him be dangerous?

If your child is allergic to something this does not mean he should not be immunized. Most of the genuine concerns are about the Measles and Mumps vaccines, as these are developed on chick embryos. The danger of an allergic reaction to egg protein in the vaccine has been exaggerated. Only if your child has shown severe allergy to egg, such as immediate swelling of the lips, difficulty with breathing, or a rash, should you avoid the Measles immunization. Very rarely a child may be allergic to the neomycin in the Measles vaccine or MMR, or to the carrying fluid in the DPT vaccine. If you are worried, consult your doctor.

it later. But all individuals run a lifetime risk of becoming infected with Hepatitis B and should be protected. The vaccine is effective, cheap and very safe. All infants should receive it.

My neighbour's child has just been given 'H.flu' vaccine (HiB). Is it necessary?

Haemophilus influenzae type B (no relation to the influenza virus) causes severe infections in young children, particularly bacteraemia, meningitis and epiglottitis. The vaccine is effective and has virtually no side effects. All infants should receive it.

What about Mumps and Rubella?

MMR has been available for many years. It is very effective and safe, though expensive. In many countries it has replaced the single Measles vaccine.

What side effects can I expect in my baby after BCG vaccination?

This vaccination is given as a shallow injection into the skin of the right upper arm. A small pimple appears at the site, reaches its maximum size four to six weeks later, and may form a small scabbed sore. It gradually fades, leaving a scar. There is often an enlarged gland in the right armpit. These are normal reactions. Sometimes the sore on the arm may be bigger or the armpit gland may form an abscess. These reactions are generally not serious, but if you are worried, return to the clinic to have the baby assessed, or consult your doctor.

If BCG prevents tuberculosis, why is there still so much TB around?

No vaccine has yet been perfected to prevent tuberculosis. The BCG vaccine, in use for over 80 years, reduces the risk of some serious forms, such as tuberculous meningitis, found mostly in very young children. BCG does not prevent the tubercle bacillus from establishing itself in the lungs, so pulmonary TB remains common.

Is immunization permanent – or does it wear off?

The immunity conferred by the Pertussis (whooping cough) vaccine wears off, but the vaccine is not usually given after the age of 18 months because whooping cough is less dangerous to children after this age.

The immunity conferred by the Measles and the MMR vaccine may wear off in later childhood, so the child should get a booster when he starts school.

Although diphtheria is now almost unknown, Diphtheria vaccine boosters should be repeated every 10 years.

Immunity following the Polio vaccine is permanent.

The immunity conferred by the Tetanus vaccine does wear off, so a booster should be given if the child has a contaminated injury (*see* Tetanus, page 50).

Are there other vaccines my child should receive?

Consult your doctor about immunization not routinely given at clinics.

The flu vaccine is effective and safe and should be given annually to children with immune deficiency or any chronic illness. Such children should also receive the heptavalent (seven strain) pneumococcal vaccine to protect against serious pneumococcal infection.

A vaccine against chicken pox is available for children with certain disorders.

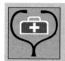 **Always consult your doctor if you are worried.**

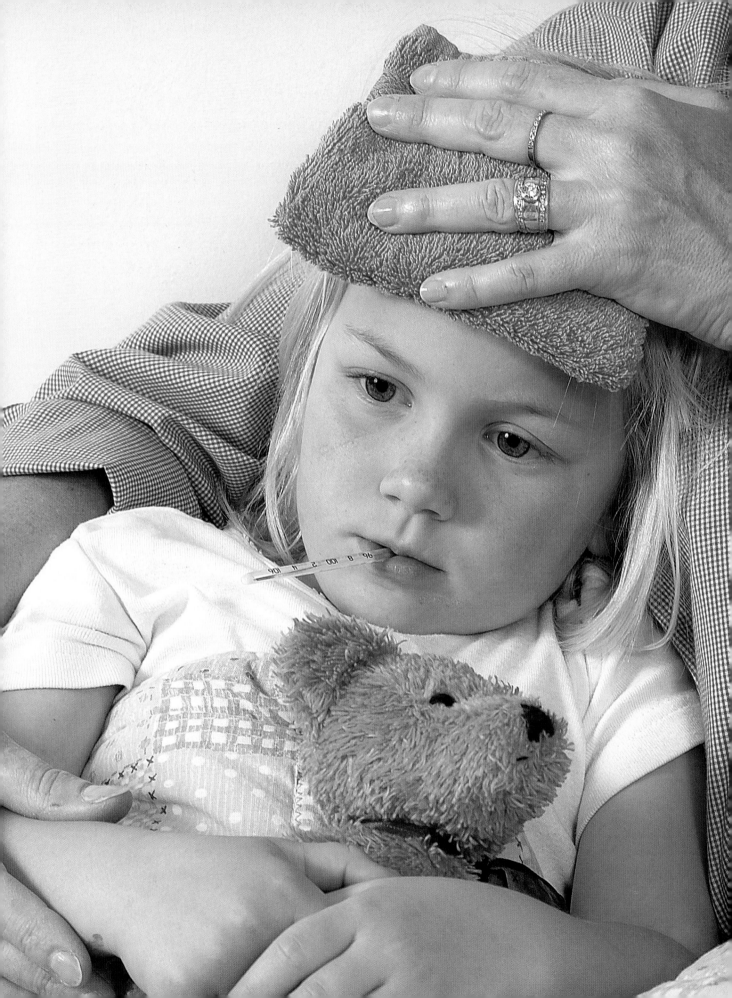

Acute Illness Table

✳ Go for it yourself

✳✳ Get a medical opinion (non-urgent)

✳✳✳ Get a medical opinion urgently

✳✳✳✳ Get medical help immediately

SYSTEM	DISORDER	SYMPTOMS	SEE PAGE	URGENCY
RESPIRATORY SYSTEM	Common cold	Watery nasal discharge, sneezing, cough, slight sore throat, maybe some fever	108	✳
	Influenza	High fever, headache, limb pains, cold symptoms	108	✳✳
	Sinusitis	Yellow nasal discharge, one or both sides. Pain over cheekbones or forehead; maybe swelling around one eye	109	✳✳
	Pharyngitis/ tonsillitis	Very painful, inflamed throat and/or tonsils, fever, enlarged tender glands below jaw angle	117	✳✳
	Nosebleeds	Bleeding from one or both nostrils; blood is often vomited up	118	✳ ✳✳✳ if it cannot be controlled
	Croup	Dry, barking cough, crowing sound on breathing in	112–113	✳✳✳

SYSTEM	DISORDER	SYMPTOMS	SEE PAGE	URGENCY
RESPIRATORY SYSTEM	Epiglottitis	High fever, malaise, difficulty breathing in and swallowing, loss of voice	113	✻✻✻✻
	Whooping cough (pertussis)	Cold and cough for one week; then regular spasms of coughing, ending in a whoop or vomiting, for up to three months	110	✻✻
	Bronchitis	Tight cough, 'phlegm on the chest' and wheezing on breathing out, usually following a cold; attacks are often recurrent	113	✻✻
	Asthma	Recurrent attacks of tight cough and wheezing, often at night or brought on by exercise; family history usually positive for asthma or other allergies	114	✻✻✻ full medical evaluation essential; then ✻ most attacks can be managed at home
	Anaphylactic shock	Increasing difficulty with breathing, shock and collapse, generalized itchy rash, swelling around the eyes.	111–112	✻✻✻✻
	Bronchiolitis	Infants under two years affected. Cold symptoms first; then slight fever, irritability, poor appetite, rapid shallow breathing	113–114	✻✻✻
	Pneumonia	High fever, cough, rapid breathing; may be chest or abdominal pain	110	✻✻✻ ✻✻✻✻ if danger signs (*see* page 110)

SYSTEM	DISORDER	SYMPTOMS	SEE PAGE	URGENCY
EYES AND EARS	Conjunctivitis	**Viral:** red eyes, irritation, watery discharge **Bacterial:** yellow discharge; eyelids matted together after sleeping Also caused by chemical irritation or allergy; both eyes almost always affected	119	✳✳ ✳✳✳ if only one eye affected, or if vision is affected, or cornea is abnormal
	Stye	Red, painful spot on eyelid which may discharge pus	120	✳ ✳✳ if recurrent
	Otitis media	Pain in one or both ears, hearing loss, maybe fever		✳✳ ✳✳✳ if severe pain
	Ear discharge	**Watery, mucoid** or **purulent (discharging pus):** ruptured drum following otitis media **Recurrent, purulent:** chronic perforation of drum **Bad smelling, purulent:** foreign body or mastoid (the hard area behind the ear) infection **Both ears, itchy:** external otitis	117–118	✳✳ ✳✳ ✳✳✳ ✳✳

SYSTEM	DISORDER	SYMPTOMS	SEE PAGE	URGENCY
NERVOUS SYSTEM	Meningitis	Headache, vomiting, stiff neck; listlessness, fever, maybe purple/red-brown spots on the skin	121	✳✳✳✳
	Fits	Temporary disturbance of consciousness with or without stiffening or jerking.	120–121	✳✳✳
DIGESTIVE SYSTEM	Oral thrush (candidiasis)	White patches on the tongue, inside cheeks or in throat; cannot be rubbed off without causing bleeding	115	✳ ✳✳ if persistent
	Gastroenteritis	Frequent loose stools, vomiting, abdominal cramps, may be some fever	125–127	✳ or ✳✳, depending on severity
	Dysentery	Frequent mucoid or blood-streaked stools, cramps and generally fever	125	✳✳✳
	Intestinal obstruction	Bouts of central abdominal pain; vomiting bile; may be abdominal distension; no stools passed	128–129	✳✳✳
	Pyloric stenosis	Recurring forceful vomiting 15 minutes after feeds, in infants one to four months old; weight loss and constipation		✳✳✳
	Intussusception	Sudden onset of bouts of severe abdominal pain in infants under two years; constipated, but may pass blood-stained mucus ('redcurrant jelly')	129	✳✳✳✳

SYSTEM	DISORDER	SYMPTOMS	SEE PAGE	URGENCY
DIGESTIVE SYSTEM	Acute appendicitis	Central abdominal pain and vomiting, pain then localizes to right lower abdomen, which is tender to pressure; may be some fever	129–130	✱✱✱✱
	Mesenteric adenitis	Central abdominal pain, fever, may be sore throat	129	✱✱✱
	Hernias: 1. Inguinal/groin (strangulated)	A lump in the groin which does not disappear on gentle pressure; maybe symptoms of intestinal obstruction as above	128	✱✱✱✱
	2. Umbilical	Swelling at the umbilicus caused by bowel herniating through a weak spot; seldom obstructs	128	✱✱
	Anal fissure	Painful passage of hard motion streaked with blood	131	✱
	Acute hepatitis	Loss of appetite, malaise, some fever; upper abdominal pain and tenderness; then urine becomes dark brown in colour; yellowness of skin		✱✱
	Worm infestation: 1. Roundworms	Worms in stool or worm is vomited	132	✱
	2. Thread (pin) worms	Anal itching	132	✱
	3. Whipworms	May cause mucoid, bloody stools	132	✱✱
	4. Hookworm	Anaemia	132	✱✱
	5. Tapeworm	Segments in stool	132	✱

SYSTEM	DISORDER	SYMPTOMS	SEE PAGE	URGENCY
URINARY TRACT AND GENITALIA	Urinary tract infection	General symptoms: fever, irritability, vomiting, diarrhoea (children under two years) In older children: frequency and burning on passing water; pains in back or abdomen, bed wetting (when previously dry); urine smoky or pink, maybe odd-smelling	133	✲✲
	Glomerulo-nephritis	Urine brown, reddish or smoky, output diminished; Swelling around the eyes, later more generalized; may be headache		✲✲
	Vulvovaginitis	Burning or itching of vulval area; vaginal discharge; discomfort on passing water	133–134	✲ ✲✲ if severe, or if molestation a possibility
	Torsion of testis	Tender tense swelling high in the scrotum	134	✲✲✲✲
	Balanitis	Swelling, itching of head of penis and foreskin; redness and white discharge	134	✲✲
	Paraphimosis	Retracted foreskin, cannot be replaced	134	✲✲ ✲✲✲ if over four years
	Phimosis	Unretractable foreskin	134	✲

SYSTEM	DISORDER	SYMPTOMS	SEE PAGE	URGENCY
MUSCLES, BONES AND JOINTS	Arthritis	Pain on movement of one or more joints; may be swelling of joint(s)		✳✳✳
	Osteomyelitis	Fever, pain, maybe swelling and redness of affected limb		✳✳✳
BLOOD DISORDERS	Anaemia	Unusual paleness of palms of hands; also of tongue, lips, eyes (conjunctivae)		✳✳
	Purpura	Tiny bleeding spots in skin or mucous membranes; unduly easy or spontaneous bruising or bleeding		✳✳✳✳
LYMPH NODES (GLANDS)	Enlarged lymph nodes	Small painless nodes (under 1cm) may be felt in healthy children in neck, below angle of jaw, in groin		✳ ✳✳ if nodes are tender, suddenly appear, or any node is larger than 1cm
INFECTIOUS DISEASES	Roseola	High fever, irritability for three days; then faint rash appears on trunk as fever subsides	135	✳✳
	Rubella	Slight fever, tiredness for a day, then spots appear	136	✳✳
	Measles	Fever, flu symptoms, maybe diarrhoea for three to five days, then rash	136–137	✳✳✳
	Scarlet fever	Fever, sore throat, headache, diffuse red rash on trunk	137	✳✳✳

SYSTEM	DISORDER	SYMPTOMS	SEE PAGE	URGENCY
INFECTIOUS DISEASES	Slapped cheek disease	Maybe slight fever and tiredness; red cheeks followed by rash on trunk; then lacy rash on limbs	138	**
	Infectious mononucleosis	Inflamed throat, enlarged glands in neck, armpits, groins, may be spotty rash on trunk	137	**
	Varicella	Crops of small blisters evolving into sores and scabs mostly on trunk; also in hair, in mouth, throat		**
	Shingles (*herpes zoster*)	Crop of blisters on one side of head or body, ending at midline; usually not painful in children		**
	Hand, foot and mouth disease	Small sores in the mouth or throat, followed by blisters symmetrically on hands, knees, feet	116	**
	Herpetic stomatitis	Fever, sore throat, painful sores in mouth; red, swollen gums		**
	Kawasaki disease	High prolonged fever; variable rash localizing to hands and feet; red lips and eyes		***
	Tick bite fever	Fever, generalized papular rash, including palms and soles; tick bite	96	***
	Mumps	Fever variable; swelling in front and below one or both ears or under chin	116	**

SYSTEM	DISORDER	SYMPTOMS	SEE PAGE	URGENCY
SKIN DISORDERS	Nappy rash	Variable rash in nappy area	139–140	✳ ✳✳ if severe or infant not thriving
	Cradle cap	Greasy, yellow crusts or scales on scalp; red, scaly patches on trunk	139	✳
	Impetigo	Large blisters developing into golden crusted scabs	140	✳✳
	Cellulitis	Spreading area of redness, swelling and tenderness, often related to a break in the skin		✳✳✳
	Boil, carbuncle, stye	Painful papule developing pus at its head	140–141, 120	✳✳
	Scalded skin syndrome	Widespread blistering with loss of skin		✳✳✳✳
	Toxic shock syndrome	High fever, shock, maybe disturbed consciousness or respiratory difficulty		✳✳✳✳
	Urticaria	Irregularly shaped itchy papules which come and go; may be other signs of allergy	143	✳✳✳
	Papular urticaria	Fixed itchy papules, usually on legs and trunk	97	✳
	Warts	Firm raised growths with rough or smooth surface on hands, feet, face or elsewhere	143	✳ ✳✳ if multiple or on awkward spots

SYSTEM	DISORDER	SYMPTOMS	SEE PAGE	URGENCY
SKIN DISORDERS	Molluscum contagiosum	Pearly, dome-shaped nodules, often with central depression		✲ ✲✲ if multiple, or on eyelids
	Scabies	Tiny very itchy papules or small lines– wrists, between fingers, armpits, sides of trunk, genitalia; may be sores and scabs from scratching	145	✲✲
	Lice	Itching and tiny red spots on scalp; nits (small white eggs) attached to scalp hairs; lice may not be seen	145	✲
	Ringworm: 1. Of scalp	Early: general scaliness (like dandruff); OR round patch of hair loss with scaly surface; OR multiple bald scaly patches; OR multiple crusted lesions with enlarged neck glands	144	✲✲
	2. Of body	Scaly, round or irregular patch with clear-cut, slightly raised edge	144	✲
	Athlete's foot	Cracked skin with itching and soreness between toes	145	✲ ✲✲ if no improvement when treated
	Pityriasis rosea	Patch like ringworm on body; then multiple oval spots, slightly scaly, appear on trunk, lasting up to two months	143	✲✲
	Pityriasis versicolor	Discoloured patches of skin, slightly scaly, usually on neck and shoulders	144	✲✲

FIRST AID

In order to be helpful and effective, first aid procedures must adhere to certain rules and be performed in specific sequences. The various do's and don'ts are covered in the individual entries dealing with medical emergencies, but ultimately, it all comes down to this: enrol for a recognized first-aid course so that you can rely on your knowledge in any emergency situation. This will enable you to know what to do and to remain calm. If there are no materials to hand, your understanding of what is required will allow you to assess the suitability of items around you in order to improvise. The best advice is: learn the basics. So, attend a recognized course and you could end up saving someone's life one day.

IN THIS SECTION

Assessing a casualty

As with most of the matters involving the human body, it is fairly predictable that no two casualties you will assist as a first responder, will be exactly the same, or require the same type of intervention. Infants are particularly prone to viral infections and to choking, while older children are more prone to asthma and severe injury and elderly people are often troubled by a combination of chronic medical problems, any one of which may cause acute breathing difficulty or circulatory collapse. However, this does not mean that you cannot provide effective first aid without knowing the precise cause of the collapse. Instead, the guidelines for first aid and resuscitation are systematically designed to deal with virtually any instance where you encounter an acutely distressed or unconscious person. The key to being an effective first responder is to follow the basic guidelines in the correct sequences that are recommended in this section of the book: SAFE (*see* below) and ABC (*see* pp164–5).

THE 'SAFE' APPROACH

Whenever you are approaching a casualty who has collapsed for any reason, you should always:

- Summon help immediately – either yourself or by sending another responsible person to call for medical assistance or an emergency service while you attend to the casualty.
- Take precautions to ensure your own safety as well as that of the injured party. This applies especially when attending to casualties injured as a result of road traffic collisions, electricity, fire, toxic inhalation, or any situation where the risk of injury still persists in the vicinity. The SAFE acronym (below) summarizes the correct approach in an easy-to-remember fashion.

S   **Shout for help:** Summon medical assistance or the emergency services immediately.

A   **Approach with care:** Check for surrounding hazards that may also be a danger to yourself.

F   **Free from danger:** Even though we recommend that casualties should not be moved if possible, this precaution must be weighed against any obvious risk, e.g. if a child has been knocked down on a busy street you must move him or her – with all possible care of course – to a safe place before commencing resuscitation.

E   **Evaluate the ABC:** Having taken the above precautions, you are now ready to assess vital functions and commence resuscitation if required.

THE UNCONSCIOUS PERSON

Someone lying motionless on the ground may not be unconscious. Check for response, i.e. establish if a person is conscious by tapping them on the shoulder, or shaking them gently by the shoulder. Call the person's name if you know it, or ask 'Are you alright?' or 'Can you hear me?' If the casualty responds and is able to speak it means that the airway is clear and that breathing and circulation are satisfactory. In this case, stay with him or her and wait for the emergency services to arrive. If the casualty is very drowsy, turn them carefully into the **recovery position** (see p167).

Some common causes of loss of consciousness are **head injury** (see pp193–5), **epilepsy** (see pp178–9), **stroke** (see pp214–5), **meningitis** (see pp180–1), and a lack of sufficient oxygen. This is commonly associated with **choking** (see pp170–1), **near-drowning** (see box on this page) or severe **asthma** (see p228).

WHAT TO DO:

· Check the response as described above. If there is none, shout for help.

· Your priority is to **check the ABC** (see pp164–5). If the airway is blocked the person will be unable to breathe so your aim is to **open the airway**, then check their breathing again (see p168).

· If the casualty is breathing and displays **signs of life** (such as movement and/or coughing) turn them into the recovery position (see p167).

· If the person has stopped breathing and shows no signs of life, administer **chest compressions** and **rescue breaths** (see pp168–9).

FAINTING

This temporary loss of consciousness results from decreased blood flow to the brain. It commonly occurs when someone is feeling very hot, not eating enough, or experiencing an emotional upset, and is caused by sudden slowing of the heart rate. This can be confirmed by checking the pulse rate at the

wrist (see **circulation** p165). Usually, the only first aid required consists of support, reassurance and a cup of sweetened tea once consciousness returns. Raising the casualty's legs may improve blood flow to the brain and hasten their recovery.

ACCIDENTS HAPPEN

Accident situations in the home are fairly common, small mishaps happen regularly, particularly if your household includes small children. A variety of sound precautions are described in this book that will help to make your home child-friendly (see p258–260).

NEAR-DROWNING

Near-drowning victims may be unconscious and will probably be unable to breathe as a result of having been under water. Children can drown in a few centimetres of water because their bodies are top-heavy and this weight, biased towards the upper body makes them overbalance more easily. Infants can drown in a few seconds. For that reason children need constant supervision anywhere near water, even in the bath. If you suspect near-drowning:

· Get the person out of the water immediately.

· Call an ambulance.

· If the casualty is not breathing or unconscious commence **rescue breathing** (see p168).

· When they are breathing normally, ensure they lie in the recover position.

· It is imperative that you get medical help in all cases of near-drowning.

Procedures for resuscitation

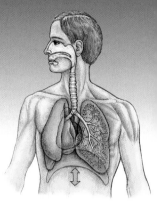

Normal breathing and blood circulation ensure an adequate supply of oxygen and nutrients to all parts of the body. Either or both of these vital functions may fail in an acutely ill or injured casualty. The brain is particularly sensitive and will suffer permanent damage if deprived of oxygen for more than four minutes. Cardiopulmonary resuscitation, a combination of rescue breathing and chest compressions refers to a set of practical skills that enable you to:

The airway, lungs and diaphragm work together to regulate breathing.

- Ensure the casualty has a clear **A**irway to breathe through, and assess the adequacy of **B**reathing and **C**irculation in someone with acute illness or injury (*see* **ABC** below).
- Provide oxygen to casualties who are not able to breathe on their own.
- Establish an artificial heartbeat in someone whose heart is not beating effectively.

The skills described in this section are not enough to turn you into an expert first-aid provider. They should, however, encourage you to enlist for a proper hands-on course offered by a professional organisation.

THE ABC (AIRWAY, BREATHING, CIRCULATION)

CHECK THE AIRWAY

An unconscious person may be unable to breathe if the airway has become obstructed by:

- Kinking, due to abnormal positioning of the head and neck

- The tongue falling back into the throat

- Misplaced dentures

- Food, blood or other foreign matter

Open the airway by lifting the casualty's chin and thus allowing an unobstructed passage to let the air flow in and out of the lungs.

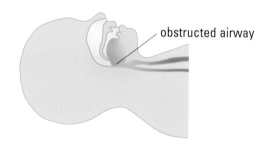

obstructed airway

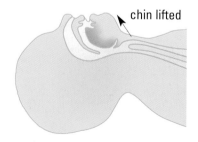

chin lifted

Tilt head back and lift the chin to create an unobstructed passage to the lungs.

RESTORE BREATHING

The normal position of the tongue and the airway can be restored using a combination of the chin-lift and head-tilt (see p164). Once the airway is cleared:

· Check the mouth for foreign bodies and remove what you can see. Well-fitting dentures that are correctly positioned need not be removed.

· To prevent injuring the person, do not sweep your fingers blindly around inside the mouth or throat.

· When you have opened the airway, the casualty may start breathing unaided. All that is necessary is to turn the casualty into the **recovery position** (see p167) and ensure that the airway remains open while you wait for help to arrive. If the casualty does not begin breathing normally, you should assume that the heart has stopped beating, and commence resuscitation (see pp166–169):

CIRCULATION

If the casualty is conscious, meaning that he or she is able to speak and respond to you, or at least able to breathe unaided, then the circulation is in order.

If the person is not responding to you and appears to be unconscious, you must establish that there are **signs of life**:

· Tap the person on the shoulder, or shake them gently by the shoulder to see if they will respond.

· Call the person's name if you know it, or ask "Can you hear me?", or "Open your eyes."

· Look for visible rising and falling of the chest (indicative that the person is breathing).

· Look for any signs of movement.

If you can detect no signs of life within 10 seconds, you should assume that the heart has stopped and commence resuscitation as indicated above. If you are a trained health care provider, you may confirm the presence of a heart beat by checking for a pulse at the following locations:

· The **radial pulse** is felt on the inside of the wrist roughly at the base of the thumb. Use two or three fingers and press down lightly.

· The **carotid pulse** is felt on the side of the throat between the windpipe and the large neck muscle.

· The **brachial pulse** (used for infants and small children) is felt on the inside of the upper arm, just above the elbow.

Normal pulse rate for an adult is between 60 and 80 beats per minute (in fit young people it can be somewhat slower); a young child's pulse is much faster at 140 beats per minute.

UNCONSCIOUS WITH A SUSPECTED NECK INJURY

If there is any possibility of a neck injury in an unconscious casualty, you must restore the airway using the jaw-thrust method. To do this:

· Kneel behind the casualty's head.

· Keeping head, neck and spine aligned, put your hands on either side of the face to support the head. Your fingertips should touch the angles of the jaw; thumbs on cheeks.

· Without tilting the head, lift the jaw forward gently with your fingers to unblock the airway. Listen and look for breathing for 10 seconds.

· If the casualty begins to breathe, maintain support of the head and check breathing and circulation regularly until help arrives. If there is no breathing, begin **rescue breathing** (see p168).

RESUSCITATION FOR ADULTS AND OLDER CHILDREN (OVER 8 YEARS)

ASSESSMENT

There are two major scenarios you may encounter. You must first assess which category the casualty falls into (for each of the 'What to do' sections, it is assumed you have classified into the relevant scenario). They may be categorized as follows:

1 unconscious
breathing
signs of life/circulation

2 unconscious
not breathing
no signs of life/no circulation

Condition	Adults and children over 8 years of age
Unconscious breathing (*see* below)	Place in **recovery position** (*see* p167) Call an ambulance Ensure airway remains open and normal breathing continues
Unconscious not breathing no signs of life/ no circulation (*see* p168)	**Open the airway** (chin lift and head tilt; *see* p168) Look, listen and feel for signs of breathing for 10 seconds Call an ambulance (if someone else is present, ask them to call an ambulance as soon as possible) Give **30 chest compressions** (*see* p169) followed by **2 rescue breaths** (*see* p168) Continue cycles of two breaths to 30 compressions until breathing resumes or help arrives Place in recovery position if breathing resumes, and monitor carefully

SCENARIO 1 unconscious   breathing   signs of life/circulation

WHAT TO DO:

· Place the casualty in the **recovery position** (see opposite).

· Call an ambulance.

· Ensure the airway remains open and that normal breathing continues.

UNCONSCIOUS ADULT (RECOVERY POSITION)

An unconscious casualty who is breathing normally alone and has normal circulation should be placed in the recovery position. You need to put the person on their side to prevent the tongue from falling back, minimize the risk of vomit being sucked into the lungs and allow you to monitor their breathing and circulation as you wait for help. For treatment **in case of suspected neck or spinal injury** see p165.

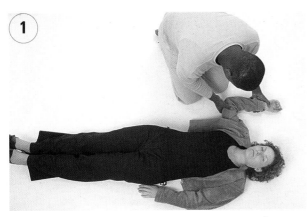

Bend the casualty's arm nearest to you at the elbow (±90°), palm up and open.

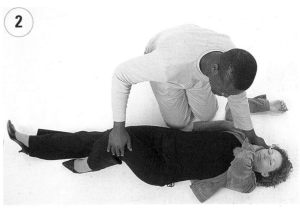

Tuck the palm of the hand furthest from you against her cheek. At the same time grasp the knee furthest from you and pull up.

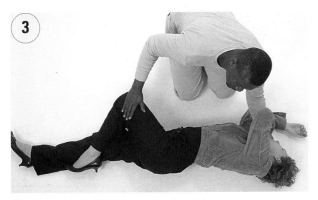

Keep her hand on her cheek, pull on her thigh to roll casualty onto the side, facing you.

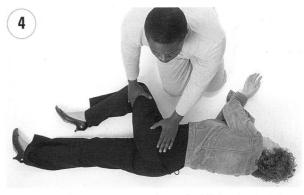

Angle her knee at approximately 90°.

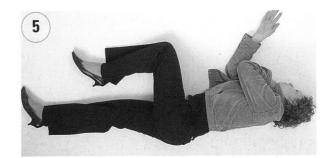

When positioning is complete, check breathing and circulation regularly until help arrives. Place a blanket or jacket over a casualty who appears pale or in shock.

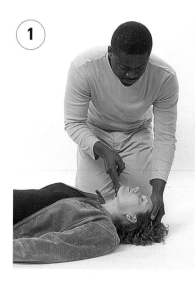

1 Support the casualty's head with the left hand, and tilt the chin up with the fingers of your right hand to open the airway.

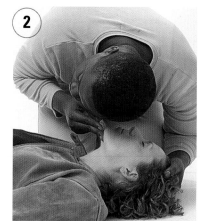

2 For 10 seconds listen for signs of normal breathing; watch for chest movement.

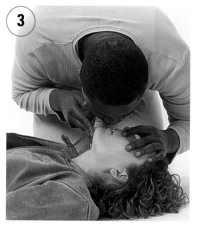

3 Maintain chin lift and pinch the nose shut.

WHAT TO DO:

- If there is another person present, ask them to call an ambulance immediately. If you are alone, call an ambulance as soon as you know that the casualty is not breathing normally (see below).

- **Open the airway** (see step 1).

- Listen and look for **signs of normal breathing** (see step 2). If there is no sign after 10 seconds:

- Position your hands in the centre of the chest (see step 5) and perform **30 chest compressions using 2 hands** as follows: keeping your arms straight, lean over the casualty and use your body weight to depress his breastbone to a depth of about 4cm (1½in). Do compressions at a rate of about 100 per minute.

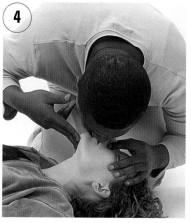

4 Cover casualty's mouth with your own. Keep the airway open. Exhale slowly and firmly. Give 2 rescue breaths.

- Give **2 rescue breaths between every 30 compressions** (*see* steps 3– 4).

- Continue cycles of **2 rescue breaths for every 30 chest compressions** until breathing resumes or medical help arrives.

- Place in **recovery position** if casualty begins to breathe unaided (*see* p167).

- If you are alone, continue resuscitation for 1 minute, call for an ambulance, and then continue with cycles of 2 breaths to 30 chest compressions.

(5)

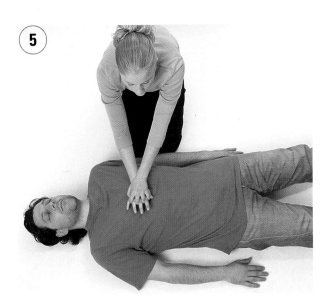

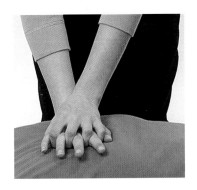

Place your hands on the centre of their chest.

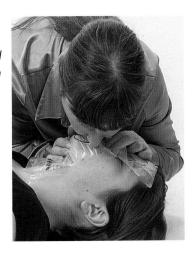

A plastic face shield may be used to prevent infection and for reasons of hygiene. It should be placed over the casualty's face, with the filter over the mouth.

Choking

Choking is caused by an obstruction of the upper airway, commonly as a result of food becoming impacted. In some cases, a coughing spell is enough to expel a foreign body from the airway. However, even small objects may lodge firmly in the narrow airway of an infant or small child, in which case you may have to use the techniques described here to clear the airway. The upper airway can also become obstructed by tissue swelling caused by **allergy** (*see* p229), or severe infection. In such cases, treatment of underlying causes is required. Techniques described here are designed to help the casualty expel a foreign body by creating a high-pressure wave inside the lungs, rather like an artificial cough. If you suspect choking in an unconscious casualty, first attend to the ABC (*see* pp164–5). Use the techniques described here only if you are unable to give rescue breaths.

Condition	Adults and children over 8 years of age
Suspected choking	If coughing, encourage cough and monitor carefully Up to 5 back blows – check the mouth and remove any obstruction Up to 5 abdominal thrusts – check the mouth and remove any obstruction Do 3 cycles of back blows and abdominal thrusts If breathing: **open airway** and remove visible foreign matter (*see* p164) place in **recovery position** (*see* p167) If unconscious or not breathing, commence **resuscitation sequence** (*see* pp164–9)

SYMPTOMS

In someone who is unconscious or struggling to breathe, you should consider choking as the cause whenever:

- a healthy adult or child has a sudden coughing spell, and then struggles to breathe.
- you find other foreign bodies, i.e. peanuts or small toy parts, near the casualty.
- a casualty who is coughing or struggling to breathe may point at his neck to indicate that something is stuck in the throat.
- resuscitation remains ineffective despite the head tilt and chin lift being correctly applied.

Common causes of airway obstruction

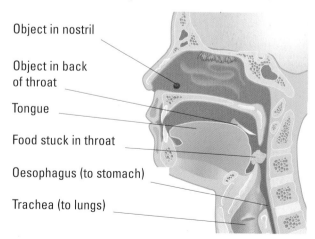

Object in nostril

Object in back of throat

Tongue

Food stuck in throat

Oesophagus (to stomach)

Trachea (to lungs)

FIRST AID FOR CHOKING ADULTS AND OLDER CHILDREN (OVER 8 YEARS)

Use a combination of back blows and abdominal thrusts for an adult or older child who seems to be choking and is unable to breathe or cough up the foreign body themselves. Do 3 cycles of the entire procedure then **call an ambulance if there is no improvement**. Continue with cycles of back blows and abdominal thrusts until help arrives, and resuscitate if necessary (see pp164–9).

BACK BLOWS
WHAT TO DO:

· Using the heel of your hand, give up to 5 firm back blows between the shoulder blades.

· Carefully check in the casualty's mouth for obvious obstructions. Do not probe blindly.

· Remove the obstruction.

· If this does not help, do abdominal thrusts too.

ABDOMINAL THRUST
WHAT TO DO:

If back blows fail to dislodge the obstruction, do up to 5 abdominal thrusts. These can be done with the person standing, seated on your lap, or – in a choking casualty who has lost consciousness – lying flat on the ground. If at any stage during this sequence the casualty begins to breathe, check the mouth and clear away any visible foreign object.

· Place one fisted hand midway between the navel and the breastbone and place the palm of your free hand over the fist.

· Using both hands, thrust firmly inwards and upwards towards the chest up to five times.

· If there is no relief after 3 cycles of back blows and abdominal thrusts, call an ambulance.

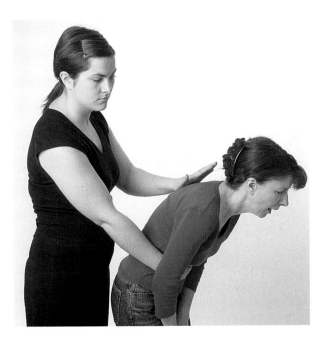

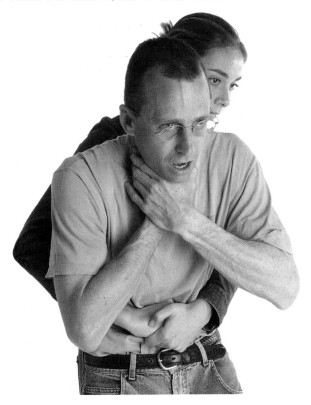

Bleeding

Bleeding (loss of blood) occurs either externally – through a break in the skin, or through a natural opening such as the mouth. Substantial or ongoing blood loss will inevitably lead to **shock** (*see* p174), with particular risk of damage to the brain and kidneys. The aim of the first-aid provider is to recognize severe bleeding and control it so that: the flow of blood is effectively stemmed, there is a minimal risk of infection and the casualty does not go into shock from loss of blood – *see also* the **DO NOT** box on page 179. It is essential to get the injured person to a doctor or hospital as soon as possible.

TREATMENT

· **Call an ambulance** if the bleeding appears to be very severe.

· For deep wounds that are free of foreign objects, **stop the bleeding** by applying firm pressure on the wound using a sterile pad or clean cloth. If blood soaks through do not remove the pad, but simply place a second one over it. If you have nothing available with which to make a pad, use your hand. Be sure to maintain the pressure until help arrives.

· Examine the wound carefully to see whether there is any foreign object, such as a shard of glass, embedded in it. If there is DO NOT REMOVE it.

TIP

Use surgical gloves to prevent infection. (HIV and viral hepatitis can be transmitted if infected blood makes contact with broken skin.) If you have no gloves, wash your hands well before and after first aid, using an antiseptic soap or solution.

Instead, place a sterile piece of gauze or cloth gently over the embedded object and bandage around it (*see* p220).

· Elevate the limb, either by holding it up, or using any handy object (such as a chair, or a rock) to support it. This elevation will reduce the bleeding by diverting blood from the wound, and will also prevent the casualty from going into shock by directing more blood towards the brain.

· Reassure the casualty and get him or her to sit comfortably or **lie down** if they appear slightly disoriented and look pale and distressed. Monitor the casualty closely for signs of **shock** (*see* pp174–5) while you attend to the wound.

· When you have controlled the bleeding, leave the first pad in position and **bandage** the wound (*see* p173). If the wound bleeds heavily through the first and second pad while you bandage, discard both pads and begin again with a fresh pad pressed firmly to the wound to staunch the flow of blood. It is imperative that you control the bleeding.

· If necessary, get the casualty to lie down. This reduces the chance of fainting by increasing the blood flow to the brain. Raise the legs to maintain blood pressure (*see* p175).

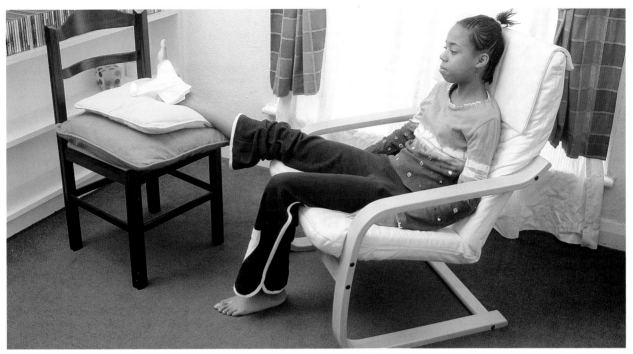

When you have stopped the bleeding and bandaged the wound, get the casualty to lie down or sit comfortably and elevate the limb.

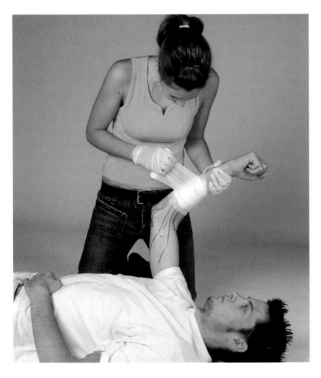

Raise the limb to decrease blood flow to the wound and increase blood flow to the brain. Apply apply direct pressure to the area.

X DO NOT

- **remove an embedded object**, such as a piece of glass, or a knife, for example. If it has punctured an organ, removing it could do more damage and increase the amount of bleeding. Make a **ring bandage** (*see* p220) around the object by using two or more tightly rolled-up bandages as supports around the embedded object to prevent it from being pressed any deeper into the wound. Once the support stays are in place, you can bandage on and around them without touching the embedded object or the wound itself, while at the same time maintaining pressure on the wound to staunch the flow of blood.

Shock

Shock results when the regular, healthy blood flow to tissues and organs is reduced to a dangerously low level. It can be caused by a variety of conditions, including sudden **bleeding** (*see* p172), **heart attack** (*see* below and pp212–3), **anaphylactic shock** (*see* p176), **burns** (*see* p186), and damage to the nervous system (**spinal cord injuries**, *see* p208) and even **head injury** (*see* pp193–5). If shock is not treated rapidly enough, vital organs, such as the heart, kidneys and brain, may suffer damage and fail. The body reacts to shock by directing blood away from the extremities and towards the vital organs. Always treat shock as an urgent medical emergency as the effects can worsen very quickly and may require **rescue breaths** (*see* p168) and/or **resuscitation** (*see* pp164–171).

SYMPTOMS

These vary, depending on what caused the shock, but may include the following:
- Paleness (pallor)
- Moist, cool, clammy skin
- Nausea and vomiting
- A rapid and/or irregular pulse that turns gradually weaker
- Shallow breathing
- Repeated yawning and/or sighing
- Blue-tinged lips and fingernails
- Agitation, anxiety or confusion
- Restlessness
- Thirst
- Fainting
- Unconsciousness
- Chest pain
- Profuse sweating

CAUSES
- Bleeding or severe dehydration following a serious injury (hypovolemic shock).
- Heart attack or heart failure (cardiogenic shock).
- Allergic reactions (anaphylactic shock).
- Spinal cord injuries (neurogenic shock).
- Loss of body fluids as a result of burns, severe diarrhoea or vomiting.

TREATMENT
- If you suspect someone may be suffering from shock, summon medical assistance immediately.

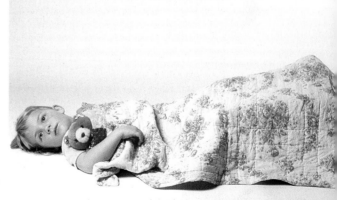

Lying the patient down with their feet raised improves blood flow to the vital organs.

Treat all obvious injuries (burns, fractures and/or bleeding) and be sure to **monitor the vital signs** (*see* pp164–7) and treat as appropriate until medical assistance arrives.

- **If the casualty is conscious** and you are sure there is no injury to the head, neck, spine or legs, lay them flat on their back on the floor with their feet raised about 30cm (12in), or above the level of the heart.

- **If a head or spinal injury is suspected**, do not attempt to move the casualty at all – they should remain in the same position as found until medical assistance arrives.

- **If a casualty vomits or drools**, turn their head to one side to prevent choking through the inhalation of vomit into the lungs. If there is an injury to the head or spine, hold the casualty's head still in relation to their body and roll them onto their side. Place supporting material under the head to keep it in the same position relative to the body.

- **Loosen tight clothing** and cover the casualty with a blanket or garment for warmth.

- **Reassure the casualty**, and give appropriate first aid for any wounds, injuries, or illnesses.

- **Do not give a shocked casualty anything to eat or drink**. Moisten the lips if they are thirsty.

PREVENTION

As with other emergencies, early recognition of the underlying cause and ensuring immediate medical care will limit the severity of shock.

Controlling external bleeding effectively in an injured person will assist the body's own mechanisms to maintain a normal blood pressure and thereby prevent shock from deteriorating to a level where the person's life is at risk.

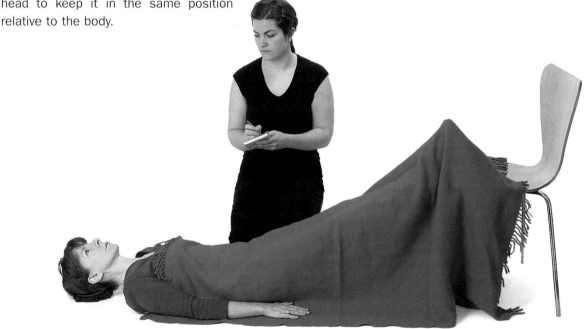

While you are waiting for medical help to arrive make the casualty is covered with a warm blanket and lying as comfortable as possible. Monitor the vital signs regularly and record your findings for rate of breathing, responsiveness and pulse.

Anaphylactic Shock

Anaphylaxis (anaphylactic shock) is a rare but severe hypersensitivity (allergic) reaction that occurs when a person's immune system recognizes a particular substance as a threat to the whole body. The reaction spreads rapidly throughout the body, causing blood pressure to drop suddenly and narrowing the airways, making breathing difficult. Anaphylaxis can be fatal unless immediate treatment is available.

SYMPTOMS

The symptoms usually develop very quickly and may include the following:
- Difficulty in breathing
- Wheezing, or abnormal, high-pitched breathing sounds
- Tightness in the chest and throat
- Itchy red skin rash
- Swollen face, lips and tongue
- Anxiety or confusion
- Light-headedness, fainting, loss of consciousness
- Abdominal pain, cramping, diarrhoea
- Nausea and vomiting
- Nasal congestion or coughing
- Palpitations (sensation of feeling the heart beat)
- Rapid or weak pulse
- Slurred speech
- Blueness of the skin, including the lips or nail beds

CAUSES

Extreme allergic reaction to a specific substance. Common allergens include insect stings; allergies to certain foods, such as shellfish, nuts or strawberries; or to specific medicines, such as penicillin (*see also* **allergies** p229).

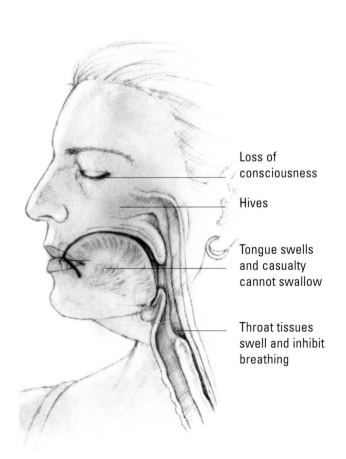

Loss of consciousness

Hives

Tongue swells and casualty cannot swallow

Throat tissues swell and inhibit breathing

TREATMENT

- **Get to a doctor or call an ambulance right away**. Anaphylaxis can be fatal unless promptly treated.
- While waiting, if the casualty is conscious, help him into a sitting position to ease breathing. If the casualty has an **Epipen** (adrenaline or epi-nephrine syringe), help him to administer it to the thigh muscle, through clothing if necessary.
- If the casualty loses consciousness, carry out **rescue breaths** (*see* p168) if necessary.
- **Do not leave the casualty alone**, except when you go to call an ambulance.

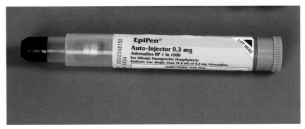

If you suffer from a severe allergy, you should always carry a pre-filled adrenaline syringe. In the event of an anaphylactic reaction, the adrenaline should be injected into your thigh muscle.

CAUTION

- If you are alone when you have symptoms that suggest you may be having an ana-phylactic reaction, contact your doctor or an emergency service immediate-ly and explain what is happening to you. Don't drive yourself to the emergency room – the symptoms may become more pronounced en route and cause you to have an accident.

PREVENTION

People who have a known sensitivity to particular allergens should always wear a medical alert tag so the correct treatment can be given in an emergency. They should also ask their doctor to prescribe an emergency kit to keep at home. (Such kits normally contain antihistamines and a syringe of adrenaline.)

The best prevention is to avoid exposure to known allergens. For example, if you are allergic to bee stings, wear long pants and long-sleeved tops when you are working in the garden or taking part in any outdoor activities.

Food allergy sufferers should read packaging labels, and enquire about the ingredients used when ordering in a restaurant, stating clearly that they are allergic to a particular food.

A clearly visible Medic Alert tag must be worn at all times. It will provide medical personnel with details of your allergies in the event that you are unable to speak for yourself. This is especially important if you are allergic to penicillin or other medications which may be given in an emergency situation .

Convulsions and seizures

A seizure can be alarming to witness: it may last anything from 30 seconds to a couple of minutes, and involve the whole body or just one part. In severe cases, there may be violent muscle contractions and relaxations triggered by spontaneous electrical activity in the casualty's brain, causing them to convulse. Nothing can be done to end a seizure. All you can do is wait it out and try to ensure that the person does not suffer an injury by slamming a limb into a table, for example. If a seizure lasts longer than two minutes or so, or one seizure follows another in quick succession without the casualty regaining consciousness between each one, you have a medical emergency on your hands, as the person will be unable to breathe normally for the duration of the seizure. Summon assistance immediately and note the duration and severity of the seizure, what movements the casualty made, and with which limbs, if there was a loss of bladder control, any eye or head movements, and whether the casualty displayed different levels of consciousness. This information will help in diagnosing the cause of the seizure and deciding on the appropriate treatment. If seizures recur and no underlying causes can be identified, a person may suffer from epilepsy which, fortunately, can usually be controlled with medication.

SYMPTOMS

Strange sensations such as noises in the ears, flashes of light, nausea, dizziness, fear or anxiety can appear before an attack. Some sufferers recognize these and know when a seizure is about to occur. During a seizure, the casualty may:

- Black out or lose consciousness and fall.
- Exhibit confused behaviour.
- Cease breathing temporarily.
- Drool or froth at the mouth.
- Experience tingling or twitching in one part of the body.
- Experience vigorous muscle spasms causing the limbs to twitch and jerk.
- Grunt and snort.
- Lose bladder or bowel control.
- The head or eyes may move erratically.

CAUSES

- Intoxication/overdose (alcohol or drugs)
- Brain infection
- Injury to the brain or the head
- Choking
- Adverse effects of drugs
- Electric shock
- Epilepsy
- Fever (young children)
- High blood pressure (particularly during late pregnancy)
- Hypoglycaemia (low blood sugar)
- Heat Intolerance
- Poisoning
- Stroke

TREATMENT

- The first priority is to **prevent injury**. Clear away furniture or other objects that could cause harm.
- **Loosen tight clothing**, particularly around the casualty's neck, if possible.
- **If the casualty vomits**, turn the head to face downwards so vomited material is ejected from the mouth and not taken into the lungs.
- If you think a **high fever** could have caused a seizure in a young child, cool him gradually using cool compresses and tepid water.
- **Many people go into a deep sleep following a seizure**; cover them with a blanket to keep them warm, check that their airway, breathing and heartbeat are normal and let them to sleep. Do not be alarmed if they are disorientated after waking.
- If an unconscious casualty is **diabetic** or you think he may be, you can place some sugar granules or liquid glucose under the tongue. In the case of a casualty who has regained consciousness, it will be safe to provide some sugar water or concentrated liquid glucose. **Note:** Attempt this only once the seizure has ended, not while it is in progress.

PREVENTION

- If you have epilepsy, take your prescribed medication regularly and wear a Medic Alert tag (*see* p177) at all times.
- Treat high fevers (39°C+), especially in children.
- Ensure that chronic medications are taken as directed, particularly in children and the elderly.

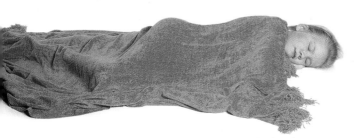

Cover casualty with a blanket to minimize loss of body heat.

SEEK MEDICAL HELP IF:

- the casualty has a seizure lasting longer than two minutes.
- he or she suffers more than one seizure in an hour.
- the casualty does not regain consciousness between successive seizures.
- there is absolutely no previous history of convulsions.
- the patient is a diabetic or suffers from high blood pressure.
- the casualty is pregnant.
- the seizure occurred in the water.

X DO NOT

- forcibly restrain the casualty; merely try to restrict the worst of the convulsions to prevent injury;
- place anything – handle of a spoon or your fingers – between the casualty's teeth during a seizure;
- move the casualty unless they are in danger or near something hazardous;
- try to stop the casualty convulsing;
- give rescue breaths to a seizure casualty, even if they are turning blue. Most seizures end well before brain damage can begin;
- give the casualty anything to eat or drink until the convulsions have stopped completely and you are satisfied that they are fully awake and alert.

Fever and meningitis

Fever is the body's response to illness and infection. Normal temperature is in the region of 37°C (98.6° F), with small variations from one individual to another. Temperature varies throughout the day, it is usually lower in the morning. Factors that influence temperature include stress, the amount of clothing worn, exercise, medication, age (children have a tendency to develop high fevers) and a woman's menstrual cycle. A low-grade fever is one of 38°C (100°F) or lower; high-grade fever is above 39°C (102°F). Most fevers are caused by infection. Fevers may peak suddenly and then subside, or come and go over a period of time. They may be accompanied by chills and shivering, as bacteria, viruses or toxins are released into the bloodstream.

 SEEK MEDICAL HELP IF:

- the fever remains above 39.5°C (103°F) after an hour or two of home treatment.
- the temperature rises above 40°C (105°F) at any time.
- the fever lasts two days or longer.
- the patient is a baby younger than six months of age.
- a child between six and 12 months has a fever for more than 24 hours.
- you think you may have taken or given the wrong medication or dosage.
- the patient develops a stiff neck, or becomes confused, irritable or sluggish.

CAUSES

- Colds or flu-like illnesses
- Ear infection, sore throat and 'strep' throat
- Upper respiratory tract infections (such as tonsillitis, pharyngitis, laryngitis)
- Acute bronchitis or pneumonia
- Viral or bacterial gastroenteritis
- Infections of the urinary tract (the bladder and the kidneys)
- Overdressing infants in hot weather or when a room is too warm

FEVER

Feverish patients send out mixed signals – the body temperature is raised, but the patient is shivering and suffers from chills. They are not cold, however, so do not cover them with blankets, you'll only raise the temperature higher. With a mild fever, all the patient needs is to rest and drink fluids. Other measures may include bathing in tepid water or sponging the patient down. Do not use cold water or rubbing alcohol as this can be easily absorbed through the skin. Some medications can be given to fight a fever or chills, but you should exercise caution. Aspirin should never be given to a child under the age of 12. If in doubt, do not provide any medication and summon medical attention.

REDUCING FEVER

Fever can be brought down by giving two paracetamol tablets to an adult (use the recommended dose of paracetamol syrup for children). Cool an adult's fever by wiping the patient down with a cool, damp cloth, and give him or her plenty to drink.

If a child's temperature is still over 39.7°C (103.5°F) one to two hours after giving medication, remove their clothing, seat them in a bath of tepid water up to the navel and gently sponge their upper body, adding more warm water to the bath as necessary, to prevent shivering. The water must not be cold. When the fever is down, pat the child dry, put on light, loose garments, give it plenty of liquids and ensure that the room remains comfortably cool.

X DO NOT

- give aspirin to children under 12 and ibuprofen to infants under six months old.
- use iced water or rubbing alcohol to reduce a child's temperature.
- bundle a feverish child in blankets.
- wake a sleeping child to give it medication or check temperature. Sleep does more good than you realize.

MENINGITIS

This inflammation of the brain membranes can be caused by a virus or by bacteria. Viral meningitis, the most common form, is milder. Most cases of viral meningitis infections occur in children under the age of five. Acute bacterial meningitis must be treated as a medical emergency, as it can result in brain damage or death.

SYMPTOMS (MENINGITIS)

- Fever and chills, panting
- Severe headache
- Nausea and vomiting
- A stiff neck
- Pink-purple rash
- Sensitivity to light
- Loss of appetite
- Confusion or decreased consciousness
- Agitation, or irritability
- In babies it may look as though the fontanelles (*see* **glossary** p294) bulge out

The 'Glass Test'

If the child has developed a pinkish-purplish rash, press the side of a glass firmly against it. If it is just a rash, then the discolouration should fade and lose colour under pressure. If it does not change colour, however, and you can still see the rash clearly through the glass, contact your doctor immediately.

MENINGITIS TREATMENT

Seek medical care immediately. Speed is often the key to a successful outcome.

METHODS OF TEMPERATURE READING

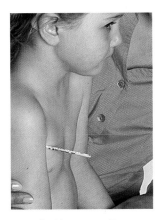
In the armpit

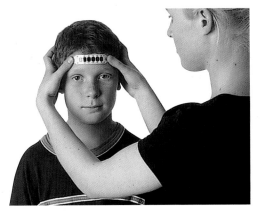
Strip against forehead

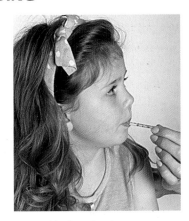
Under the tongue

Poisoning

If a person suddenly becomes ill for no apparent reason, consider whether they might have ingested or inhaled poison. Household products, plant matter, decaying food, pesticides, chemicals and narcotics can all result in poisoning. In addition, many medicines designed to be beneficial in small quantities, can be very dangerous when taken in excess.

Speed is absolutely crucial, so contact the nearest poison information centre or hotline, or your local emergency services, immediately you suspect poisoning. Look for containers from which the contents may have been consumed. The label should contain essential information which will be required by the doctors. Even if the label is partially destroyed, take the container along with you to the emergency room. Small children are particularly at risk, as they cannot distinguish poisonous substances from those that are not harmful, and they naturally put things into their mouths. Ensure that potentially dangerous items are, at all times, kept in locked cupboards or on high shelves.

SYMPTOMS

Affecting the stomach, appearance and general sense of wellness:

- Nausea and vomiting
- Abdominal pain
- Fever
- Headache
- Skin rash or burns
- Diarrhoea
- Loss of bladder control
- Irritability
- Loss of appetite
- Lips have bluish hue
- Unusual breath odour

Affecting breathing, circulation and the nervous system:

- Shortness of breath
- Dizziness
- Heart palpitations
- Chest pain
- Double vision
- Confusion
- Muscle twitching
- Drowsiness or stupor
- Numbness or tingling
- General feeling of weakness
- Seizures
- Unconsciousness

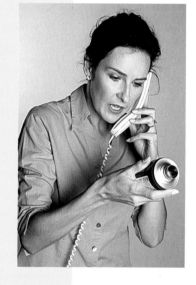

Above: In order to prescribe the correct treatment, your doctor will need to know the contents of the poisonous substance inhaled or consumed.

CAUSES

Ingested (swallowed):

- Food poisoning (such as botulism) caused by eating food that has become contaminated.
- Accidental or deliberate overdosing on medicines, either prescribed or over-the-counter.
- Eating poisonous plants. If you are not sure what the plant is, take a piece to the emergency room for identification
- Accidentally drinking solvents that were stored in cool-drink bottles.
- Overdosing on narcotic drugs, either by swallowing or injection.

Inhaled:

- The fumes or vapours from household cleaners or chemicals.
- Insecticides, pesticides or weedkillers can be inhaled while working in the garden.
- Carbon monoxide gas (from furnaces or motor vehicle exhausts).
- Abuse of solvents, adhesives and other substances to get 'high'.

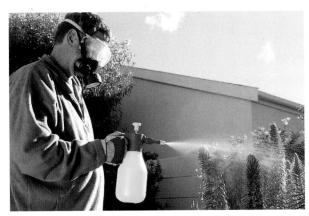

When spraying plants, wear a mask and goggles to prevent yourself from inhaling the chemicals.

Contact poisons:

- Exposure to household detergents, cleaners and chemicals.
- Exposure to toxins (venom) produced by some snakes and spiders.

TREATMENT

If the casualty is conscious and breathing normally, the first step is to contact your nearest doctor or emergency room. They will tell you what to do until help arrives. Ask the casualty what they ingested or inhaled. If they are unable to give a coherent reply, look for anything that may give a clue, such as empty containers. Try to ascertain the type of poisoning by checking for burns around the mouth, unusual breath odours, vomiting or laboured breathing.

Ingested (swallowed) poison:

- If the casualty is unconscious and not breathing, check the **vital signs** (*see* p293) and begin **rescue breaths** (*see* p168) and **chest compressions** (*see* pp164–9). Monitor until medical help arrives. While waiting and as soon as casualty is breathing unaided, place them in the **recovery position** (*see* p167) and keep calm and comfortable.
- Never induce vomiting (unless told to do so by the poison control centre).
- If the casualty vomits, clear the airway (use one finger wrapped in a cloth). Save as much of the vomitus as you can in a container. If the casualty ate part of a plant, fragments in the material will aid identification, and the same goes for pills that might have been consumed.
- If **convulsions** (*see* p178) begin, protect the casualty from injury and give appropriate first aid.
- Clothing soaked in a chemical or toxic substance should be removed and the affected body area washed with water. For poison in dry powder form, brush off (away from the face) as much as you can, remove clothing and wash the affected area.

Inhaled poison:

- The first step is to remove the person and yourself from the source of the poison. If you are uncertain of the source, or you suspect fumes are still present, try to have someone else on stand-by, in case you also succumb.
- Take deep breaths of fresh air, hold your breath, cover your mouth and nose with a wet cloth and drag the casualty into the open air. If you cannot do that, open doors and windows, or use a fan.

- Once out of the danger area, check the casualty's **vital signs** (*see* pp164–5 and p293). Begin **rescue breaths** (*see* p168) and/or **chest compressions** (*see* pp164–9) if required.
- An inhaled poison, such as an insecticide, might have affected the eyes or skin. Check these and administer the appropriate first aid (*see* **eye injuries** p196).
- If the casualty vomits or convulses, treat as indicated above.

PREVENTION

The average home contains many substances that can be highly dangerous when taken or used incorrectly. One of the easiest ways to prevent accidental poisoning at home is to educate your children, as soon as they are old enough, not to touch any substances that have not been approved by you.

In the home
- Keep all medicines, household cleaners, garden products, and solvents locked away, and keep the keys kept out of reach of children.
- Never use food or soft-drink containers to store anything other than food or drinks.
- Keep hazardous substances in their original containers. If a container starts leaking, transfer the contents to a new non-food/drink container and label it clearly. If possible, remove the old label, or photocopy it and use it to identify the new container. Transfer safety warnings as well.

- Always wash fruits and vegetables thoroughly before use.
- Prepare and cook food in hygienic conditions and discard any items that might have gone off or be contaminated in some way.
- Be aware of food allergies. Someone allergic to peanuts, for instance, can develop breathing difficulties if nut products are used in a dish (*see* **anaphylactic shock** p176).
- Check food when purchasing to ensure the 'sell by' date has not been reached.

DO NOT

- give an unconscious casualty anything by mouth.
- induce vomiting unless instructed to do so by medical personnel (any poison that burned on the way down will do so again on the way up and increase the damage).
- try to neutralize the poison, unless told to do so by a medical expert.
- give any emetics (such as Ipecac).

In the garden
- Remove toxic plants from your garden.
- Never eat wild berries, mushrooms or any other plants unless you are absolutely certain that they are safe.
- When using insecticides or garden sprays, remember that even a light breeze could blow the mist back onto your face or body, or through an open window into the house. If the kitchen windows are open, food could easily be contaminated.
- Keep pets out of the way when you are working with garden sprays and other chemicals.

CARBON MONOXIDE POISONING

Carbon monoxide is a colourless, odourless gas. It is produced during combustion in vehicle engines, charcoal-burning barbecues, portable propane heaters, or portable or non-ventilated natural gas appliances such as a shower-head water heater. Under normal circumstances, when you inhale, you take in air containing oxygen. Carbon monoxide interferes with the blood's ability to carry oxygen, thereby progressively starving the tissues of oxygen, leading to the symptoms mentioned below.

SYMPTOMS

- Headache
- Nausea and vomiting
- Impaired judgement
- Hyperactivity
- Irritability
- Abnormal or rapid heart beat
- Rapid breathing
- Shortness of breath
- Low blood pressure
- Fainting
- Chest pain
- Convulsions
- Coma, followed by unconsciousness and death

CAUSES

Carbon monoxide poisoning occurs in confined or non-ventilated spaces, so be careful when using any appliance that involves combustion in its operation.

Carbon monoxide poisoning may occur accidentally, by working on a vehicle engine and keeping the garage door closed in cold weather, for example; or deliberately, by running the engine in the same conditions in order to commit suicide.

Because you cannot smell carbon monoxide, poisoning can occur more easily than if you could detect its presence.

TREATMENT

Get the casualty into fresh air, as this will immediately halt the level of contamination. If the carbon monoxide levels are very high, you could be in danger yourself, particularly if breathing hard from anxiety or exertion.

- Take three deep breaths, hold your breath, enter the area and get the casualty out into fresh air. Drag them out by their clothing, legs or whatever, if this will reduce your exposure. Leave the door open to ventilate the area.
- Call for medical assistance immediately. If possible, inform the dispatcher of the casualty's condition, age, weight and the length of time they have been exposed to the carbon monoxide.
- If the casualty has ceased breathing and there is no pulse, administer **resuscitation** (*see* pp164–171) while awaiting the arrival of medical assistance.
- Recovery is usually slow and, depending on the severity of the attack, there may be permanent brain damage with impaired mental ability. If the latter is still apparent after two weeks, complete recovery is not very likely. Even though the victim may seem free of symptoms, impaired mental ability can appear within a week or two of the incident.

PREVENTION

Install carbon monoxide detectors in areas in which gas appliances are used, such as the kitchen, bathroom, garage and workshop.

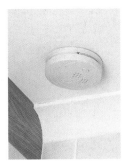

Carbon monoxide detector.

Burns and scalds

Burns are among the most common injuries, although fortunately, the vast majority are comparatively minor. They are graded in severity (see box). Providing the appropriate first aid can reduce the consequences of a burn injury but medical attention is vital if the burn is serious (second- or third-degree), does not heal properly, or complications, such as infection, set in afterwards. When in doubt as to a burn's severity, always treat it as serious. Be particularly alert if the burn is not painful – this could mean a severe burn in which the nerves have been destroyed. (*See* p187 for information on **treating minor burns and scalds**.)

SYMPTOMS

Airway burns:
- Burns on the head, neck or face, including a charred mouth and/or burned lips
- Coughing and wheezing
- Carbon-stained mucus or saliva
- Laboured, difficult breathing
- Singed nose hairs or eyebrows
- Voice change

(Note: Severe airway burns can occur in the absence of any surface burn, for example, if a person is caught in a smoke-filled room.)

Surface burns:
- Blisters
- Pain (in the absence of pain, suspect a severe burn)
- Peeling skin
- Red skin
- White or charred skin
- Swelling around the affected area
- **Shock** (*see* p174) – signs include pale, clammy skin, bluish lips and fingernails, weakness, disorientation and decreasing alertness

A NUMBER OF FACTORS DETERMINE THE SEVERITY OF A BURN

- **Size** – the extent of the body covered.
- **Locality** – burns on face, hands, feet and genitalia tend to be more serious because of possible loss of function, either while the burn heals, or permanently.
- **Degree and type of heat** (i.e. flame, electricity, or hot oil). Burns from a chemical or toxic substance may result in other complications.
- **Length of time** the casualty was exposed to the heat source (brief or prolonged exposure).
- **Age** – children under four and adults over 60 years old tend to develop complications more readily than other age groups.

CAUSES

- Thermal burns are caused by dry, radiated heat such as from a fire, hot surface (heaters or stoves), or the sun.
- Scalding is caused by hot liquid or steam.
- Chemical burns come from skin contact with chemicals, including some household products.
- Electrical burns result from contact with a live wire or current.
- Friction burns are common in sports injuries or motorcycle accidents.
- Smoke, super-heated air or toxic fumes can cause burn injuries to the airways.

TREATMENT OF MINOR BURNS AND SCALDS

The prime objective is to reduce the heat that still remains in the tissue.

- **Remove the source of heat**.
- **Reassure the casualty**.
- **Remove watches and rings** as well as other restricting items before swelling begins.
- **If the skin is intact**, gently run cool (not ice-cold) water over the burn area or soak in a basin of cool water for at least 10 minutes.
- **Once the burn area has been cooled, cover it with a clean cloth or sterile bandage**. Try not to subject the burn to friction and do not tie the dressing too tightly.
- If necessary **use a mild over-the-counter pain medication to reduce the pain**. Minor burns do not usually require further treatment, other than a change of dressing.

TREATMENT OF MAJOR BURNS AND SCALDS

Always treat these as serious and call for immediate medical assistance.

- **Remove the casualty from the heat source**, so if someone's clothing is on fire, pour water over them or hose them down (use a gentle spray).
- If water is not available, wrap the casualty in a thick coat or blanket made of natural fibres, such as cotton or wool, to **smother the flames**. (Do not use items made of synthetic fibre, such as nylon, as they could ignite).
- Lay the casualty flat and roll him on the ground.
- **Ensure all smouldering or burning garments are fully extinguished**.
- **Do not remove items of burnt clothing unless they come off easily**.
- **Ensure the casualty is breathing** before attending to the burn. If the airway is blocked, open it. If breathing does not restart spontaneously, begin **rescue breaths** (*see* p168).
- **Place a cool, moist, sterile bandage, or kitchen clingfilm (pvc wrap) over the burn area**. Do not use a blanket or towel as fibres may get into the burn and cause complications later.
- If fingers, feet or inner surfaces of the legs have been burned, **keep injured surfaces separated** with dry, sterile, non-adhesive dressings. A pillow slip or plastic shopping bag can be tied around burnt hands or feet.
- **Raise the burn area**, protecting it from being subjected to pressure and friction.
- **Prevent shock** by lying the casualty down and raising their feet about 30cm (12in) unless a head, neck or back injury is suspected. Keep them warm by covering with a coat or blanket.
- **Monitor the casualty's vital signs** until medical help arrives.

A minor burn or scald can be soothed by holding it under cool running water before it is loosely bandaged in sterile dressing, or cling wrap to avoid infection of the affected area.

TYPES OF BURNS

- **First-degree** (superficial) – minor burns to the outer skin layer look like mild to moderate sunburn (reddish, hot skin).
- **Second-degree** (partial thickness) – deeper burns that damage both the outer and underlying skin layers result in pain, redness, swelling and blistering. If precautions are not taken, blisters can become infected.
- **Third-degree** (full thickness) – serious burns affecting both outer and underlying skin layers, causing extreme pain, redness, swelling and blistering. Third-degree burns extend into deep tissues, causing brown or blackened skin that may be numb.

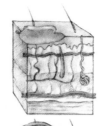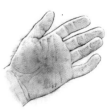

First degree burn

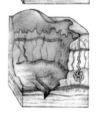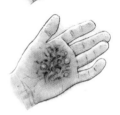

Second degree burn

Third degree burn

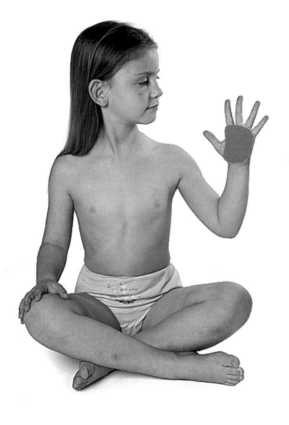

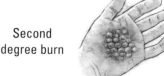

⚠ CAUTION

Call for emergency medical assistance if:
- a burn is large, severe or there is any difficulty with breathing.
- any burn affects the face, hands or groin.
- a child under two years of age is burnt.
- it is a chemical or electrical burn.
- the casualty shows signs of **shock** (*see* p174).
- treat a second-degree burn as a major burn if it is greater than 50–75mm (2–3in) in diameter, or is on the hands, feet, face, groin, buttocks, or a major joint.

The surface area of a burn may be estimated using the hand as a measure. The palm is equivalent to 1% of Total Body Surface Area (TBSA). As a rule, any burn involving more than 1% TBSA requires medical attention.

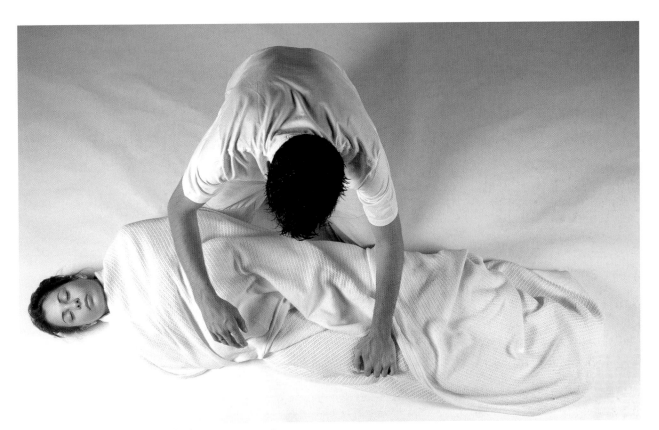

If clothing catches fire, roll the person up in a blanket made of natural fibre, such as cotton or wool, to smother the flames.

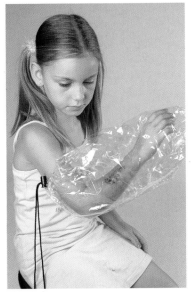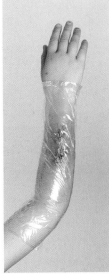

To prevent infection, loosely cover a severe burn with a clean plastic bag or cling wrap.

✕ DO NOT

- apply an adhesive bandage, cotton wool or fluffy cotton dressing, ice, medication, oil, ointment or any household remedy to a burn, as they can prevent proper healing, and possibly cause an infection.
- apply cold compresses or immerse a severe burn in cold water; this can cause reduced circulation and delay healing.
- breathe or cough on the burn.
- burst or puncture a blister.
- disturb or attempt to remove blistered or dead skin.
- give a severely burnt casualty anything by mouth.
- place a pillow under the casualty's head if there is an airway burn and he or she is lying down. This can restrict the airway.

PREVENTING BURN INJURIES

The easiest way to avoid being burned is to not go near hot things, but this is rarely possible in the normal course of daily living. Ovens and stoves, heaters and radiators, open fires and a host of small appliances are things we take for granted, and cannot imagine living without. While adults usually get burnt out of carelessness, children tend to burn themselves because they are ignorant of the dangers involved. It is every parent's duty to try and keep their children out of harm's way, by removing or reducing the potential for accidents or injuries to occur.

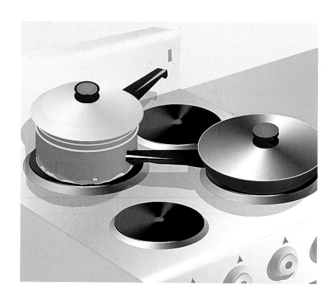

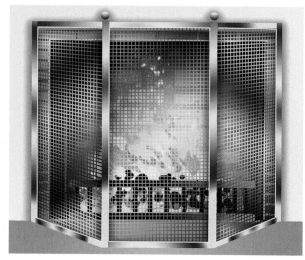

Install fireguards around open wood, coal or gas fires. Do not hang clothing or anything else on the fireguard – this only creates a hazard.

KITCHEN

More domestic fires start in the kitchen than anywhere else, making it the room with the greatest potential for burn-related accidents.

- Never leave anything unattended on the stove or under the grill. If you leave the kitchen, turn off the heat and/or move the pot to a cold plate.
- Use your oven timer to remind you when something needs to be removed from the oven.
- Make sure your oven gloves and pot holders are in good condition. It is easy to burn your hands if there are holes or gaps in the fabric.

- Turn pot handles away from the edge of a stove or countertop and make use of the back plates.
- When lifting the lid off a boiling pot, don't bend over it, or you could scald your face as the steam escapes.
- Watch your hands when doing the ironing, a lapse in concentration can result in burnt fingers.

BATHROOM

A child left in the bath unattended could turn on the hot tap and suffer severe **burns** (*see* p186) in a very short space of time.

BEDROOM

Electric blankets account for thousands of fires every year. Don't use a blanket that has worn or frayed wiring, or shows signs of scorching. Ensure plug and control connections are secure and don't leave it switched on for hours. Turn the blanket off when you get into/out of bed. Consider replacing electric blankets that are more than 10 years old.

OUTDOORS

Summer is barbecue time, which means flames, hot coals and the potential for burns. Prevent children from playing around the cooking area, keep some water on hand to douse any flare-ups and dispose of hot coals safely, not where some little foot could stand on them.

Chemical burns and injuries

Most chemical burns are the result of accidental contact with an abrasive substance. The inadvertent ingestion of such a substance (*see* **poisoning** p182) can cause severe internal damage. The degree of injury depends on the amount of chemical involved, where on (or in) the body it landed and the length of time the casualty was exposed to it. Certain chemicals, including battery acid, common household bleach and swimming-pool acid, can cause problems ranging from relatively mild effects (including burns), to much more serious reactions. Immediately suspect exposure to a chemical if an otherwise healthy person (or pet) becomes ill for no apparent reason. See whether you can find a chemical container nearby.

SYMPTOMS

These vary, depending on the chemical to which the casualty was exposed, and the amount and duration of the exposure.

Chemical poisoning:
- Abdominal pain
- Breathing difficulty
- Convulsions (seizures)
- Dizziness
- Headache
- Hives, itching, swelling
- Nausea or vomiting
- Weakness resulting from an allergic reaction
- Unconsciousness

Burns:
- Bright red or bluish rash on the skin and lips
- Pain where the skin has made contact with a toxic substance
- Blisters, burns on the skin

CAUSES
- Chemical burns are caused by accidental skin contact with a toxic or corrosive substance.
- Poisoning results from either the ingestion of too much medicine or taking the wrong medication (accidental overdose), or from deliberately swallowing medicines or chemical substances, as in a suicide attempt.

TIP

If possible, keep the chemical container and hand it to the paramedic or doctor. The information on the container will assist the medical personnel with an approproate diagnosis and suitable treatment.

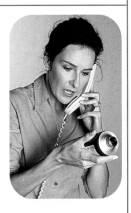

TREATMENT

Minor surface chemical burns will generally heal without further treatment. However, if there are second- or third-degree **burns** (*see* p188), call for medical assistance immediately. Medical help should also be obtained without delay in the case of a chemical being ingested.

- If possible, **remove deposits of the chemical from clothes or skin**, doing your utmost to avoid contact. If the chemical is dry, brush it off. If there is a breeze, brush away from the eyes and downwind, covering the casualty's eyes and protecting your own to avoid contamination. If a chemical does get into the eyes, flush them with water for at least 15 minutes and call for medical help.
- Remove **contaminated clothing**, including jewellery (a watch or ring, for instance, could trap deposits of the chemical).
- **Flush away any remaining chemical residue on the body**, using cool running water for at least 15 minutes. (*See* below.)

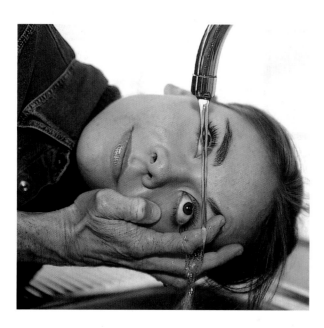

- Treat the casualty for **shock** (*see* p174) if they appear faint or pale, or if their breathing sounds shallow or rapid.
- Apply cool, wet compresses to relieve pain.

- **Dry the burn and cover it with a dry sterile dressing or clean cloth**. Protect the burn from pressure and friction.
- **Watch carefully for systemic reactions** and treat the casualty accordingly while awaiting medical assistance.

PREVENTION

- Toxic products are found in many household products and incorrect use can be dangerous. Always follow the manufacturer's instructions and observe any precautions.
- Keep exposure to chemicals to a minimum – over time, even low-level contamination can cause health problems.
- Select products that are contained in child-proof, secure containers, keep them in those containers and with labels intact.
- Keep chemicals away from food, children and pets, as well as kitchen surfaces.
- Re-seal the container immediately after use and store securely in a lockable cupboard or on a high shelf, out of the reach of toddlers.
- Never mix chemicals – the result could be dangerous. The concoction might produce harmful fumes, or even explode.
- Always handle substances that produce fumes (such as paints, solvents and ammonia) in well-ventilated areas.
- Never put chemicals (solvents for example) into cool-drink bottles or food containers.

X DO NOT

- allow the chemical to contaminate you as you give first aid.
- try to neutralize a chemical without getting medical advice from your nearest poison control centre or doctor.
- disturb a blister or remove dead skin.
- apply any ointment or salve.

Head injuries

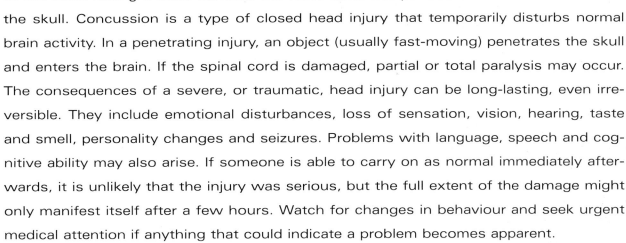

Head injuries are classified as either closed or penetrating. In a closed injury, usually caused by a blow to the head or due to the head hitting a solid surface, the force does not penetrate the skull. Concussion is a type of closed head injury that temporarily disturbs normal brain activity. In a penetrating injury, an object (usually fast-moving) penetrates the skull and enters the brain. If the spinal cord is damaged, partial or total paralysis may occur. The consequences of a severe, or traumatic, head injury can be long-lasting, even irreversible. They include emotional disturbances, loss of sensation, vision, hearing, taste and smell, personality changes and seizures. Problems with language, speech and cognitive ability may also arise. If someone is able to carry on as normal immediately afterwards, it is unlikely that the injury was serious, but the full extent of the damage might only manifest itself after a few hours. Watch for changes in behaviour and seek urgent medical attention if anything that could indicate a problem becomes apparent.

SYMPTOMS

Not all head injuries are cause for concern. The list below is intended to assist you in diagnosing the seriousness of the injury yourself before medical help arrives:

Scalp
- bruising at the site of impact
- a small cut at the site of impact

Skull
- accumulation of blood under the scalp soon after the accident could indicate a skull fracture
- headache
- clear or blood-stained fluid leaking from the nose or ears

Neck
- pain or stiffness in the neck
- a feeling of weakness, or pins-and-needles sensations in the arms or legs could indicate injury to the spinal cord
- severe neck injury may be accompanied by breathing difficulties (resulting from paralysis of the diaphragm and chest muscles)

Brain
- *mild concussion* is indicated by headache, irritability, nausea and vomiting (especially in children)
- *severe concussion* is indicated by a temporary loss of consciousness. Convulsions (fits) are possible, as is nausea

CAUSES

One of the most common causes of head injuries is vehicle accidents, and children are particularly vulnerable if they are not suitably restrained in safety seats. Accidental blows to the head, or falls sustained during sports and other recreational activities also common causes of head injuries.

TREATMENT

In the case of a minor bump on the head, observe the person for a few hours (checking their level of consciousness, heart rate and respiratory rate regularly). If no symptoms develop, the injury was mild and no treatment is required other than a painkiller or cold compress.

If the casualty exhibits any of the following symptoms, summon immediate medical assistance without delay:

- **If the casualty is unconscious** but their breathing and pulse is satisfactory, treat as for a **spinal injury** (*see* pp208–9). Stabilize the neck by placing both hands on either side of the head and keep it in that position until help arrives.
- **Stem scalp bleeding** by firmly pressing a clean cloth on the wound, without moving the casualty's head. Place a second cloth over the first if the latter becomes soaked.
- **Do not apply direct pressure** to an injury if you think the skull may be fractured.

- **Do not remove any debris** from a wound. Cover it with a sterile gauze dressing and wait for medical help to arrive.
- Apply ice packs to bruises under the scalp.
- If the casualty is vomiting, do not turn the head (in case there is a spinal injury). Instead, roll the head and body as one, supporting the head and neck in the same relative position to the body, to

✗ DO NOT

- move the casualty unless necessary.
- shake a dazed casualty in an attempt to get a response.
- pick up a fallen child when there is any sign of a head injury.
- remove any object sticking out of a head wound.
- remove a motor cyclist's helmet if you suspect a head injury (unless breathing is compromised). This really needs two people to execute, otherwise you could aggravate a neck injury.
- wash a head wound that is very deep or bleeding profusely.
- consume alcohol within 48 hours after suffering a head injury.

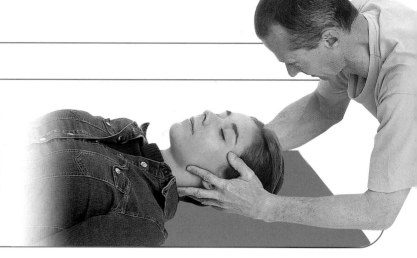

CAUTION

- In the case of serious head injury, you should always assume that the cervical spinal cord has been injured. Ensure that the casualty's head and neck are well stabilized and well protected until medical help arrives.

prevent choking. Children often vomit once after sustaining a minor head injury, but if there is repeated vomiting, or if the child becomes drowsy, contact a doctor.

In all of the above instances, the sooner help arrives the better. While you wait, check the vital signs (*see* p293) and begin **rescue breaths** (*see* p168) and/or **chest compressions** (*see* p169).

PREVENTION

- Wear the correct seat belts when in a vehicle.
- Reduce your risk by not drinking and driving or allowing yourself to be driven by someone you suspect is drunk.
- Wear protective headgear when riding a bicycle, motorcycle or horse, or when mountain climbing, and an approved hard hat on construction sites.
- Ensure your child's play area is safe, and super-vise them at play.
- If walking or jogging after dark, wear light-coloured clothing to make yourself more visible.

SKULL FRACTURE

If the skull undergoes severe trauma it can fracture, leading to possible brain injury, which can only be confirmed by an X-ray or brain scan. Fractures take a variety of forms:

- Simple – a break in the skull; no skin damage.
- Linear – a break resembling a thin line, with no splintering, depression, or distortion of the skull.
- Depressed – a 'crushed' portion of the skull, resembling a dent, is depressed inwards.
- Compound – a splintered fracture where the skull bones are broken at the site of the trauma.

FRACTURES OF THE JAW

It takes a lot of force to fracture the upper or lower jaw. However, you should suspect this injury if:

- you notice marked swelling or bruising of the gums, in the floor of the mouth or around the lower half of the face.
- the casualty is unable to open or close the mouth normally.
- you notice that the upper and lower sets of teeth

do not meet each other normally.
- two or more teeth appear displaced.

TREATMENT

- Ensure that the airway remains open by letting the casualty lean forward so that blood can drain from the mouth. Loose teeth can be kept and given to the doctor or emergency service.
- Let the casualty support the injured jaw by gently holding a soft cloth against it.
- Ensure that you get the casualty to a doctor or to a hospital as soon as possible.

INJURIES TO THE NOSE

A blow to the nose will often cause no more than a little swelling and some bleeding from one or both nostrils. Fractures of the nasal bones are usually caused by assault and will result in severe bruising and heavier bleeding. The fracture can only be con-firmed with special X-rays of the face. The 'bones' of a child's nose are mostly soft, pliable cartilage until they begin to harden with calcium in the early teens, so true fractures of the nose are uncommon in young children. If you suspect a broken nose:

- Control the bleeding (*see* p172).
- Control bruising/swelling with a cold compress.
- Use a mild painkiller if necessary.

Seek a medical opinion when:

- the nose appears crooked after the swelling has gone down.
- there is persistent or recurrent bleeding from one or both nostrils.
- the casualty seems to have difficulty breathing through either nostril.
- the outer edge of the nostril has been lacerated.

TREATMENT

- Treat the bleeding nose (see pp222–3).
- Reduce the swelling by holding a cold, wet cloth loosely against the nose.
- If you suspect a more serious injury or fracture. ensure that you get the casualty to hopsital or to a doctor as soon as possible.

Eye injuries

Loss of sight can affect just about every aspect of your life, so treat as an emergency anything which could lead to loss of vision if left untreated – this includes ridding the eye of a foreign object but then experiencing persistent discomfort or pain. Have it checked!

Eye injuries can be caused by airborne objects, and can include cuts, scratches, burns, or a blow to the eye. Chemical injuries result from direct exposure when droplets splash into the eyes, or from fumes given off by household cleansers, pesticides, weedkillers, solvents, acids, alkaline substances and more. The workshop is particularly dangerous, as particles can fly into the eye at speed, either penetrating it or severely damaging its delicate surface. Sports injuries or fights can leave one with a black eye, when bleeding under the skin causes bruising or a dark discolouration of the surrounding area. This will disappear with time, but eye injuries should always be checked by your doctor.

SYMPTOMS

- Bleeding or bruising in or around the eye
- Double vision, or loss of vision
- Itching, stinging or burning eyes
- Pupils of unequal size
- Redness (bloodshot eyes)
- Scratchy feeling in the eye
- Sensitivity to light

TIP

Over-the-counter (OTC) eye drops contain mild vaso-constrictors (decongestants) and should only be used in the case of mild allergies or eye irritations. They should never be used to treat an injury or when there is any chance of an eye infection.

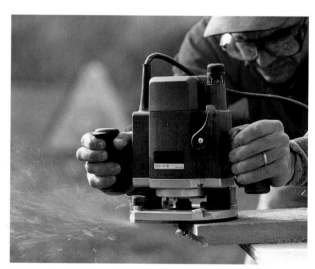

Protect your eyes by wearing plastic goggles whenever you are working with power tools, to prevent sawdust or metal shavings from shooting up into your eye. A foreign body in the eye can cause unpleasant irritation, and in some cases lasting damage. If you do get something in your eye, rinse with water immediately. If the irritation persists, see a doctor.

CAUSES
- Blow to the eye socket
- Foreign object in the eye
- Injury to the eyeball itself
- Chemical injury
- Medical conditions (i.e. infection or glaucoma)

TREATMENT

Object on the surface of the eye:
- If blinking or shedding tears do not expel the object, go to a well-illuminated area and check the eye as the casualty swivels their eyes from left to right and up and down until you spot the offending object.
- If you don't spot the object, gently pull the lower lid out and down to expose the fold between the eyelid and the globe of the eye. You may need to do the same to the upper lid.
- Once you spot the object, gently wash it out with water or a damp cotton-tipped swab; use the latter as a last resort and keep it away from the pupil.
- Do not try to remove an object embedded in the eyeball. Make an eye cup out of the bottom half of a styrofoam cup and secure this over the eye with strapping or plaster (*see picture at right*) to avoid aggravating the injury or inflammation.
- If you cannot find or remove the object, and the casualty still has discomfort or blurred vision, cover the eye and seek medical help.

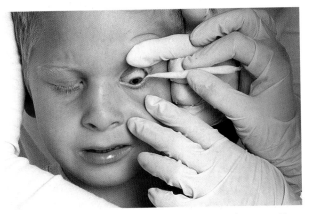

To remove a foreign body, moisten a clean cotton bud or piece of cotton wool. Lift the lid up and get the child to look down.

Object embedded in the eye:
- Do not apply any pressure to the object or try to remove it, and stop the casualty from rubbing or touching the eye.
- If the object is large, cut out the base of a paper or foam cup and place the cup over the injured eye, taping it into position (*see picture below*). If the object is small, cover both eyes with a clean cloth or sterile dressing to discourage eye movement.
- Keep the casualty quiet, calm and reassured until medical assistance is available.

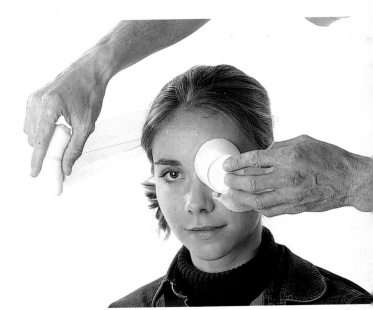

Bandage a paper cup in place to protect an injured eye until medical help can be obtained.

Chemical injury to the eye:
- Irrigate the eye immediately with tap water. Turn the casualty's head so the injured eye is down and to the side, hold the eyelid open, and run water in and over the eye for at least 20 minutes or until you have medical help.
- If the chemical has got into both eyes, get the casualty into the shower and hold their eyes open-

with their head tilted back. Do not run the shower full-blast as powerful droplets of water could add to the discomfort.

- Remove contact lenses, only after the eyes have been rinsed.
- Cover both eyes with a clean dressing and avoid rubbing the eyes.
- Get medical help urgently.

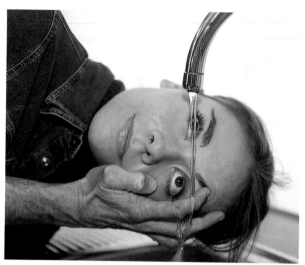

In the case of a chemical injury, wash the eye with cold water for at least 20 minutes.

Burns

- Gently pour cool water over and into the eyes (unless it is painful to do so) to reduce swelling and relieve the pain.
- Apply a cool compress to the eyes, but avoid applying pressure.
- If there is swelling in or around the eyes, if the lashes or lid skin is burned, or if there is any change in vision, seek medical help.

Cuts, scratches and blows to the eye

- Seek medical assistance immediately if the eyeball has been injured.
- Do not apply pressure to the eye.
- Gently apply cold compresses to reduce swelling and help stop bleeding, but do not apply pressure to control bleeding.

- If blood is pooling in the eye, cover both eyes with a clean cloth or sterile dressing to reduce eye movement. Get medical help immediately.
- Small cuts to the eyelid (less than a few millimetres long) should require little more than cleaning and dressing. However, if the eye can't be closed, or the cut is larger or deeper, or goes over the edge of the lid, cover the eye with a sterile pad and seek medical attention.

Double vision (diplopia)

This is a very serious symptom following an eye injury, as it may result from the displacement of the eyeball and traction on the delicate optic nerve. If a casualty complains of 'seeing double', seek urgent medical attention.

Stye

An infection of tiny glands situated on the lower edge of the upper and lower eyelid, causing very localized pain and redness of the lid. Styes usually disappear spontaneously, but see a doctor if pain persists.

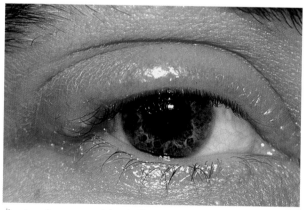

A stye is caused by inflammation of one of the hair follicles from which eyelashes grow. The condition, while not very serious, is unpleasant and unsightly. The eye itches and the movement of the eye lid causes discomfort. Cool the inflamed lid with a cold cloth and visit your doctor. The treatment is relatively quick and effective and may include a salve and eye drops.

DO NOT

- let the casualty rub the eye; this is a natural reaction to discomfort, but may make the condition worse.
- press on an injured eye.
- remove contact lenses unless rapid swelling is occurring, or you can't get prompt medical help.
- remove a foreign body that is resting on the cornea (the clear surface of the eye through which we see), or that appears to be embedded in any part of the eye.
- use dry cotton wool, cotton swabs or sharp instruments (such as tweezers) near the eye.
- risk contamination of a burn by breathing or coughing on it.

PREVENTION

- Wear protective goggles or safety spectacles when working with power tools or striking tools (such as hammers), to prevent objects flying into your eye.
- Only use garden sprays on a calm day, and wear protective goggles when spraying.
- When cutting trees or bushes, wear protective goggles as the sap of some plants can produce severe discomfort if it lands in your eyes.
- When working with toxic chemicals or any other substances that produce fumes, work in well-ventilated areas and wear protective goggles which seal the eye area.

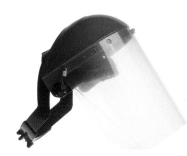

A full face mask will not only protect the eyes but the face as well.

Conjunctivitis (pink/red eye)

This an eye infection, as opposed to an environmentally based allergy or irritation. Conjunctivitis is characterized by severe burning and redness, with or without swelling of the eyelids and a yellow or greenish discharge. All eye infections are serious and should be seen by a doctor as soon as possible. In the interim, wash the eye with cool water and cover the closed eye with a cool cloth to help relieve the discomfort.

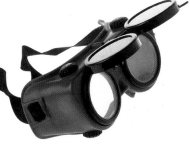

Welding goggles shield the eyes from the brightness and the danger of the sparks.

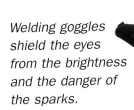

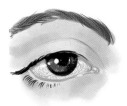

Viral conjunctivitis is also commonly known as 'pink eye'.

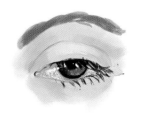

Bacterial conjunctivitis causes gummy, sticky eyelashes.

SEEK MEDICAL HELP IF:

- the eyeball appears scratched or has been penetrated by an object.
- a chemical has splashed into the eye.
- there is persistent pain and/or nausea.
- there are any vision problems.

Chest injuries

Chest injuries generally fall into two categories: penetrating or open wounds (where the skin is broken), and closed wounds (internal injuries). Treat them both as serious if the casualty is experiencing severe discomfort and/or shortness of breath

CAUSES

Closed chest injuries can occur when a motorist's chest hits the steering wheel as a result of an accident, for instance, or when a large heavy object, such as pipe or length of timber, slams into the casualty's chest. Such an accident can cause serious damage to the ribs, breast bone, heart or lungs.

Penetrating injuries include gunshots, stab wounds or penetration by other sharp objects.

SYMPTOMS

Closed chest injuries
- Pain
- Difficulty in breathing
- Shock due to loss of blood/oxygen
- Deformity or abnormal chest movement during breathing
- Bruising

Penetrating chest injuries
In addition to the above, these symptoms may also be present:
- A sucking sound as the casualty inhales
- Bubbling as the casualty exhales
- Bubbles in the blood around the wound

TAKE NOTE

- If an injury results in ribs being broken in more than one place, so that rib segments are able to move independently to some degree, the injured part of the chest wall tends to move abnormally (in when the casualty inhales, and out when they exhale). This is called a paradoxical chest movement and it makes breathing very difficult and painful.
- In extreme cases, an injury may cause one or both lungs to collapse; this condition, called pneumothorax, is life-threatening and must be treated as an emergency. This can happen with minimal trauma, and can occur spontaneously, in people with an inborn weakness or defect in their lungs (spontaneous pneumothorax).

TREATMENT

Call for an ambulance. Chest injuries are medical emergencies and must be assessed by a doctor.
- **Close off the wound to stop the flow of air through it**. If you do not have an airtight sterile dressing available, improvise with whatever is at hand, such as a clean plastic bag, or sandwich wrap for instance. Make a patch to cover the wound and tape it down on three sides only (*see* picture on p201). This will close when the casual-

ty inhales, admitting more air to the chest, and open when he or she exhales.

- Do not move the casualty if you suspect a head or spinal injury.
- If you have no reason to suspect a head or spinal injury, move the casualty into a semi-reclining position by propping them up. Lean them slightly towards the injured side so that the uninjured side is higher.
- If an embedded object (such as a piece of glass) caused the injury, do not remove it as you could do more damage. If feasible, support the object with a **ring bandage** (*see* p220).
- If a large object has caused a crushing chest injury, keep the casualty immobile while you wait for medical assistance.
- Loosen tight clothing, including belts or waistbands.

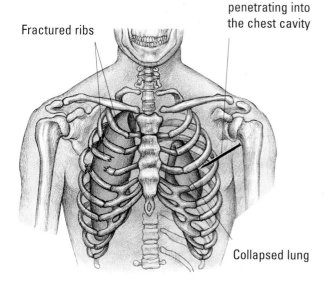

Sharp object penetrating into the chest cavity

Fractured ribs

Collapsed lung

This illustration depicts two causes of chest injuries: on the right is a penetrating injury with a collapsed lung, while the left side depicts fractured ribs.

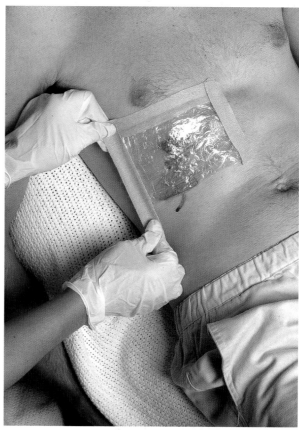

For an open chest injury, such as this puncture wound caused by an unfortunate fall, tape down the dressing on three sides. Leave one side open.

X DO NOT (also for p38)

- apply a tourniquet to control bleeding.
- lift the pad to see if bleeding has stopped, or replace a blood-soaked dressing. Just place a new one on top of it.
- probe an injury or try to remove a foreign object such as a knife.
- try to clean a large wound. This can cause heavier bleeding.
- try to clean an injury after you get the bleeding under control.

Fractures

A fracture is an injury to bone. A break results from the application of a force or stress that causes the bone to split or break. Stress fractures, usually small breaks, result when bone is subjected to repeated stress. A compound, or open, fracture occurs when the end of a broken bone breaks the skin and protrudes, or when the fracture results from a penetrating crush injury. Compound fractures must be treated immediately to prevent infection. As we age, our bones become brittle, which is why elderly people are more prone to fractures than younger people.

SYMPTOMS

- Limitation or unwillingness to move a limb
- Numbness and tingling
- Intense pain
- Bruising
- Swelling
- Inability to bear weight on a leg or use an arm
- Visibly out-of-place or misshapen limb or joint
- Bleeding or laceration (open fracture)

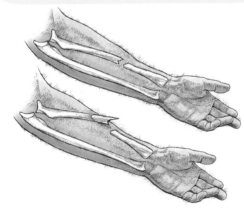

In a closed fracture (top), the bone does not penetrate the skin, as it does with an open, or compound, fracture (bottom).

CAUSES

- Direct blow to the bone.
- Falls, either from a height or on a slippery surface.
- Motor vehicle accidents.
- Excessive pressure.
- Stress fracture, from repetitive sports activity, for example.

TREATMENT

- In the case of a serious accident with the likelihood of broken bones, first **check the casualty's vital signs**. If it is necessary, begin **resuscitation** (*see* pp164–71), and control **bleeding** (*see* p172). Check for other life-threatening injuries, then keep the casualty still, provide reassurance, and call for medical help.
- **Keep the casualty warm**. Raise the feet about 30cm (12in), but do not move the casualty at all if a head, neck, or back injury is suspected.
- **In the case of an open, or compound fracture** try to gently rinse away any pieces of grass, bits of dirt and suchlike, but do not probe the wound, breathe on it or subject it to a vigorous scrubbing or flushing to remove the debris.
- **Cover open wounds with clean dressings** before immobilizing the injury (use a proprietary splint or improvise one from a rolled-up newspaper or piece of wood). Immobilize the area both above and below the injured bone, leaving it in the position in which it ended up.

SPLINTING FRACTURES BELOW THE ELBOW

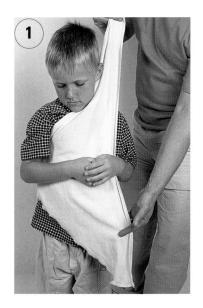 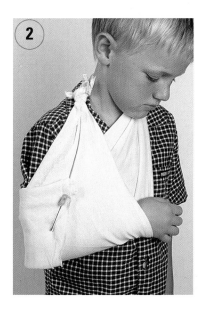

1. *Prepare a triangular bandage while the child supports the injured arm. Always apply the sling or bandage to the arm in whichever position you find it. Then tie the ends securely so that the knot does not rub against and irritate the back of the neck.*

2. *Do not bend the elbow beyond 90 degrees as bone fragments can press on the nerves and vessels that run just in front of the elbow and may interfere with blood flow. For the same reason you should never apply any sling or dressing that encircles the arm tightly at any point.*

- **Check that circulation is still healthy below the fracture**. For instance, in the case of a broken arm, press your fingertip on the casualty's finger for five seconds. The area should turn pale and then regain its normal colour within three seconds. If it does not, or there is numbness, lack of a pulse and pale or blue skin, the circulation is inadequate. Splint the fracture in the position in which you find it and get the casualty to a hospital as soon as possible.
- If an open fracture is bleeding, place a clean, dry cloth over the wound. **If the bleeding continues, apply direct pressure** to the site of bleeding, taking care not to apply any pressure to the protruding end of the bone.
- **Summon medical assistance** as soon as possible. In the case of a broken ankle or arm, get the casualty to an emergency room.

PREVENTION

- Wear the recommended protective gear while engaged in an active sport or pastime.
- Create a safe environment for young children and supervise them properly no matter how safe the situation appears to be. Help children learn how to look out for themselves and teach them basic safety techniques.
- Avoid falls by taking care when walking on wet, slippery or icy surfaces, and observing posted warnings.
- Use handrails when going up and down stairs and getting on and off escalators.
- Ensure that ladders are secure when doing household maintenance or gardening.
- Some people are reluctant to use a cane or walking aid, but it is far better to suffer some loss of dignity than deal with the aftermath of a broken limb or hip.

EASY SLING FOR FRACTURES ABOVE THE ELBOW

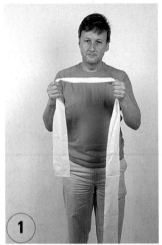

1 Grab a 1m (3ft) length of flannel or linen. Hold it away from the centre in such a way that you have one long end and one shorter end.

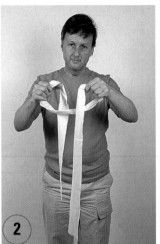

2 Fold two loops as shown; the longer one looping behind and the shorter one in front of the central piece.

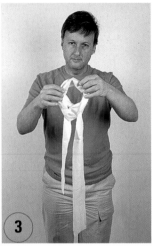

3 Superimpose the two loops (fold them together) to form a clove hitch.

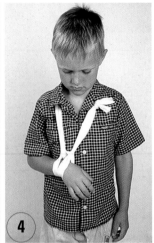

4 Place the double loops around the wrist of the injured arm and tie the ends together.

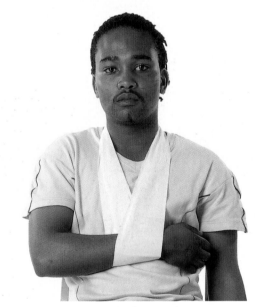

An alternative method of strapping an upper limb. Use a triangular bandage and a strip of flannel or linen to immobilize an arm or shoulder injury until the casualty can be taken to an emergency room.

✗ DO NOT

- move the casualty if a head, spine or back injury is suspected. In the case of a fractured hip, pelvis or upper leg, move the casualty only if absolutely necessary (for example out of harm's way following a road accident). Do so by pulling the casualty by their clothing, not by any limbs, which could also be injured.
- move the casualty unless the injury is completely immobilized. Never try to reposition a suspected cervical spine injury.
- try to straighten a misshapen bone or joint, or change its position.
- test a misshapen bone or joint for loss of function.
- give the casualty anything by mouth.
- apply a tourniquet to the extremity to stop the bleeding. Apply direct pressure.

SPLINTING FRACTURES BELOW THE KNEE

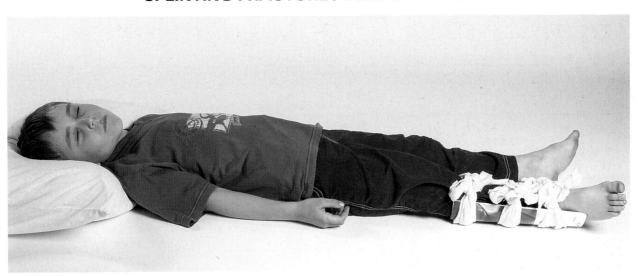

If you have called the ambulance, simply support the calf with a pillow, a rolled-up towel or blanket. If you have to transport the child yourself, you can splint the lower leg with a rolled magazine, newspaper or any sturdy object which extends a few inches above the knee and below the ankle. Foot injuries do not need splinting, particularly if the child is small enough for you to carry.

Pain relief – Pain at the fracture site is mostly due to the broken bone ends rubbing against each other. This can be minimized by splinting the limb and letting the child move as little as possible.

SPLINTING FRACTURES ABOVE THE KNEE

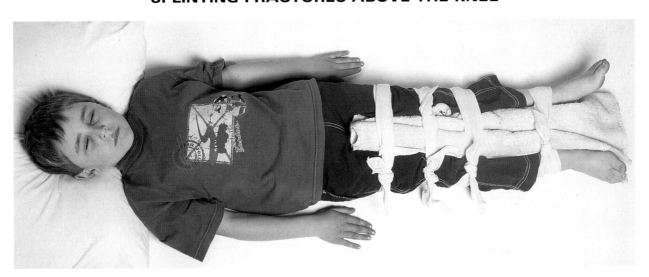

Splint the injured leg to the opposite limb using four 1m (3ft) lengths of linen, flannel or adhesive plaster. Do not move the casualty; wait for the ambulance to arrive and allow the ambulance staff to move him.

Sprains and strains (muscle, tendon and ligament injuries)

The terms 'strain' and 'sprain' refer to injuries caused by overstretching or tearing a muscle, tendon or ligament. These are uncommon before adolescence because the developing bones of children are more susceptible to injury than the neighbouring soft tissues. Consequently, strains and sprains should only be diagnosed in children once fractures or joint injuries have been excluded beyond doubt by X-ray examination. The fully developed bone of adults is reinforced with calcium, so that injury to the muscles, tendons and ligaments occur more frequently, particularly in an active person who frequently indulges in a variety of sports, exercise or exertion. (*See also* **fractures**, p202).

SYMPTOMS

- Sudden severe pain or cramp at the site of injury
- Aggravation of pain by any degree of movement at the site of injury
- Swelling directly over the injury. This is greatest with torn muscle which has a rich blood supply, however bruising only becomes visible in the days after injury

Ligaments are short, fibrous bands which run between neighbouring bones, to reinforce joint capsules. They may be stretched and damaged by forcibly moving a joint beyond its normal range, or as part of a deeper joint injury caused by a fall, sports injury or motor vehicle collision.

CAUSES

Even at rest, low-level nerve impulses ensure that muscles and their tendons remain semi-taut and in a state of readiness, prepared to act in response to the body's needs.

Any sudden, violent movement for which the muscles or tendons are unprepared, can cause them to tear, causing bleeding, pain and loss of function. This happens most frequently during vigorous exercise or contact sport, or if a fall onto an outstretched arm or leg results in sudden, involuntary stretching or bending of the limb.

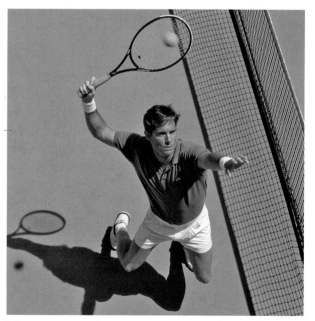

Vigorous exercise can cause a tendon or ligament to stretch or tear.

HOW TO MAKE A COLD COMPRESS

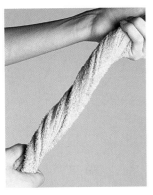

1. *Wring out a wet hand towel.*

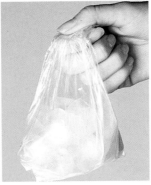

2. *Fill a bag with ice.*

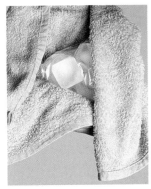

3. *Wrap the ice in the damp towel.*

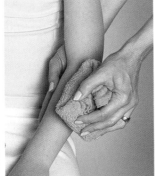

4. *Apply the compress to the affected area.*

TREATMENT

- Let casualty sit or lie down.
- Follow the **RICE** principle: rest the affected limb; apply a cold compress and keep it in place for 10 minutes. Repeat if necessary. Elevate the injured limb, supporting it in the most comfortable position by using a pillow or rolled-up item of clothing.
- **Use splints** to keep movement of the injured limb to a minimum (*see* **fractures** p202).
- If pain persists despite splinting, **a painkiller may be administered** orally (500mg for older children, 1000mg for adults).
- **Seek medical attention** to confirm the diagnosis and provide definitive treatment. Sprains and fractures may occur together, so suspected injuries should be X-rayed.

- Do not delay application of a **cold compress** for the sake of rubbing on ointments or lotions. With a sprain, nothing is quicker or more efficient than ice to keep swelling and bleeding to a minimum.
- Do not treat sprains and strains with just an elasticated bandage around the injured area, as this will do little to limit movement. Torn ligaments and tendons may require rigid immobilization in a plaster cast or even surgical repair. A doctor must take the decision regarding the correct management of the injury.

PREVENTION

- Sports participants should ensure that they are sufficiently fit for their sport. Being a good runner doesn't mean you won't suffer an arm or shoulder injury if you play a vigorous game of tennis.
- Always warm up properly before beginning any exercise or sport, and take care not to get chilled during exercise.
- If you sustain a sprain or strain during sport or exercise, allow time for complete healing to take place before you become active again. Continued aggravation may turn a minor injury into a major one, while repeat injuries can result in delayed or incomplete healing, or even permanent weakness of the tendon or ligament. Once the injury has healed, start slowly and build up gradually before returning to your previous level of activity.
- When working up a ladder, or at any height above ground level, ensure that you are securely positioned at all times to prevent yourself from falling (*see* p273).

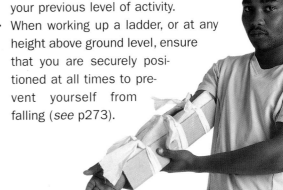

This forearm splint has been improvised from cardboard and soft dressing materials.

Neck, back and spinal cord injuries

The spine, or vertebral column, has two important functions: it is the central 'strut' of the skeleton around which all movement occurs, and it encases and protects the spinal cord along which nerve impulses are conducted to and from the brain to all parts of the body. It is this second function which concerns us most in the event of injury. Any fracture or displacement of one or more vertebrae can compress, tear or sever the spinal cord, causing partial or total paralysis of the body below the level of injury. When providing first aid, always consider the possibility of spinal injury and take the necessary precautions to avoid aggravating any injury which may already be present.

SYMPTOMS

- Unconscious casualty: always assume a spinal injury at first, particularly if there is also evidence of a head injury.
- Conscious casualty: may complain of pain at the site of a back injury; in the case of neck injury they may hold their neck rigidly to one side.
- Damage to the spinal cord may cause weakness of all or some muscles below the level of the injury, giving a sense of numbness (pins and needles).
- Damage to the spinal cord in the neck region may cause paralysis of the chest muscles and diaphragm, making it difficult for the casualty to breathe normally.
- Blood vessels below the level of spinal cord injury lose their normal tone, so that blood pressure drops. This is known as 'spinal shock', and should be suspected in any casualty who appears to be paralysed.
- Severe spinal cord injury may affect bladder functioning.

CAUSES

Most spinal injuries in young people result from high-velocity impact, such as car accidents, contact sports and falls from a height. However, the spine may also be injured in accidents which occur around the home, such as falling off a ladder or diving into a shallow swimming pool. Elderly people can sustain spinal injuries from relatively minor trauma such as a fall, purely because their vertebrae and the discs between them are more brittle and less able to absorb the shock of even a minor impact.

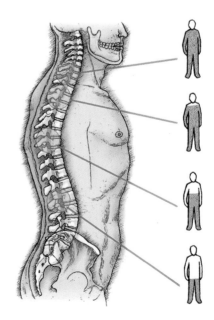

Depending on the site of an injury to the spinal cord, different parts of the body are affected.

TREATMENT

- **If you suspect a spinal injury**, call for an ambulance or the emergency services immediately.

- **If the casualty is unconscious**, assess the **ABC** (*see* pp164–5) and then commence **resuscitation** (*see* pp164–71) if necessary.

- If providing resuscitation, steady the neck with the same hand which pinches the nostrils closed. **Always maintain the neck in whichever position you find it**.

- If you have a second person to assist with first aid, they should stabilize the neck with two hands while you proceed with resuscitation.

- **A casualty who is conscious and breathing, but complains of neck or back pain**, should remain on his back until the emergency services arrive. Support the neck using a solid, heavy object, such as a brick placed on either side of the head. If something solid is not available, continue to support the head and neck gently but firmly with your hands.

⚠ CAUTION

- Don't give the casualty anything to eat or drink as they are likely to vomit it up.
- Don't try to straighten the spine if you find the casualty lying at an angle; you may cause more damage.
- Be extremely cautious about raising the legs to treat shock, particularly if there is any sign that the pelvis or lower back may be injured. Raising the legs may aggravate the injury and also cause severe pain.

PREVENTION

- Any child under eight years old should be supervised by an adult when near any body of water.
- Do not permit children to dive into shallow pools, or any water where the depth, or the presence of submerged objects, is unknown.
- During home DIY activities, ensure that your ladders are in a good state of repair, securely positioned on level surfaces, and long enough for the job in hand to be performed safely.
- Elderly people, particularly those with failing vision or who may be unsteady on their feet, should be escorted, or use walking aids when negotiating unfamiliar territory, especially steps or staircases.
- In contact sports such as rugby football, gridiron and ice hockey, neck injuries are less likely if the teams are appropriately matched, and if referees strictly apply the rules of the game.

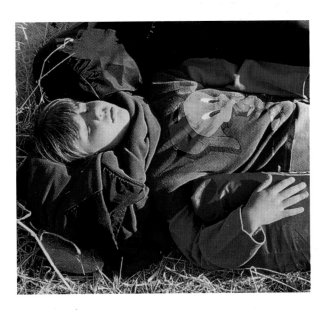

If the neck is stiffly held in one position, leave it as it is. Carefully support the neck by placing a heavy object on either side until the patient is fully awake. Do not force him or her to straighten a stiff neck, as this may well aggravate an underlying injury.

HOME CARE

The ability to provide effective first aid in the home may save you a visit to a hospital or doctor's rooms when minor injuries or illnesses occur. In this section, we describe a range of basic skills and techniques which, together with a well-stocked first aid kit (*see* pp14–7), will enable you to treat a range of minor conditions with confidence. You will also learn which symptoms are serious enough to require medical assistance.

In any family group, it is the very young and the elderly who are most vulnerable to injury, and who create the greatest anxiety when they are unwell. This section covers a range of minor childhood problems, but the scope of our recommendations is limited by the fact that no two children react identically to the same illness. Symptoms and signs may vary, therefore, if doubt exists regarding a diagnosis or suitability of home care, we urge the first-aid provider to seek medical advice without delay.

Managing injuries in small children requires patience and steady nerves. Some are so distressed that any attempt at first aid risks becoming a battle of wills. In such cases, prudence is certainly the better part of valour, and medical assistance should be sought.

Elderly family members are prone to injury due to failing eyesight, brittle bones and unsteady gait, or may require ongoing home nursing. Rather than attempt to cover the full range of medical conditions which may trouble the elderly, we offer practical suggestions on day-to-day home nursing and frail care in the final chapter of this section.

IN THIS SECTION

Chest pains

Not all chest pain signifies a heart attack, but a systematic first aid approach will allow you to determine whether a particular type of chest pain signals a life-threatening episode, and how best to react. Chest pain is not an uncommon occurrence, but it creates justifiably more cause for concern in adults – particularly those with a family history of heart disease and those known to be exposed to certain risk factors (i.e. high blood pressure, or smoking). Chest pain that occurs without warning may be a symptom of a variety of conditions. The significance of the pain depends not only on its severity, but on the presence or absence of associated symptoms (see panel below).

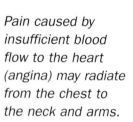

Pain caused by insufficient blood flow to the heart (angina) may radiate from the chest to the neck and arms.

SYMPTOMS

In all cases of chest pain it is advisable to seek medical help immediately.

- Severe, prolonged pain which does not go away with rest, or causes the casualty to go into **shock** (*see* p174), strongly indicates the likelihood of a heart attack.
- Sharp, sudden pain in the upper chest or back, accompanied by signs of shock, may be due to blood leaking from a diseased aorta.
- A sense of pressure or heaviness over the breastbone that is triggered by either physical exertion or emotional stress is likely to be angina.

- A stabbing pain felt in any part of the chest wall, and aggravated by deep breathing or coughing, may be due to an inflammation in the chest cavity, especially if the person also has a mild fever.
- Burning pain in the lower chest, especially after meals, may signify acid reflux associated with hiatus hernia. It is often relieved by antacids.
- Sharp, stabbing pains in the lower chest after persistent or violent bouts of vomiting may indicate a tear in the oesophageal lining, particularly if streaks of fresh red blood appear in the vomit.

- Sudden, deep discomfort while eating solid food, sometimes accompanied by difficulty breathing and excess salivation, could be due to abnormal or delayed peristalsis (the normal movement of the oesophagus) or by food becoming impacted at any point in the mid- or lower oesophagus.
- If chest pain is caused by an injury to the chest wall (by blunt or penetrating trauma), emergency first aid should follow the recommendations for **chest injuries** on p200.

CAUSES

- **Cardiovascular** Chest pain may signify heart strain (angina), from early or advanced coronary artery disease, heart attack, infection or inflammation of the heart muscle (myocarditis) or the thin sac surrounding the heart (pericarditis), or leakage of blood from the aorta.
- **Respiratory system** Although pain is seldom a major feature of lung or airway infection, severe chest pains experienced during breathing may be caused by an infection spreading to the pleura (the thin membrane covering each lung and lining the chest cavity).
- **Digestive system** Chest pain may be caused by stomach acid leaking into the lower oesophagus (gullet), a frequent symptom in people with hiatus hernia. Simply eating too fast may cause solid food to impact on the mid- or lower oesophagus, with temporary pain or discomfort. Repeated vomiting for any reason can tear the delicate lining of the oesophagus.
- **The chest wall** The muscles of the chest wall may be torn or sprained by physical exertion, causing either immediate discomfort, or chest pain which only becomes obvious after a few hours. Certain viruses, which cause flu-like illnesses, may cause an inflammation of the intercostal muscles (between the ribs), resulting in sharp, localized pain on breathing, two to five days after other symptoms of the illness have disappeared.

TREATMENT

Although it helps to establish the likely cause of chest pain if possible, the focus of first aid is to recognize what – mainly cardiovascular – causes are life-threatening, then to call for assistance, and to provide supportive treatment while you wait for help.

If you suspect that the casualty has had a heart attack – and until an ambulance or your doctor arrives – you can:

- Give them 1 soluble disprin to dissolve slowly under the tongue.

 DO NOT

- give the casualty anything by mouth, other than prescribed heart medication.
- leave the casualty alone, except to call an ambulance.
- wait to see if the symptoms disappear without intervention.

 SEEK MEDICAL HELP IMMEDIATELY:

- If the casualty loses consciousness or stops breathing. Commence resuscitation (see pp164–71) and continue until help arrives.
- If the casualty shows any signs of shock (see p174) or has trouble breathing. Cover him with a blanket to reduce heat loss and wait for help to arrive. Calmly comfort and reassure an anxious person if necessary.
- If the casualty is known to suffer from heart disease or has had a previous heart attack.
- If pain which appears after effort, and which is possibly cardiac in origin, does not improve immediately with rest.
- If blood is coughed or vomited up after the onset of pain.
- If the casualty suffers from a heart condition and has medication handy, provide assistance to take it (usually a tablet that is placed under the tongue). The pain should subside within three minutes of taking the medication and resting; then summon medical assistance immediately.

PREVENTING HEART DISEASE

You can reduce the risk of heart disease by:

- Avoiding smoking.
- Keeping your weight within the recommended range for your height.
- Maintaining a balanced, low-fat diet.
- Moderating your alcohol intake.
- Engaging in physical activity three times a week for 20 minutes.
- Having annual check-ups and blood cholesterol measurements from age 40 onwards.
- Having annual check-ups from age 30 if heart disease is prevalent in your family.

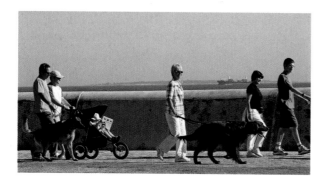

COMMON HEART CONDITIONS

- **Angina,** an inadequate supply of blood to the heart muscle, causes pain that radiates to the neck, shoulder, or arms, accompanied by sudden fatigue, shortness of breath or palpitations. Angina usually improves with rest, or by placing isordil nitrate tablets under the tongue.
- **Hiatus hernia** is a protrusion of the stomach into the chest cavity. This common condition can be successfully treated with weight loss, medication or 'key-hole' surgery. See your doctor if persistent symptoms occur after meals, or interfere with routine eating habits.
- **Hypertension,** persistent high blood pressure, puts strain on the arteries and heart, resulting in damage that occurs over time. Termed the 'silent killer', it has no symptoms.

Regular exercise such as walking or jogging will tone your body and reduce the likelihood of heart disease.

Stroke

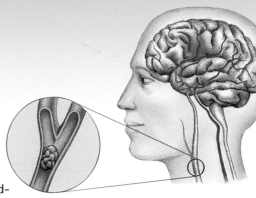

Strokes are a major cause of death in many developed countries, and result in significant disability among survivors. Also known as cerebrovascular accidents (CVAs), strokes can be caused by a haemorrhage (bleeding) from an artery in the brain (a process called cerebral thrombosis), or when atherosclerosis plaques (fatty deposits and blood clots) migrate from another part of the body and lodge in the carotid artery that supplies blood to the brain (*see* illustration). A stroke is therefore an interruption of the blood supply to any part of the brain. If the interruption is longer than a few seconds, brain cells can die resulting in permanent damage.

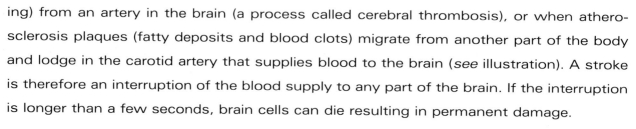

The symptoms depend on the severity of the stroke and the part of the brain that is damaged. Some may even be unaware that they have suffered a minor stroke. In others, both symptoms and long term effects are severe. Generally, the symptoms develop suddenly:

- Loss of movement (paralysis) or co-ordination of any body area, including the face
- Numbness, weakness, loss of sensation or tingling in the limbs, particularly on one side of the body
- Dizziness or vertigo (a sensation of movement), possibly leading to a fall
- Impaired vision, drooping or uncontrolled eye movements
- Drooling or swallowing difficulties
- Loss of ability to identify certain stimuli
- Slurred speech or the inability to speak, or understand speech
- Changes in levels of consciousness (e.g. sleepy or lethargic, comatose or faint)
- Loss of memory

CAUSES

Strokes often result from atherosclerosis. Blood platelets and fatty deposits collect on the artery walls and, over time, obstruct the flow more and more. If the deposit stays where it formed and blocks the artery, it is known as a thrombus. If it breaks free and blocks a vessel elsewhere, it is called an embolus.

Heart disorders such as an irregular heart rate, may cause a stroke, depriving the brain of blood and oxygen. Ailments such as diabetes and hypertension can also contribute to the onset of a stroke.

Although men are generally more at risk, certain factors increase a woman's risk over the age of 35.

Most notably, these include a combination of smoking and taking certain birth control pills, or other medication that promotes clot formation.

TREATMENT

If the casualty does not lose consciousness, or the symptoms are transient:

- Reassure the casualty.
- Avoid any physical exertion; keep the casualty sedated and monitor the heart beat.
- Do not administer any medication, whether prescribed or otherwise.
- Observe the casualty until all of the symptoms are totally resolved.
- Seek medical advice without delay.

If the casualty is unconscious, has difficulty breathing or is unable to move:

- Call for medical help immediately.
- Check their airway (remove loose dentures, food or any other obstruction in the mouth).
- If the casualty is not breathing, commence **resuscitation** (*see* pp164–71) and continue until help arrives.
- Ensure that all known information regarding regular medications is conveyed to the hospital via the emergency staff.
- Do not give the casualty any food or drink, as the swallowing mechanism may be paralysed, risking aspiration into the lungs.

PREVENTION

Lead a healthy lifestyle and modify your habits to reduce high alcohol consumption, excessive smoking and lack of exercise. Take prescribed medication for conditions such as high blood pressure, diabetes or high cholesterol. If you are over the age of 40 ensure that you have regular medical assessments annually. Begin this earlier if you have a known family history of conditions such as high blood pressure, high cholesterol, heart attacks or strokes. (*See also* Preventing Heart Disease p214.)

Preventing infection

Once the protective skin barrier that surrounds the human body is disturbed or broken, bacteria can invade and there is a risk of infection. In order to prevent infections you must ensure that wounds are cleaned thoroughly and all germs and dirt removed using an antiseptic dilute (chlorhexidin or povidone-iodine). Do your best to keep a fresh wound free of moisture for at least 48 hours. It is not necessary to change the dressings every day unless they become soiled; in any event, doing so may do more harm than good because it can disturb the scar and thus cause delayed healing. Dressings that remain clean and intact can be removed after seven days, and need only be replaced if the wound still appears raw. Wet, bloody or tattered dressings should be replaced swiftly to prevent infection.

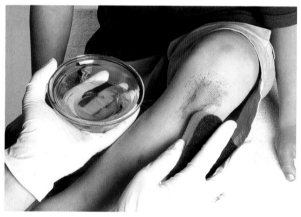

To reduce the risk of infection, wash all wounds thoroughly with a mild antiseptic solution.

TIP

Always wash your hands thoroughly before you begin any first aid. To guard against the risk of infection, use surgical gloves when blood or bodily fluids are involved.

TREATMENT

· **Stop the bleeding:** Many small wounds stop bleeding on their own. More vigorous bleeding can be controlled with direct pressure for a few minutes, using a clean dressing or cloth. Wash all open wounds with water and a dilute antiseptic solution. Even if the wound appears clean to your naked eye, you can safely assume that dirt is present and must be washed out. Injured hands, feet and limbs can be washed under cold water for two minutes. Wounds on other parts of the body can be washed with a clean cloth dipped in antiseptic solution.

· **Cleaning:** Carefully remove all dirt and foreign matter still visible in the wound after washing. Wipe the wound gently but firmly with a soft clean kitchen sponge dipped in dilute antiseptic solution. Then use a clean pair of tweezers or forceps to pick out any ingrained dirt which remains. If a flap of skin has been lifted over the cut, be sure to wash and clean well underneath it. Wounds with deeply ingrained soil or dirt that is difficult to remove may require cleaning under a local anaesthetic. In such cases, cover the wound with a clean dressing or cloth and go to see your nearest hospital or emergency room.

DRESSING WOUNDS

Dressings should protect a fresh wound from re-injury and infection. Tiny cuts and abrasions which are not actively bleeding may be left open, lightly dabbed with antiseptic ointment or cream (such as Dettol, Savlon or Betadine) or simply covered with an adhesive plaster.

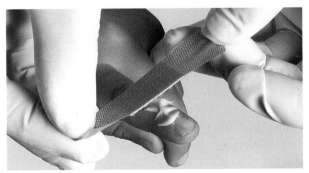

The mildest injury requires only a dab of antiseptic ointment and an adhesive plaster.

All dressings consist of two components: a non-sticky pad or swab to cover the wound, and a secure bandage or adhesive plaster to keep the pad in place. Paraffin-impregnated gauze (Jelonet) is a versatile dressing for any raw or burnt area of skin. A single layer of paraffin gauze is sufficient to cover most wounds.

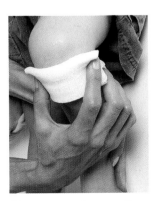

Place a swab over the wound then ...

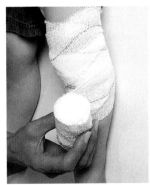

... bandage to keep the swab in place.

 DO NOT

- use cotton wool to dress raw wounds, as the fibres will become embedded in the scar, making removal very painful.
- apply powdery substances, foodstuffs or household cleaning agents to an open wound. Use only what is recommended, or nothing at all.

SEEK MEDICAL HELP IF:

- Wounds have not been washed and cleaned within six hours of injury.
- Wounds appear infected: surrounding skin is red and puffy; there is increasing pain; there is a yellowish discharge.
- It is a puncture wound, particularly if an animal or human bite has broken the skin.
- The wound requires stitches.
- A penetrating wound has occurred below the wrist (risk of tendon or nerve injury).
- Lips or the eyes are wounded.
- There is bruising around the eye socket.
- A wound continues to bleed despite adequate pressure (*see below*).

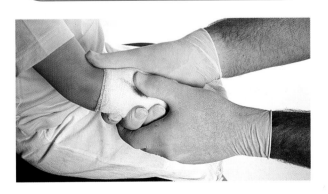

Cuts, grazes, bruises and lacerations

Cuts, grazes and bruises are everyday occurrences, particularly with children, but can easily be treated at home with the help of antiseptic cleaning agents, dressings and bandages. Most cuts heal quickly and completely, but a common complication is infection, which can delay healing and cause scarring. Therefore, the priority for first-aid treatment is to clean all wounds as quickly and thoroughly as possible, using basic principles of hygiene.

SYMPTOMS

- **Cuts, lacerations and puncture wounds:** These may be clean cuts or ragged injuries. With deeper cuts particularly, there is a risk of infection if the wound is not properly cleaned. Pain, swelling, or a yellowish discharge are all signs of infection.

- **Abrasions:** The scraped area of skin is painful and appears dark pink or red. Bleeding varies according to the depth of the abrasion. Dirt may be embedded in damaged skin, depending on what surface was scraped against.

- **Bruises:** A fresh bruise is very tender to touch, and may or may not cause swelling under the skin. As it heals, a bruise changes colour from reddish-purple to green to yellow over a period of five to seven days, disappearing within 10 days.

TREATMENT FOR CUTS AND GRAZES

- **Wash** with mild soap and warm water, or a solution of mild antiseptic liquid and water, to remove any obvious loose debris or dirt from a superficial injury (one that affects the surface of the skin only).

- **For grazes** (not for cuts), pat **dry and apply antiseptic ointment**, and **dress** with a plaster or sterile dressing

- **For cuts**, pat **dry**, and **dress** with a plaster or sterile dressing

- **Do not probe** a wound for embedded objects or debris. You may cause more damage. Rather leave it as is and get it treated immediately.

- If muscle, tissue or bone have been exposed, do not push them back into place. Simply **bandage or dress** the wound and get the casualty to an emergency room.

- If you suspect a deep wound may require stitches, **take the patient to a doctor** or hospital room as soon as possible.

- Consult your doctor if an infection is not cured or becomes worse.

CAUSES

- **Cuts and lacerations:** A cut is an injury in which the skin has been opened. Cuts have clean edges, lacerations are jagged wounds or tears.
- **Puncture wounds:** These can be from scissors, pins, or splinters, for instance, to those caused by large objects such as tools or kitchen utensils. Animal bites can result in deep puncture wounds.
- **Abrasions:** The superficial outer layers of the skin may be accidentally scraped as a result of a fall or a slide along any rough surface.
- **Bruises:** Usually caused by blunt force such as a fall, bumping into something, being hit by a moving object. The skin remains intact, but damage to blood vessels causes bleeding under the skin.

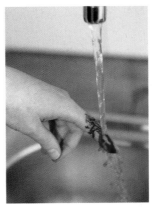

Wash a cut under a running tap to remove blood and dirt.

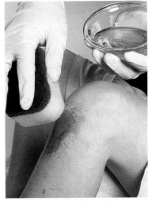

A graze can be cleaned with a sponge dipped in diluted antiseptic.

✕ DO NOT

- clean a large wound or try to clean it if bleeding has stopped. In the first instance you may make the bleeding worse, and in the latter, you may restart it.
- attempt first-aid remedies that may have to be undone before proper treatment can take place. If you suspect that a wound will require stitches, simply apply a clean, lint-free bandage or dressing to contain the bleeding and get the casualty to the doctor or emergency room.
- encircle a finger, arm or leg with any tight plaster or bandage which could interfere with the blood supply.

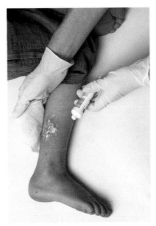

Only use antiseptic ointment on grazes before dressing.

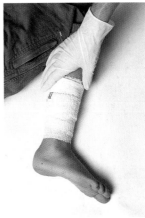

Dress a cut or graze with a plaster or a clean bandage.

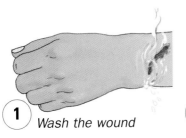

1 Wash the wound

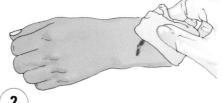

2 Clean carefully and gently.

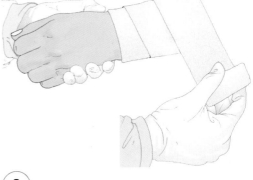

3 Apply dressing.

Cuts, grazes, bruises and lacerations

LACERATIONS

- Rinse, then wash the wound thoroughly with mild soap and water.
- Control **bleeding** (*see* p172).
- Cover the wound with a butterfly bandage.
- If the laceration looks serious, consult your doctor.

PUNCTURE WOUNDS

- Rinse and then clean the wound with mild soap and flowing water – to try to wash out any fragments of whatever caused the injury.
- Apply a clean bandage.
- Get medical assistance.

EMBEDDED OBJECTS

- Apart from splinters and objects of a similar size, do not remove an object that is embedded in the skin, particularly one that has penetrated deeply – doing so can cause more damage and initiate bleeding if the object has penetrated a major blood vessel.
- Make up a ring bandage, place it over the object without touching it, and bandage it into position to prevent it from moving laterally. Do not move the object or apply any downward pressure to it. You will need to carry out this manoeuvre extremely carefully as the object should be kept absolutely still with relation to whatever part of the body it has penetrated.
- Call for assistance or get the casualty to a hospital or doctor immediately.

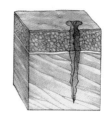

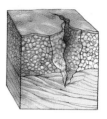

The entry of a puncture wound is neat, but the wound can go deep into the muscle.

Lacerations are usually fairly shallow but have wider openings and jagged edges.

TETANUS

Tetanus, sometimes known as lockjaw, is a life-threatening infection. The bacterial organism responsible is particularly widespread in manure and other animal waste. Once tetanus bacteria enter the body through an open wound, they target the spinal cord, releasing a toxin that causes severe spasms and difficulty in breathing. If left untreated, death can occur from heart or lung failure. Tetanus is extremely difficult to treat once symptoms appear as it does not respond to antibiotics. Children are routinely immunized by standard vaccination schedules.

APPLYING A RING BANDAGE

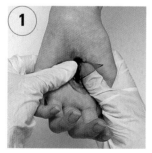

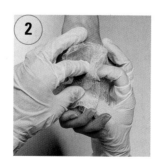

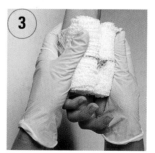

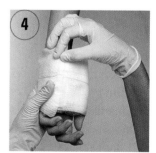

1. *Pinch the edges of the wound together to stem the bleeding.* **2.** *Cover the area with gauze.*
3. *Support the embedded object with pads on either side.* **4.** *Bandage lightly over padding and secure.*

SPLINTERS

- Use a clean pair of tweezers to remove the splinter at the same angle that it entered the skin.

_...se it is under
...it to gently lift
...tainless steel
...t over a burn-_

...ve dressing if

...iate.

_...g a cold com-
...ave an ice
...he bruise_

_...nay result
...er the nail,
...ot drained
...e replaced
...nce of the
...inlessly as
...in a flame
...end of the
...blackened
...remove the
...through the
...ve drainage._

_...wounds can
...knives, scis-
...tools. Keep
...oung children
...o understand,
...items._

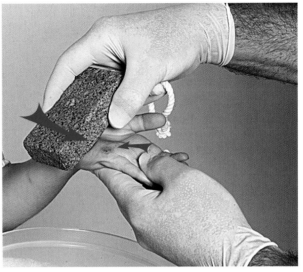

Use a pumice stone in the opposite direction the splinter entered to ease it out.

REMOVING A SPLINTER

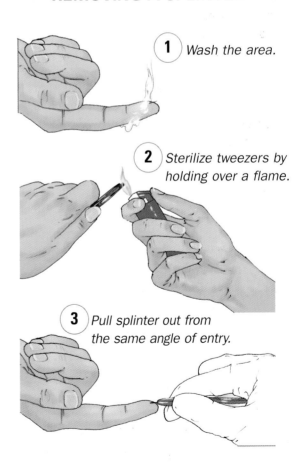

1. Wash the area.

2. Sterilize tweezers by holding over a flame.

3. Pull splinter out from the same angle of entry.

Bleeding from the mouth and nose

Because the mouth and nose are important sensory organs (taste and smell), both have an extremely rich blood supply. As a result, even small wounds inside the mouth or nose can bleed dramatically. Such injuries are most common in children, although nosebleeds can occur at all stages of life. Most injuries to the mouth and nose can be safely managed at home with the first-aid measures recommended below. Small injuries usually heal rapidly with minimal, if any, scarring, thanks to the excellent blood supply in these areas.

SYMPTOMS

- Bleeding due to any injury will usually be obvious within seconds, and accompanied by immediate pain.
- The site of bleeding from the mouth may be easy to confirm if the injury involves the lips, teeth and tongue, or gum margin. A small flashlight is useful for spotting injuries further back in the mouth cavity, such as puncture wounds caused by foreign objects.
- Blunt injuries may cause visible swelling of the injured area as well as bleeding.
- Spontaneous nosebleeds can occur at any time, but may be precipitated by sneezing, nose blowing or picking at dried secretions inside the nostril.

CAUSES

Bleeding from the mouth is common in children, usually a result of falls, or puncture wounds caused by solid objects e.g. pencils, ice cream or lollipop sticks carried in the mouth.

Children who are distracted while eating can accidentally bite into the tongue or lip, producing a painful, bleeding injury. The mouth and nose may be injured at any age by assault. Loosening or loss of a tooth will cause vigorous bleeding from the gum and tooth socket.

Spontaneous nosebleeds are common after colds and other viral infections which cause drying of the mucous lining, or as a consequence of repeated nose-blowing, or overuse of decongestant nasal sprays which interfere with normal mucus production.

PREVENTION

- Children should be discouraged from sucking on sharp or solid objects, and certainly from walking or running with such objects in their mouths.
- At mealtimes, children should be encouraged to eat slowly, and discouraged from speaking while chewing on solid food.
- Don't allow the inside of the nose to dry out, particularly after viral infections. If drying occurs, a twice-daily dab of petroleum jelly to each side of the septum will reduce the risk of nosebleeds.
- Limit use of decongestant nasal sprays to one or two days, if at all. Prolonged use dries out the nose and will also aggravate a blocked nose due to the 'rebound' effect of the medication.

TREATMENT

- Stem bleeding from the lips by applying a clean gauze pad soaked in iced water, and gently pinch the wound between your fingers. In a cooperative patient, the same technique can be used for small tongue injuries.
- Control bleeding in the mouth cavity by giving the casualty ice cubes to suck, or by rinsing and gargling with iced water. The water should be spat out, as swallowed blood may irritate the stomach and cause vomiting.
- Soak a lost tooth (or portion of a broken tooth) in milk or saltwater to preserve (so it can be reinserted by a dentist). A gauze swab soaked in very cold water can be pressed gently against the bleeding tooth socket.
- To stop a nosebleed, pinch together the soft part of the nostrils until bleeding ceases. While this constant pressure is being applied, hold the head slightly forward so that excess blood drips into the mouth and can be spat out.
- Persistent pain after injury can be treated with a mild painkiller.

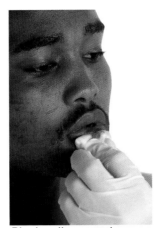

Pinch a lip wound together with a swab soaked in cold water.

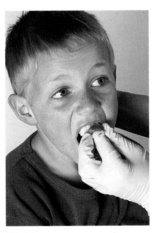

Hold a gauze swab against the tooth socket to stem the bleeding.

AFTERCARE

- Anyone with a mouth injury should avoid spicy or acidic foods for five days afterwards.
- Twice-daily teeth-brushing and rinsing the mouth after meals will reduce the risk of wound infection. If teeth or gums have been injured, twice-daily gargling with an antiseptic mouthwash can be done in place of teeth-brushing for the first few days.
- After blunt injury, the crooked appearance of a broken nose may only be obvious once the swelling settles down. If this happens, seek a medical opinion.

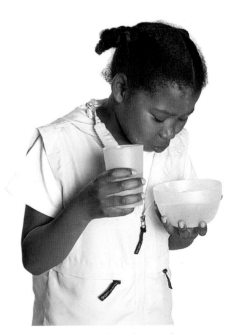

Rinse the injured mouth with water and antiseptic gargle, after every meal.

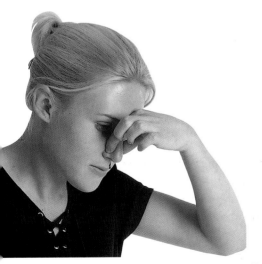

Gently pinching the nostrils will usually stop a nosebleed within 10 minutes.

Coughs, colds and croup

Upper respiratory tract infection (URTI) is an unfortunate part of life that most people have to endure at some time or other, particularly during the colder months, and certainly in countries that experience cold, wet winters. The incidence and severity of URTI are particularly higher in smokers. Most 'common' colds are mild, self-limiting and require nothing more than symptomatic treatment. However, the risk of complications and related illness may be greater in babies, infants, elderly people, and anyone with chronic lung disease, or other illnesses or conditions that interfere with the body's normal immune response to infection.

SYMPTOMS

- Common colds typically present with mild fever, cough, nasal discharge and persistent sneezing, with or without a sore throat. Fever is more marked in infants and children than in adults. Muscle aches, high fever and chills are more typical of influenza than a common cold.
- Cough, due to post-nasal drip following an URTI, may be accompanied by a sore throat, an offensive taste in the mouth, and yellow-green sputum produced by coughing.
- The typical 'wheeze' (prolonged exhalation of air) differentiates a bout of asthma from URTI. (See **asthma** p228).
- Prolonged fits of coughing followed by a 'whoop' as a child struggles for breath, typify whooping cough. Symptoms may persist for up to three months and can recur.
- Croup presents as a barking or crowing sound when a child coughs. It is usually worst at night.

CAUSES

- Most URTI are caused by viruses, although bacteria may prolong or aggravate an existing illness.
- Chronic sinus infection causes post-nasal drip, where infected secretions leak into the windpipe and lungs, resulting in a persistent cough, with or without mild fever.
- When coughing is a dominant symptom, it may be difficult to distinguish URTI from asthma, although the two conditions do co-exist, often in children.
- The bacterium *Bordetella pertussis* causes whooping cough (*see* p110) which can be prevented by immunization.
- Croup describes the typical barking cough heard in children between six months and three years of age. It is most commonly caused by a viral infection involving the area just below the larynx (voice box). A severe form of croup is caused by *Haemophilus influenza*, a bacterium which causes swelling of the epiglottis (epiglottitis), leading to high fever, drooling saliva and difficulty with swallowing foods.
- An isolated cough may have many non-infectious causes, including the side-effects of medication, such as drugs used to control blood pressure, foreign bodies impacted in the respiratory tract, lung tumours or tumours elsewhere in the chest.
- Suspect an inhaled foreign body in a child with chronic cough, shortness of breath and fever, particularly if a course of antibiotics has been given without success.

TREATMENT

- **Common colds may be safely treated at home**. Rest, drink plenty of fluids and take paracetamol or aspirin to bring down fever. That is usually all that is necessary. Medicated lozenges are ineffective against viruses and are no better than warm drinks and glucose or boiled sweets for soothing a sore throat.
- Like aches and pains, **a cough is a warning symptom, not a diagnosis**. It serves to expel infected secretions or other harmful agents from the respiratory tract. Therefore, medication which suppresses the cough reflex may do more harm than good, and is not recommended as first-line treatment for adults or children. The priority is to identify and treat the cause, not just the symptom.
- Both **whooping cough and viral croup** may be treated at home, but always in consultation with your doctor, in case complications arise.

SEEK MEDICAL HELP IF:

- cold symptoms do not clear up within three to four days, or become worse, suggesting bacterial infection.
- there is a cough or a breathing difficulty (with or without fever) in a child under six months of age.
- symptoms are suggestive of asthma.
- symptoms are suggestive of either whooping cough or croup.
- a cough persists even after the other cold symptoms have disappeared.
- a cough produces infected-looking sputum or blood.
- persistent dry coughing occurs as an isolated symptom.

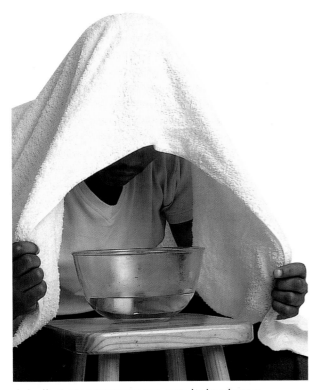

Inhaling steamy vapours can help clear a blocked nose and relieve congestion.

PREVENTION

- You can reduce the risk of colds and other viral infections by protecting your immune system, particularly during the colder months of the year. Avoiding overexertion or stress, maintaining a healthy balanced diet, and ensuring that you are protected against extreme temperatures does not guarantee you won't contract viral infection, but certainly makes it less likely.
- Do not smoke! However many (or few) cigarettes you smoke each day, your risk of respiratory infection and many other diseases, will be greater than the average non-smoker.
- Ensure that your child is immunized against the bacteria which cause whooping cough and epiglottitis (*Haemophilus* influenza).
- Keep small objects such as toy parts, coins, pins, clips and bits of jewellery away from infants and toddlers. Peanuts should not be given to children under the age of five years, due to the risks of choking and aspiration into the lung.

Headaches and migraines

Although millions of people worldwide suffer from headaches, most attacks are mild and do not require medical attention. Primary headaches are those which have no specific cause, but may be triggered by certain stimuli. Tension headache is by far the most common variety of primary headache, particularly in women. Cluster headaches, which are less common, but extremely painful, occur more frequently in men. Secondary headaches may be a symptom of a serious underlying illness or injury, where treatment is aimed at the cause, rather than the symptom. Migraine is a syndrome, of which headache is a common feature. However, the treatment and prevention of migraine are similar to that for other primary headaches.

SYMPTOMS

- Tension headache is a mild to moderate ache, or a band of pressure affecting both sides of the head and is often felt behind the eyes, with or without tension in the neck muscles. It may last a few hours, or build gradually during the day. It almost always comes on during daytime and seldom affects sleep. Most sufferers have one to two tension headaches per month.
- Cluster headaches typically strike with distressing frequency over a period of weeks, then disappear for months before returning. They can occur several times a day – often at night. They begin without warning and are agonizingly painful, but seldom last longer than an hour. They are usually felt on one side of the head, although not always the same side. The eye on the side of the pain often becomes inflamed and watery and the nostril may be blocked.

CAUSES

Many things can trigger primary headaches and avoiding these can do much to stop a headache from occurring in the first place.

Common triggers include stress, depression, fatigue, nicotine, caffeine, foods like ice cream, eye strain, hormonal variations due to menstruation, and some medications. Chronic use of painkillers for headache may precipitate withdrawal headaches. Alcohol often triggers cluster headaches.

Secondary headache may be a symptom of infection, head injury, disorders of the blood circulation, brain tumours, or chronic illnesses such as diabetes.

Mild headaches commonly occur in the early stages of viral and other infections.

Migraine is thought to result from the liberation of a chemical known as serotonin around blood vessels in and around the brain. Migraine attacks vary in severity from person to person and are typically preceded by warning symptoms such as mood changes, tingling sensations or visual images like zig-zag lines or flashing lights. The headache is usually one-sided, and may be accompanied by nausea and vomiting.

Migraines seldom last more than an hour, but a feeling of exhaustion or general illness may persist for longer. In children, migraine may present as abdominal pain with no headache.

TREATMENT

Wherever possible, trigger factors should be identified and avoided (*see* Prevention).

- Tension headache and mild migraine usually respond well to mild painkillers such as asprin or paracetamol/acetaminophen, and these should always be the first treatment option. Non-steroidal anti-inflammatory drugs may be helpful for some people, but should only be used after consultation with a doctor.
- Cluster headaches usually require prescription drugs, many of them not specifically intended for this purpose. Always seek a medical opinion if you suspect that you may be suffering from cluster headaches.
- The duration of all headaches may be limited by rest and relaxation until the pain wears off.

PREVENTION

The key to reducing primary headaches is recognizing and avoiding the trigger factors.

- If your headaches recur frequently, keep a diary to record and identify possible trigger factors.

CAUTION

- Secondary headache can occur at any age. It occurs 'out of the blue' in someone not normally prone to headache
- A headache following head or facial trauma requires urgent medical attention
- A headache associated with fever, persistent nausea or vomiting, drowsiness, lossed or blurred vision, convulsions, speech disorders, muscle weakness or abnormal behaviour, could indicate a serious underlying disorder and requires medical attention.

SEEK MEDICAL HELP IF:

- If headaches cause persistent pain for more than 15 days each month.
- If headaches persist for more than 24 hours without relief.
- Mild painkillers don't help.
- You suspect a cluster headache.
- There are symptoms which suggest a secondary headache (*see* above).
- If the patient is a child, and if the headache is associated with fever, drowsiness and/or the appearance of purplish spots on the body. These may indicate meningitis and require immediate investigation and treatment.

- If you suffer from cluster headaches, avoid alcohol during attacks, and limit your intake during attack-free intervals.
- Headaches experienced while in any static position may be related to bad posture or muscle strain. Consult a physiotherapist or occupational therapist.
- Headaches accompanied by burning or itching eyes, particularly while reading or working at a computer, suggest eye-strain or visual disorders, and require the opinion of an optometrist.
- If you take regular medication for a chronic condition, ask your doctor whether headache is a possible side-effect of the medication.
- Your doctor may prescribe drugs to reduce the frequency of cluster headaches or migraine, if attacks are frequent enough to interfere with your lifestyle.
- If you suffer frequent headaches, be careful about increasing your pain-relief medication, as overuse can cause withdrawal headaches. Consult a doctor about alternative methods of pain relief or headache prevention.

Asthma

Asthma is a disease in which the airways become narrowed as a result of inflammation, reducing airflow and causing the wheezing, coughing, shortness of breath and tight chest which one normally associates with this condition. It is also known as bronchial asthma, exercise-induced asthma, or reactive airways disease (RAD). Asthma is incurable, but ongoing treatment and self-discipline can enable sufferers to lead a normal life. Treatment involves long-term medications which are used on a regular basis to combat the condition, plus quick-relief measures to combat an attack. In children, the condition may improve or disappear as they grow older.

SYMPTOMS

Asthma attacks usually begin suddenly. Symptoms include:

- Breathing that requires greater effort
- Shortness of breath aggravated by exercise
- Tight chest
- Wheezing or coughing with or without the production of sputum (phlegm)
- Abnormal, laboured breathing pattern in which breathing out takes more than twice as long as breathing in

CAUSES

- Air pollutants such as wind-borne dust or cigarette smoke
- Animal hair and skin flakes (dander)
- Bee stings (also bites or stings from other insects)
- Cold air
- Dust mites
- Exercise
- Foods, especially nuts and shellfish
- Emotional stress
- Medications
- Moulds
- Plants and pollens

TREATMENT

If an asthma sufferer has an attack, get them their medication and help to administer it; calm them and give them space and air. In the case of a first-time attack, or if they don't have an inhaler with them, and they continue having difficulty breathing, call for assistance.

PREVENTION

Sufferers, particularly children, should use their medication before exercise to prevent attacks. Sufferers should try to minimize their exposure to factors that can trigger attacks. Many of the principles apply for asthma as for the prevention of **allergies** (*see* p229).

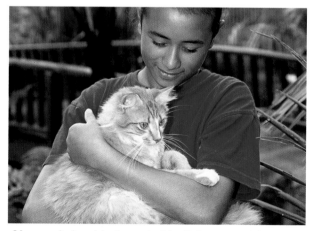

Above: *Animal hair and skin flakes can trigger allergic reactions in susceptible individuals.*
Left: *Asthma sufferers usually carry an inhaler to help relieve symptoms.*

Allergies

Most people with hay fever and other outdoor allergies think of their home as a haven where they can escape their allergies. Wrong! Houses and apartment buildings harbour and trap their own allergens, making them impossible to avoid. An allergic reaction is a response by your body's immune system to a foreign invader (a substance, such as dust or pollen, that is not native to your body). Exposure to this invader, or allergen, triggers the allergic reaction. Reactions to allergens vary from mild to severe. They might appear immediately on exposure to an allergen or after repeated exposure.

When the immune system becomes sensitized to a specific invader, it overreacts to it. This overreaction to an often-harmless substance is known as a hypersensitivity reaction and sets in motion the release of chemicals, or mediators, such as histamine. It is the effect of the mediators on cells and tissues that causes the symptoms of an allergic reaction. Severe allergic reaction, or anaphylaxis, is rare but can be life threatening, as it causes shock and narrowing of the airways, making breathing difficult.

SYMPTOMS

The symptoms of indoor allergic reactions are those of many other allergic reactions:
- Watery nasal discharge
- Sneezing
- Itchy, stuffy nose (*see also* p226)
- Itchy, watery, swollen or bloodshot eyes
- Scratchy, swollen throat
- Difficulty in breathing
- Tightness in the chest or throat
- Unexplained wheezing or shortness of breath
- Rapid or irregular heartbeat
- Hives (also known as urticaria or nettle rash), is the formation of itchy red or white raised patches on the skin

CAUSES

Pet dander (skin particles): Contrary to popular belief, an allergic reaction to an animal is not caused by hair or fur, but by substances in dander (dead skin flakes) that become loosened from the animal's skin when it licks or scratches itself. The allergens are released into the air, where they join the other components of house dust. Furred or feathered animals, such as cats, dogs, hamsters and birds, are most likely to cause allergic reactions, which may be triggered by the following:
- Playing with the animal, especially indoors.
- Cleaning animal beds, cages, or litter boxes.
- Exposure to furniture, carpets, bedding, clothing, animal beds or cages, and pet's toys where allergens might be present.
- Being in an indoor area with another person whose clothes carry the allergens.

Moulds: Moulds, a type of fungus that is generally found outdoors, are a common trigger of hay fever symptoms, as their method of reproduction results in millions of spores being released into the air. Being so tiny, moulds are impossible to keep out of a home and there is virtually no surface on which they will not thrive. All mould needs is water, or even just humidity greater than 50 per cent, hence the proliferation of mildew (a type of mould) in showers, bathrooms or any poorly ventilated space.

Cockroaches: 'Roaches' are a fact of life in homes all over the world and although they are not a major source of allergens while alive (apart from their waste when it dries), when they die their remains dry and disintegrate, adding to the house dust.

Foods: Genuine food allergies, which affect the immune system, should not be confused with food intolerance, which affects the digestive system. One of the most widespread food allergies is to nuts, especially peanuts (ground-nuts). Other foods which can cause a severe allergic reaction include are seafood, eggs and strawberries. Many children are allergic to cow's milk, and wheat or wheat-based products can cause a condition known as coeliac disease.

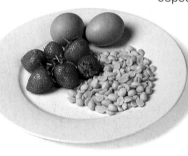

Strawberries, eggs and nuts are common allergy triggers.

SEEK MEDICAL HELP IF:

In some cases, a severe reaction to certain foods can cause **anaphylactic shock** (*see* p174), leading to difficulty in breathing, dizziness, or loss of consciousness. **This is a medical emergency and requires immediate attention.** If your symptoms suggest an anaphylactic reaction, get to an emergency room immediately. Do not drive yourself, as the symptoms may become more pronounced en route and you could have an accident.

Symptoms include:

· Tightness in the chest or throat
· Difficulty in breathing
· Dizziness, light-headedness or fainting
· Loss of consciousness
. Hives (*see* symptoms below)

including food, insect bites and plants. The raised, red rash of acute urticaria usually disappears within a few hours, but chronic urticaria can persist for days or weeks and both forms can recur.

TWO COMMON MANIFESTATIONS

Allergic rhinitis (hay fever), an inflammation of the membranes lining the nose and throat, occurs when airborne substances (allergens) are inhaled and come to rest in the linings of the eyes, nose or airway of a susceptible person. Allergic rhinitis can be perennial (occuring all year round) as a result of house dust, dust mites, animal dander, feathers or mould spores. Seasonal allergic rhinitis is caused by grass, tree or flower pollens. It occurs mostly during spring and summer, when pollen counts are high, hence the common name, hay fever.

Urticaria, also known as hives, is an itchy rash that results from exposure to a variety of allergens,

TREATMENT

Seek medical attention if the symptoms become more pronounced over a day or two, or if they fail to improve after the source of the allergen has been removed. The elimination of an allergen is obviously the best course of remedy. Unfortunately, when it comes to house dust, the best you can do is to limit the amount of dust with a suitable housekeeping routine, and treat the symptoms.

If your symptoms do not improve, your health-care provider may prescribe one or more medications, either for the treatment of an allergic 'attack' or as a prophylactic (preventative medication), to dampen the allergic response.

Self-care at home: Antihistamine medications can be taken to reduce itching and watery eyes. Some are long-acting and can be taken over the long-term.

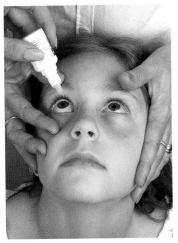

Decongestant eye-drops help to soothe itchy eyes.

Certain antihistamines may make you too drowsy to drive or operate machinery safely. In the case of children, their schoolwork may be affected, but the effects of the sedation can be reduced by using slow-release antihistamines.

Calamine lotion is useful for treating urticaria (hives) and decongestant eye drops help to soothe scratchy eyes. Nasal decongestants are to be used sparingly as there is a risk of a rebound effect if they are used too often or for longer than 24 hours.

Remedial therapy: In cases where a single allergen can be identified as the trigger for allergic rhinitis, the doctor may prescribe a course of injections that will result in desensitizing the patient over a period of time (immunotherapy). Severe seasonal rhinitis can be relieved by nasal spray and eye drops containing cromolyn sodium. Topical steroid nasal sprays are also effective.

PREVENTION

The single best thing you can do to stop the reaction is to reduce your exposure to the allergens. In the case of a much-loved family pet, the choice can be a very difficult one – to keep it or get rid of it. In any event, it can take months for the symptoms to disappear. An alternative is to keep the pet outdoors and/or have another member of the family take care of it so that your contact is reduced as much as possible.

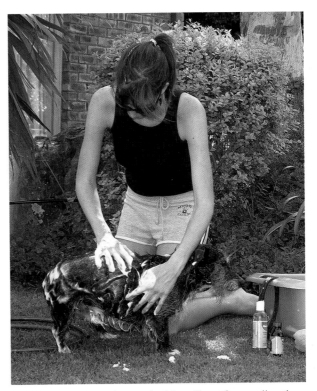

If anyone in your household suffers from allergies: regular grooming may help to reduce your pet's hair loss and thus prevent an allergic reaction.

Regular, frequent grooming of the pet might also help, but beware of causing skin problems which can actually exacerbate the problem. It helps to avoid long-haired animals, as they tend to shed greater quantities of hair than short-haired cats and dogs.

Fabric surfaces are ideal temporary traps for small particles so the fewer carpets, curtains, drapes and cloth-upholstered chairs you have, the better. Where possible, substitute tiles or wood for carpeting, fabric upholstery with leather and curtains with blinds. Ensure surfaces are kept clean and dust-free and that bedding and clothing are laundered regularly. Your pet's bedding should also be washed frequently and aired in the sun whenever possible.

Deal with mould and mildew by ensuring good ventilation in bathrooms and kitchens. Mould on ceilings can be kept in check by wiping with dilute bleach (sodium hypochloride) or using paint impregnated with fungicide.

Bites and stings

Bite injuries can be divided into those that affect mainly the skin and soft tissues (such as those from a dog, a cat and human bites) and those where there is an injection of venom or poison (from spiders, snakes and marine creatures). In the case of animal-inflicted injuries, the risk of infection is often more of a concern than the damage caused by the bite. Human bites should always be treated as an emergency, however minor they might seem. Non-venomous insect bites are usually harmless, causing local discomfort, itching and swelling, but the venom injected by some insects and the bites of certain snakes and spiders can cause a systemic reaction (affecting the whole body), which may require life support and antivenom.

 SEEK MEDICAL HELP IF:

- there are breathing difficulties. Check **ABC** (*see* pp164–5 and p293); start life support; continue until medical help arrives (*see* **rescue breathing** p168; **anaphylactic shock**, p176).
- the casualty has been seriously bitten, particularly if the attack involved a wild or unknown animal.
- the wound needs stitches. (Especially facial and hand wounds require urgent medical attention.)
- the casualty has not had a tetanus shot in the last five years.
- any bite has broken the skin.

ANIMAL BITES

With animal-inflicted bites, the skin is usually broken and bleeding, and there may be puncture wounds, crush injuries and/or bruising. Minor bites can be treated with thorough washing, cleaning and dressing with a dab of antiseptic ointment, but all bites on the hand or face require medical attention. Cat bites carry a higher risk of infection than dog bites. Unless you have recently had a tetanus shot, you should get one within 24 hours of any skin break.

 DO NOT

- let a snake bite-victim move around. Keep them still to prevent the spread of venom and, if necessary, carry them to safety.
- apply a tourniquet or other constricting device over a snake bite, or attempt to cut the wound or apply any form of suction to 'remove' the poison.

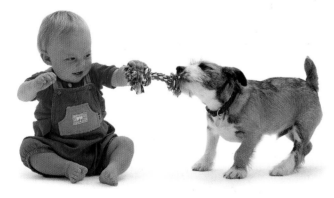

Sharp canine teeth can inflict a painful wound on a child's delicate skin, so don't let play become too boisterous.

BITE INJURIES

CAUSES

Pets are the most common cause of animal bites. Children are most at risk, and the decision to keep pets when there are toddlers in the home must be carefully taken.

Cage birds, too, can inflict a nasty bite, so children should be discouraged from sticking their fingers through the bars.

PREVENTION

- Teach your children to treat animals with respect, and not to tease or provoke them.
- Do not approach strange animals, and teach your children not to do so either.
- Choose pets carefully, particularly if you have small children, and buy from a reputable breeder. Females are less aggressive than males; some breeds are more tolerant than others.

TREATMENT FOR ANIMAL AND HUMAN BITES

- Calm and reassure the casualty.
- To prevent contamination, wear latex gloves, and wash your hands thoroughly with soap before and after attending to any wound.
- Wash the wound thoroughly using mild soap and running water. Cover with antiseptic ointment and bandage with clean dressing.
- If the bite is bleeding heavily apply direct pressure with a sterile pad or clean, dry cloth until the bleeding subsides. Do not remove the first pad if it becomes soaked, place a second one over it. If possible, elevate the area.
- All animal bites that break the skin carry the risk of tetanus. Visit a doctor for an antitetanus booster unless your immunization is up to date.
- Seek immediate medical attention for all human bites. If you have not had an antitetanus shot within the last five years, get one after any injury in which the skin is broken. It is a good idea to have a booster every 10 years.

TETANUS AND RABIES

Tetanus is caused by toxins that live in soil and in the intestines of humans and animals and act on the nerves controlling muscle activity. Symptoms usually appear five to 10 days after infection and include fever, headache, and muscle stiffness in the jaw (lockjaw), arms, neck and back. Painful muscle spasms may affect the throat or chest wall, leading to breathing difficulties. If you suspect tetanus, seek medical assistance without delay.

Rabies, a potentially fatal infection of the nervous system, is transmitted in saliva from the bite of a rabid animal. Early symptoms are flu-like, progressing to facial paralysis, thirst, throat spasms, disorientation and coma. If treated early, the chance of recovery is good. Rabies is rare in developed countries, but any bite should be followed by a visit to the doctor for a vaccination.

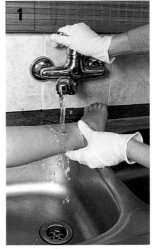 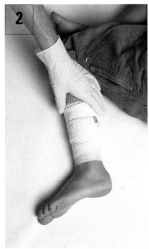

1. *Run the bite wound under the tap for three to five minutes to wash it.*
2. *Cover the wound with an antiseptic ointment and a clean dressing.*

INSECT BITES AND STINGS

Flying insects:
- A sting from a flying insect usually causes a painful red swelling which gets better within 24 hours. The only danger is if there are multiple stings and a large amount of venom is injected, which can cause toxic reactions such as fever, vomiting, and kidney malfunction. Anyone who is allergic will have a more severe reaction

Crawling insects:
- The bite of the brown spider causes local pain, swelling and a slow-healing, blister-like sore. Black widow, button and funnel web spiders inject venom which attacks the nervous system, causing muscle paralysis and breathing difficulties
- Most scorpion stings cause severe local pain and sensitivity to touch, heat and cold, but some can cause muscle pains or spasms, a general sense of weakness, coma and convulsions

There are more insects and spiders on earth than just about any other life form and, while most are harmless, or at best an irritation, there are some that are harmful, being able to deliver a bite or sting that is painful or potentially deadly. If bitten or stung by an insect, try to capture or kill it (if this can be done safely), so that it can be identified.

CAUSES

Flying insects sting anything or anyone who disturbs them or their nests or hives. The risk is generally highest in summer, particularly if you are active outdoors. Crawling insects sting when disturbed, often by lifting a rock or piece of wood. Even seemingly 'dead' insects can sting, so warn children not to pick them up.

Flying insects:
- Bees (honeybee, bumblebee).
- Wasps, hornets and yellow jackets.

Crawling insects:
- Spiders (black widow, brown recluse/violin spider, funnel web, button), scorpions.
- Ticks, fleas, ants and bedbugs.

PREVENTION

- Don't provoke the animals and avoid rapid, jerky movements around hives or nests.
- Use appropriate insect repellents on all exposed skin and/or protective clothing.
- Be vigilant when eating outdoors, especially with colas or sweetened beverages, which attract bees.

EMERGENCY DRUGS

If anyone in the family is known to be allergic to insect bites or stings, your doctor may advise you to keep a pre-packed adrenaline pen or syringe in your first aid kit. Given into the thigh muscle, this may be life-saving in the event of a severe allergic or anaphylactic reaction, but it must be given correctly. Follow your doctor's advice, and read the package instructions carefully before use.

KNOW YOUR INSECTS

Bees

A honeybee's stinger usually remains in the skin. Do not try to remove it using your fingers, as you will probably squeeze the poison sac and inject more venom. Instead, scrape the blunt edge of a knife-blade or a credit card across the stinger to remove it without injecting more venom. An alternative is to use a pair of fine tweezers, grasp the stinger as close as possible to the skin and not by the poison sac.

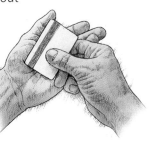

Ticks

These parasites attach themselves to a person's skin and suck their blood. Ticks can be as tiny as a pinhead or a large as a fingernail. They live in areas of dense forest, in shrub and in tall grass, and can adhere to any part of your body, from your feet to your arms and head.

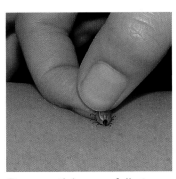

Remove ticks carefully to prevent mouth parts remaining embedded in the skin.

The unpleasant symptoms of tick-bite fever include a red rash around the area of the bite, a feeling of tiredness, raging headache and flu-like fever. Make an appointment to see your doctor if you suspect that you may have contracted tickbite fever.

Some ticks can cause Lyme disease, an infection that, if untreated, results in muscle and joint pain and can affect the heart and nervous system.

The best way to prevent a tick bite is to cover as much of the body as you can when walking in long grass or the bush. Wear closed shoes or boots with long socks, and tuck long pants into your socks. Light-coloured clothing makes it easier to spot a tick. When you return home, shake out your clothing before putting it into the wash, checking that no ticks fall to the floor. Thoroughly check your body, paying attention to the scalp, groin, armpits and the back of knees. Because ticks are sometimes hidden by swelling around the bite, it is important to check any lumps carefully.

TREATMENT

Complications from insect bites and stings include reaction to the toxic venom, infection at the site of the bite, and shock. Allergic reactions to insect bites or stings usually occur within minutes. Severe allergic reactions (known as **anaphylaxis**, *see* p176), can cause breathing difficulties and can be rapidly fatal if untreated.

- Check ABC (*see* pp164–5). Begin **rescue breathing** (*see* p168) or **chest compressions** (*see* pp164–71) if necessary. Call for emergency assistance.
- If the casualty has a severe reaction or has been stung inside the mouth or throat, call immediately for medical assistance.
- Keep the casualty calm and still, as anxiety and movement will speed the distribution of the venom through the body. If appropriate, treat for **shock** (*see* p174). Remain with the casualty until medical help arrives.
- Remove watches, rings and constricting items because the affected area may swell.
- If the pain is severe or does not subside within a few hours, get the casualty to a doctor. In the interim, keep the casualty immobile to reduce the spread of the poison. If breathing becomes compromised, begin rescue breathing.
- If emergency assistance is not required, wash the bite or sting site with soap and water and cover it with a clean, cold compress, ice pack, or a clean, moist dressing to reduce swelling and discomfort.
- Take a mild analgesic to relieve the pain.
- Over the next 24–48 hours, observe the site for signs of infection (such as redness, swelling, ulceration or increasing pain).

SPIDERS, SCORPIONS AND SNAKES

SPIDERS

Most spiders bite if they are disturbed, so avoid breaking or brushing against webs, and take care when working in the garden, as spiders often live under rocks and in any handy crevice. Many bites occur at night, when someone rolls onto a nocturnal invader in their sleep. Spider venom is neurotoxic (it affects the central nervous system). In severe cases, bites can cause breathing problems and an irregular heartbeat, leading to loss of consciousness and death.

SCORPIONS AND CENTIPEDES

Although scorpions and centipedes can deliver a painful sting, few are lethal, unless the casualty is a child. As with spiders, scorpions attack if they are disturbed in their natural habitat, so be careful when lifting stones or pieces of wood. Scorpions are nocturnal and spend the daylight hours under rocks, logs and in places that provide shade and protection. If you are camping in areas where scorpions are found, check your boots before putting them on in the morning!

SNAKES

Some 300 of the 2000-plus species of snake are dangerous to man. Depending on the species, snake venom is neurotoxic, haemotoxic, or cytotoxic. Regard all snake bites as a medical emergency, and get the casualty to an emergency room as quickly as possible, as the administration of the right anti-venom can save a life. Because of their small body size, children are at higher risk for complications or death. Most people know when they have been bitten but, in the event that someone is found unconscious, symptoms to look out are puncture marks in the skin made by the fangs, swelling or skin discoloration at the site of the bite, difficulty in breathing and a rapid pulse. A conscious casualty may experience numbness and a general sense of weakness, blurred vision, fever, nausea, dizziness, fainting, and loss of muscle coordination, along with excessive sweating, convulsions and increased thirst.

TREATMENT

- Obtain medical help immediately. Meanwhile, keep the casualty calm and restrict movement, as exertion will cause the venom to circulate faster through the body. Keep the affected area below heart level to reduce the flow of venom.
- Monitor the casualty's vital signs (pulse, breathing, and blood pressure). If there are signs of shock lay the casualty flat, raise the feet about 30cm (12in), and cover him with a blanket.
- If a bite is on the hand or arm, remove rings, watches etc., as the limb may swell.
- Apply a large, overlapping pressure bandage to the bite site and up the full length of the limb. Move the limb as little as possible, and use a splint to keep it still.
- Venom can cause partial blindness, so if any enters the eyes, rinse them immediately with water. Wipe away venom near the eyes and prevent the casualty from rubbing the eyes, even though they will want to.
- Don't remove venom on unbroken skin as it can be analyzed to identify the snake, if identification is not possible by other means.

Apply a firm, overlapping bandage from below the bite up to the armpit.

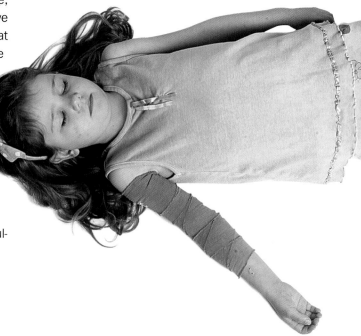

MARINE CREATURES

Several animals and organisms living in the sea are capable of delivering a variety of bites and stings. Encounters with coral, sea urchins, cone shells and a variety of molluscs can result in scratches and lacerations. And the nematocysts that are found on the tentacles of jellyfish and on sea anemones are capable of delivering nasty injuries.

The bigger fish such as barracudas, eels, rays and sharks can give a severe bite, while the venomous spines of stonefish and scorpion fish can inflict a painful wound. Electric eels are capable of delivering severe electrical shocks. Even one's dinner can fight back, and there are probably few anglers who have never been on the receiving end of a sharp bite from a fish that looked dead!

The most common reason for a bite or sting is that the marine creature has been disturbed in its natural habitat. Children who are busy exploring rock pools, and snorkellers leisurely inspecting a coast line or reef are most at risk, but swimmers and fishermen can also fall victim if they happen to have an unexpected encounter. As with all wildlife, the best remedy is to give marine creatures a wide berth and respect their habitat and environment.

TREATMENT

- If there is a trained life guard on the beach – call him or her to come and help you.
- Wear gloves when removing stingers to avoid getting stung yourself.
- Keep the casualty quiet and still to reduce the movement of toxins around the body.
- Pour vinegar or dilute acetic acid (5–10%) over the site to deactivate the stinging cells.
- Once the stingers are deactivated, remove tentacles by lifting them off with a stick – wiping them off can cause further stinging.
- Rinse the affected area with sea water to wash away any nematocysts that have remained on the skin.
- A sunburn preparation containing lidocaine or benzocaine will act as a mild anaesthetic to reduce the pain.
- Use cold compresses (ice blocks) to reduce inflammation, itching and redness.
- If the casualty develops persistent muscle spasms, seek medical attention.
- Seek medical attention if vesicles (blisters) form, as they can result in infection.

SYMPTOMS

- Localized pain, burning, swelling, redness
- Weakness, faintness, dizziness
- Difficulty in breathing or painful breathing
- Cramps and muscle weakness
- Fever and sweating
- Pain in the groin and armpits
- Nausea, vomiting or diarrhoea
- Runny nose, excessive tears
- Irregular pulse
- Paralysis

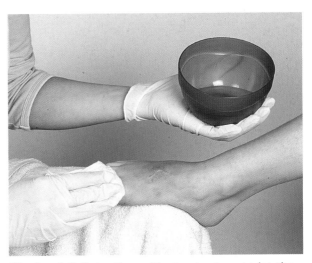

Wash a jellyfish sting with vinegar to restrict the poison from being fired from the tentacles.

Aches and pains

Although pain is an experience most people would choose to avoid, it does serve an important function, warning us that all is not well in some area or system of the body. Pain occurs when specialized nerve endings, known as pain fibres, which are distributed widely throughout the body, are irritated, damaged, or come under pressure. Pain is an early warning sign of illness or injury, telling us that we need to pay attention to the cause, as well as taking a painkiller for relief.

SYMPTOMS

- Pain associated with acute injury will resolve as the injury recovers. Large bruises or blood clots under the skin may be tender for several days.
- An irritation or obstruction of the digestive tract causes a cramping sensation which comes and goes. Infants and small children are not able to describe this, but it should be suspected if a child cries lustily, drawing up their legs periodically, with quiet intervals in between.
- Sudden sharp pain in the knees, hips or lower back, brought on by physical exertion, or lifting heavy objects, may be due to complications of osteo-arthritis, particularly in older people.
- Lower back pain that radiates down the back of a leg may be caused by nerve compression from a 'slipped' disc between the vertebrae.
- Severe pain which affects the joints of the foot, particularly at night, may be due to gout. Typically, the affected joint is swollen, and the skin is red and very tender to touch.

CAUSES

- Injury is by far the most common cause of aches and pains, which may come on abruptly after a specific injury, or increase over time through repetitive injury to bones, joints, ligaments and tendons as a result of sport or physical exertion.
- Pain is frequently a symptom of infection, obstruction, chemical irritation or stretching of the digestive, respiratory, urinary or genital tracts.
- The wear and tear of degenerative bone disease, which occurs with advancing age, may cause bones in the weight-bearing parts of the skeleton (hips, knees and lower back) to slip out of alignment with one another, or press on nerves, causing pain associated with movement, as well as stiffness on getting up in the morning.
- Any enlarging mass inside a confined space, for example a tumour, may cause varying degrees of pain, depending on the rate of growth, and the room available for expansion. Therefore, a tumour inside the skull will often cause severe headache, while a tumour of similar size inside the abdomen may cause no discomfort at all.
- Infection in any part of the body may become localized to form an abscess, which can cause persistent excruciating pain, disrupt sleep, and may be associated with fever. Superficial abscesses are red, tender swellings, but some may be deep-seated and difficult to spot.
- Localized head pain may be caused by a **headache or migraine** (*see* p226).
- Adolescents can experience 'growing pains' during the growth spurts that take place during puberty.

TREATMENT

- Treatment of aches and pains should consist of symptomatic pain relief, while ensuring that the underlying cause is identified and dealt with.
- For pain relief, always use the mildest possible analgesic. Over-the-counter painkillers such as paracetamol/acetaminophen and aspirin are generally safe, and should always be used as a first option. Cramping pain caused by disorders of the gut or urinary tract may require medication which only a doctor can prescribe. Bone or joint pain often responds best to anti-inflammatory medication, such as ibuprofen, which should be taken in consultation with a doctor due to the risk of stomach irritation and other potential side-effects.
- The severe pain of an abscess will only be relieved by surgical drainage of the pus.
- Toothache usually implies tooth decay or infection and should be investigated by a dentist as soon as possible.
- Acute gout can be prevented by avoiding certain foods and taking medication that blocks the production of uric acid. See your doctor about a long-term treatment plan.

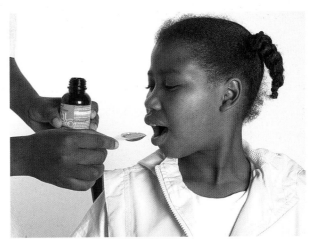

Syrup-based painkiller is best for young children and those who cannot swallow tablets.

PREVENTION

Pain is a normal physiological response to both illness and injury, and an important warning symptom which should be heeded in good time. In most instances, pain can't be prevented, but you can ensure that the cause of the pain is diagnosed and treated appropriately before a mild condition develops into a serious one.

By all means, treat a single episode of pain with a painkiller, but do not hesitate to see a doctor if pain persists, recurs, or does not respond to over-the-counter drugs.

SEEK MEDICAL HELP IF:

- there is pain in any part of the body for 24 hours or more, or pain that recurs on a regular basis.
- painkillers have to be taken with increasing frequency, or in increasing doses.
- there are abdominal cramps associated with vomiting or changes in bowel habits.
- there is a cramping pain in either side, particularly if there is blood in the urine.
- there is a painful swelling.
- a lower back pain begins to radiate down the back of the leg.

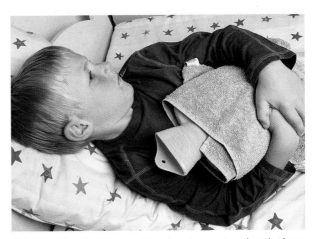

A hot-water bottle and bedrest are good solutions to easing a nagging pain.

Heat exhaustion and heatstroke

Heat exhaustion and heatstroke usually result from a combination of hot environmental conditions and physical exertion. In hot weather we sweat, resulting in a loss of fluid and salts, which causes the body to become dehydrated, resulting in heat exhaustion. If preventative steps are not taken, blood pressure can drop and the pulse rate can slow, causing a casualty to faint. If there is continued exposure to heat, the body may not be able to cool itself by sweating. The result is a rapid rise in body temperature – a life-threatening condition known as heatstroke. Both heat exhaustion and heatstroke can be avoided by taking a few precautions. Children, the obese and the elderly are most at risk, but even an athlete in peak condition can succumb if warning signs are ignored.

SYMPTOMS

Although heatstroke may be preceded by a headache, dizziness and fatigue, it often comes on quickly, bringing fever, a high temperature (above 40°C/104°F), and rapid pulse rate (over 160 beats per minute). Untreated, heatstroke can result in coma, brain damage and, in extreme cases, death due to kidney failure. Early signs are:

- Excessive sweating
- Fatigue
- Muscle cramps
- Dizziness and faintness
- Headache
- Nausea and vomiting

If exposure to heat continues, the following may develop:

- Increase in body temperature
- Increased pulse rate and rapid, shallow breathing
- Hot, dry and red skin
- Feelings of anxiety and confusion
- Weakness, light-headedness
- Irrational behaviour
- Seizures

CAUSES

- Continued exposure to very hot weather (external temperatures above 35°C/95°F), particularly when coupled with high humidity (averaging 50 per cent or more).
- Performing physical labour or exercising excessively in hot weather.
- Engaging in endurance or competitive sport, particularly when physically unfit.
- Wearing too much clothing in hot weather.

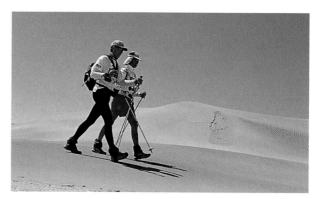

Remember to drink plenty of fluids in hot weather.

TREATMENT

HEAT EXHAUSTION

The condition will usually resolve itself with rest in a cool place and the intake of fluids (non-alcoholic, non-carbonated beverages). Avoid drinks containing caffeine. Encourage the casualty to drink small quantities every hour or so until they feel recovered. Removing unnecessary clothing and sponging the body with tepid water will lower the temperature.

Summon medical assistance immediately if the casualty's condition does not improve, deteriorates or their level of alertness changes (they become confused, or unconscious or suffer from seizures).

TREATMENT FOR HEATSTROKE

While waiting for help to arrive:

- Lie the casualty down in a cool area, feet raised about 30cm (12in).
- Apply wet cloths to the skin, soak in tepid water, or apply cold compresses to the neck, armpits and groin. Use an electic fan, or a magazine or board, to create a flow of cool air around the casualty.
- If the casualty is alert, provide cool non-alcoholic, non-carbonated drinks or administer salt solution (*see* p242) every 15 minutes. If you don't have either, plain cool water will do.
- Administer first aid for **shock** (*see* p174).
- If **seizures** (*see* p178) occur, protect the casualty from injury, and administer first aid.
- If the casualty is **unconscious** (*see* p164–71), give appropriate first aid.
- Be aware of complications if the casualty has medical problems such as high blood pressure.

CAUTION

Heatstroke is a medical emergency and requires hospitalization. **Call for assistance without delay**.

X DO NOT

- use an alcohol rub to cool the casualty.
- underestimate heatstroke or heat exhaustion as they can be serious, particularly in children, the elderly or injured.
- provide medication, such as aspirin, that is used to treat fever.
- provide anything at all by mouth if the casualty is vomiting or unconscious.
- permit someone suffering from heatstroke to resume physical activity as soon as they feel better.

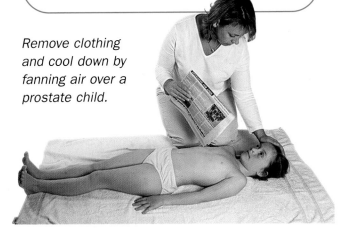

Remove clothing and cool down by fanning air over a prostate child.

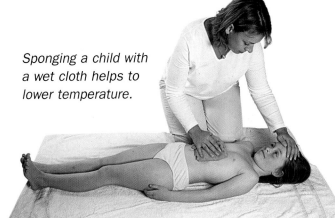

Sponging a child with a wet cloth helps to lower temperature.

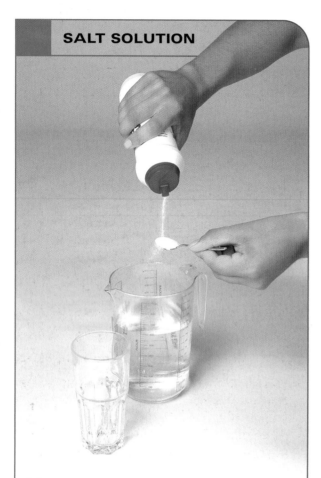

SALT SOLUTION

Mix one teaspoon of salt to one litre/two pints of water and give the casualty about half a cup (125ml) every 15 minutes. If you don't have cool drinks or salt available, plain cool water is better than nothing.

Place a child suffering from heat exhaustion in the shade and give her a drink of water.

PREVENTION

· Increase both salt and fluid intake when exercising in hot weather.
· Rather drink too many fluids than too few, but beware of overhydration.
· Avoid strenuous outdoor activity in the heat of the day. If you work or play sport in a hot and humid environment, take regular rest periods in cooler areas, either indoors or in the shade.
· Wear light, loose clothing and a hat with a broad brim. This applies particularly to children playing outdoors in very hot weather.
· If you are elderly, obese or on medication that impairs your body's heat regulation mechanism, avoid overheating.
· Tourists are often at risk of heat exhaustion. If you are travelling to the tropics, allow yourself time to acclimatize before you exert yourself.

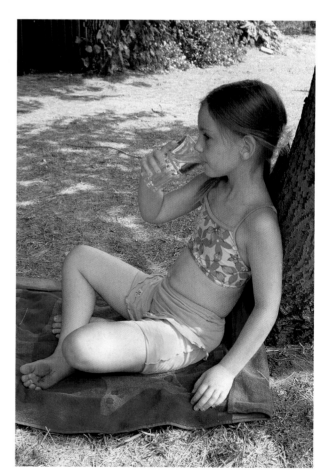

Hypothermia

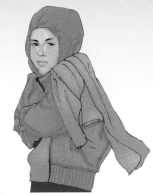

Hypothermia occurs when the body loses more heat than it can generate, usually by being exposed to cold for an extended period. It is characterized by a low body temperature, below 35°C (95°F). The symptoms of hypothermia develop relatively slowly, affecting the person's mental and physical state, leading to apathy, lethargy and drowsiness. This means the casualty might not detect hypothermia and may fail to take preventative measures either soon enough, or to the necessary degree.

Generally, people with a chronic illness, such as a heart or circulation problem, the very old or very young, and those who are tired, malnourished, or under the influence of drugs or alcohol are at risk of hypothermia when subjected to conditions which could bring it about.

SYMPTOMS

- Pale and cold skin
- Apathy, lethargy and drowsiness
- Weakness
- Slurred speech
- Confusion
- Shock
- Slowed breathing or heart rate
- Coma
- Cardiac arrest
- The casualty might shiver uncontrollably but shivering can stop when the body temperature is extremely low

CAUSES

Factors that contribute to hypothermia include the following:
- Cold weather, particularly when accompanied by wind, which causes a chill factor that lowers the body temperature further than it would drop in similar calm conditions.
- Immersion in cold water.
- Exposure to excessive cold by being outside without sufficient protective clothing.
- Continuing to wear wet clothing for an extended period of time in cold, wet and/or windy conditions.

 CAUTION

Hypothermia needs prompt treatment as it can be fatal. The most extreme symptoms – cardiac arrest, shock and coma – can set in if initial first aid measures are ineffective or are not carried out promptly.

- Heavy exertion outdoors in cold weather.
- Continual exposure to cold conditions while under the influence of certain medications or alcohol.
- Poor circulation resulting from excessively tight clothing or from lying in one position for too long. Fatigue, alcohol consumption, certain medications and smoking can all impede circulation.
- Insufficient consumption of suitable hot foods and liquids to 'fuel' the body in very cold weather.

TREATMENT

- Get the casualty into a warm environment as quickly as possible and summon medical assistance.
- Remove wet clothing. If garments are dry, loosen tight cuffs and collars – not forgetting the legs and the ankle area.
- Place the casualty on a blanket or coat to insulate against a cold floor and cover with blankets. Much body heat is lost via the top of the head, which is richly supplied with blood, so keep the head and neck region well covered.
- Apply warm compresses to the neck, chest and groin area, and keep the head warm.
- If the casualty is conscious, alert and able to swallow without choking, give warm non-alcoholic sweetened fluids to speed up the warming process.
- If it is very cold and you cannot get the casualty to a warm place, at least get them out of the wind and into a relatively sheltered area. Cover them warmly and be sure to protect them from the cold ground.
- Remain with the casualty until help arrives.

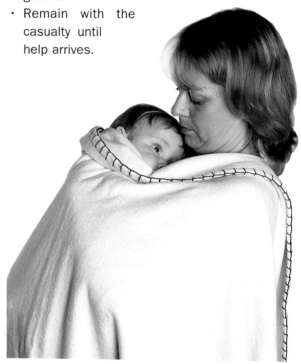

Use your own body heat and a blanket to rewarm

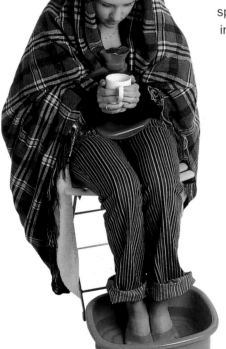

People suffering from hypothermia should not only be warmed from the outside, serve a warm drink to warm them inside.

> ## ✕ DO NOT
>
> - assume that a person found motionless in the cold is dead. Get the inert body to shelter, begin **rescue breathing** (*see* p168) and/or **chest compressions** (*see* pp164–71) if necessary, and provide the above-mentioned first aid measures.
> - try to warm the casualty by applying direct heat such as hot water, a heating pad or a heat lamp. If the casualty's senses are so dulled that they do not react, your actions could result in burns.
> - give the casualty alcohol to drink, even after recovery.

STAGES OF HYPOTHERMIA

MILD
Core temperature 35°C–32°C
(95°F–92°F)

- Complains of severe cold
- Poor judgement, confusion, irritability
- Slurred speech, stumbling
- Uncontrollable shivering
- Cold, blue hands and feet
- Stiff muscles
- High urine production leading to dehydration

MODERATE
Core temperature 32°C–28°C
(90°F–82.4°F)

- Decreased level of consciousness
- Shivering may stop
- Muscles are stiff and rigid
- Irregular heartbeat

SEVERE
Temperature below 28°C
(82.2°F)–Core temperature

- Deeply unconscious
- Slow breathing
- Slow, irregular heartbeat
- Heart may stop

is much easier to spot a car than a person. If you decide to abandon your vehicle, leave a prominently displayed message giving your departure time, direction of travel, mobile phone number and any other information that might aid those looking for you.

- Take care that babies and small children are adequately insulated and protected from the cold, especially at night. If there is any doubt, rather let them sleep with you.
- While hiking, make a mental note of landmarks and potential shelters along the way.

PREVENTION

- Wear head gear to keep your head warm and slow the loss of heat from the top of the head.
- Wear mittens rather than gloves, and gloves rather than nothing.
- Wear suitable clothing and protect exposed, sensitive areas. Clothing should be wind-proof and water-resistant, and preferably, multilayered.
- Avoid wet or constricting clothing – beware of tight cuffs, leggings, or footwear that impede circulation to the extremities (often at greater risk anyway).
- Wear two pairs of socks (cotton next to skin, wool next to footwear) and water-resistant footwear that provides protection at least to the ankles. Warm and dry feet in cold conditions are important.
- Beware of going out in extremely cold conditions, and wear suitable gear when diving, surfing or taking part in other water-related activities.
- If you are on medication, check with your doctor, as some medicines might interfere with your blood circulation and/or blood pressure.
- If your vehicle breaks down or gets stuck in unfamiliar terrain, stay with it. In adverse conditions, it

WAYS OF PRODUCING HEAT

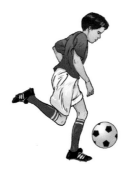

Physical activity

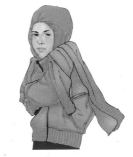

Warm clothing

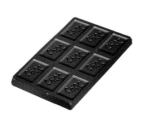

High-energy food

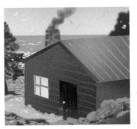

Heated shelter

Frostbite

Frostbite is the damage extreme cold can do to the skin and underlying tissues. It usually occurs on the extremities (face, nose, ears, hands, fingers and feet), which tend to be more exposed. As with many conditions, the duration and extent of exposure determine the extent of the damage. The pressure of wind chill, together with low temperatures, increases the risk of frostbite as well as **hypothermia** (*see* p243).

SYMPTOMS

- A sensation of 'pins and needles' is the first symptom.
- Numbness, throbbing or aching may follow, after which sensation (feeling) is lost completely as the affected part starts to feel like a 'block of wood' and the skin becomes hard, pale and cold.
- As the tissue affected by early frostbite thaws it becomes red and painful.
- In extreme cases, the skin will become numb and turn white as the tissue freezes. This may be accompanied by blisters and gangrene (blackened dead tissue). Bone, tendons, muscles and nerves might also be damaged.

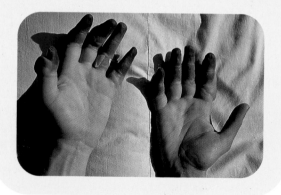

CAUSES

Anyone who is exposed to freezing cold for a prolonged period can get frostbite. Inadequate clothing and insufficient protection for the head, hands and feet exacerbate the problem; as do external factors like wind chill.

With adequate shelter and protection, most people can survive just about any weather condition, but the risk is increased by certain factors, such as taking beta-blockers (which decrease the flow of blood to the skin), smoking, being inebriated, and chronic conditions like diabetes and low blood pressure.

PREVENTION

- When venturing outdoors in icy weather, wear wind- and waterproof clothing with multi-layered upper-body protection; mittens or gloves; and a hood, scarf or woollen cap (you lose most body heat via the top of your head). Ensure cuffs are snug but not so tight they constrict the flow of blood to your hands.
- Choose well-fitting, water-resistant footwear and wear two pairs of socks: cotton next to your skin, then wool.
- If caught outdoors in very cold weather or snow, find shelter or increase physical activity to maintain body warmth.
- Be aware of factors that affect the blood vessels, such as smoking, alcohol, medication, and conditions such as low blood pressure or diabetes.
- If bad weather threatens when you are hiking, make a note of potential shelter along the route; if a storm strikes, you will know where to find refuge.

TREATMENT

- Get the casualty into warm surroundings and protect them from further cold. Remove wet or constricting clothing and jewellery, substituting it for something warm and loose. Blankets are ideal if no warm, dry clothing is available.
- Look for signs of **hypothermia** (*see* p243) and treat accordingly .
- Wrap the affected parts in sterile dressings (wrap toes and fingers individually to keep them separated) and get the casualty to a medical facility for further care.
- When medical care is not immediately available, immerse the affected areas in warm, not hot, water (about 40–42°C/104–108°F), or repeatedly apply warm cloths to the frostbitten area for about 30 minutes.
- When immersing the frostbitten area, circulate the water with your hand as this will aid the warming process. The casualty may experience severe burning pain and swelling, and the affected part may change colour during warming. Warming is complete when the skin is soft and sensation has returned to the affected area.
- Provide warm, sweetened drinks.
- If there is a chance that frostbitten parts may freeze again and you are far from medical help or warm shelter, then delay first aid procedures until the chance of refreezing has been eliminated. Tissue damage can be exacerbated if frostbite thaws and then refreezes, whereas if it is kept in a steady state and thawed once only, the damage may be lessened.
- Always have frostbite checked by a doctor, even if you have made a complete recovery. Seek medical assistance if recovery is not complete or new symptoms develop. (These include fever, malaise, discolouration of the frostbitten area and seeping or oozing of fluids from the area.)

X DO NOT

- disturb blisters on frostbitten skin.
- immerse a frostbitten area in hot water as the scalding would increase the risk of tissue damage (use warm water only).
- rub or massage a frostbitten area.
- smoke or consume alcohol during recovery, as this can interfere with blood circulation and slow the recovery process.
- thaw a frostbitten area if it cannot be kept thawed, as refreezing may make tissue damage even worse.
- use direct dry heat (from sources such as hair dryers or heating pads) to thaw the frostbitten areas, as you may apply excessive heat, burning the skin and causing more damage.

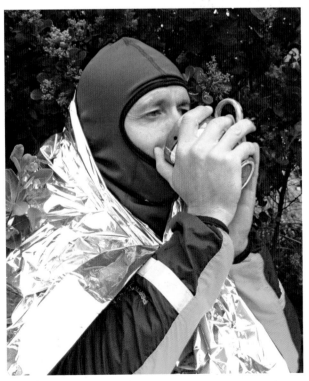

Rewarm a frozen person with a survival blanket and a warm beverage.

Electrical shock

An electrical shock occurs when the body, or part of it, becomes a conduit for electricity from a strong source to an area of lower electrical energy. The extent of the injury is determined by the size and duration of the shock, the level of conductivity between the body and whatever it is touching, and the route the current took as it travelled through the body. Depending on its severity, an electric shock can cause damage to nerves, muscles and other tissues, as well as thermal burns ranging from comparatively minor to very serious. Even if an electrical burn looks slight, the shock could have resulted in internal damage to the heart, muscles, or brain, which can result in cardiac arrest.

SYMPTOMS

- Sudden, unexplained loss of consciousness, particularly when the shock was not witnessed by another person
- Skin burns
- Muscular pain
- Numbness, tingling
- Muscle contraction with residual pain, for a while at least
- Headache
- Weakness
- Hearing impairment
- Irregular pulse
- Seizures
- Respiratory failure
- Unconsciousness
- Cardiac arrest

CAUSES

- Accidental contact with exposed wiring or unearthed parts of electrical appliances
- Incorrect connection of appliance plugs or wiring
- Children chewing on electrical cords, or poking metal objects into an electrical outlet, such as a plug socket
- Lightning strikes
- Laying electrical cords under rugs, resulting in damage to the insulation
- Accidentally cutting underground power cables while doing maintenance work
- Exposure to unearthed power tools or machinery
- Flashing (electric arcs) from high-voltage power lines

TREATMENT

- Once the casualty is free from the source of electricity, check their ABC (see pp164–5). If any funcations have ceased or seem dangerously slow or shallow, initiate **resuscitation** (see pp164–71).
- If the casualty has a burn, remove any clothing that comes off easily, cool the injury in running water until the pain subsides and administer first aid for **burns** (see p186).
- If the casualty is showing signs of **shock** (see p174), lie them down with the head slightly lower than the body and the legs elevated, and cover them with a blanket.
- If the shock has caused the casualty to fall (off a

ladder, for instance), there could be internal injuries. If you suspect a spinal injury, avoid moving the casualty's head or neck. Administer appropriate first aid for wounds or **fractures** (*see* p202).
· Stay with the casualty until professional medical help arrives.

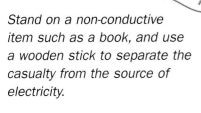

Stand on a non-conductive item such as a book, and use a wooden stick to separate the casualty from the source of electricity.

Or use a towel or rope to pull the person out of harm's way.

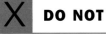

X DO NOT

● touch the casualty with your bare hands while the person is still in contact with the source of electricity.
● get within 6m (20ft) of someone who is being electrocuted by high-voltage electrical current until the power is turned off.
● move a casualty unless he or she is in any immediate danger.

PREVENTION

· Always treat electricity with respect and teach your children about the dangers of electricity.
  · Keep electrical appliances and cords out of children's reach and make sure they never play with any cord – even a piece you have discarded. Next time it might be attached to a wall socket.
· Use child safety plugs in all outlets.
· Never touch electrical appliances while touching taps (faucets) or water pipes.
· Follow the manufacturer's safety instructions when using electrical appliances or tools. Avoid using electrical appliances while wet, or when standing in a wet or damp patch – for instance in the early morning when dew is on the ground.
· If working up a ladder and using a power tool, choose a wooden rather than an alumimium ladder. Wood is a poor conductor of electricity.
· If you do not know how to wire an electric plug, then don't! Get a handyman or electrician do it.
· Always wear rubber-soled footwear when operating power tools.

SWITCHING OFF ELECTRIC CURRENT

Before you deal with the casualty, **switch off the electric current**. Use a piece of wood (broomstick or wooden spoon) to reach the switch. Do not put yourself at risk! If the current can't be turned off, use a dry non-conducting object such as a broom, chair, rug, or rubber doormat to push the casualty away from the source of the current. Don't use anything wet, damp or metallic. You may need to be rough – if the casualty has gripped the appliance, only a sharp tug or blow might break that grip and the contact. If possible, stand on something dry and non-conducting, such as a wooden plank, folded newspapers or a rubber or coir doormat while doing this.

Nausea and motion sickness

Nausea, the sensation of wanting to vomit, is a common symptom that usually does not require urgent medical attention. If, however, the condition is persistent, severe and/or prevents you keeping any food or drink down, then it may be a sign of something more serious. One of the main complications of vomiting is dehydration. The rate at which you become dehydrated depends on your size (infants can quickly become dehydrated as a result of persistent vomiting accompanied by diarrhoea), the frequency of the vomiting, and whether it is accompanied by diarrhoea.

SYMPTOMS

- An urge to vomit
- Actual vomiting
- A general feeling of unease or queasiness, particularly when at sea

CAUSES IN ADULTS

- Food allergies or food poisoning
- Viral infections
- Medications
- Seasickness or motion (car, air) sickness
- Morning sickness during pregnancy
- Accidental or deliberate ingestion of a drug or poison
- Alcoholism
- Bulimia
- Migraine headaches
- Chemotherapy

CAUSES IN INFANTS UP TO SIX MONTHS

- Overfeeding
- Being bounced excessively just after being fed
- Food allergies
- Milk intolerance
- Infection, often accompanied by fever/runny nose
- Intestinal obstruction, or a constriction in the outlet from the stomach, causing recurring attacks of vomiting and crying or screaming as if in great pain
- Poisoning
- Gastroenteritis
- Vomiting is a common sign of many infectious illnesses, including meningitis

TREATMENT

Whatever the cause of the vomiting, lost fluids should be restored as soon as possible; if not, dehydration can lead to other problems. Give water or diluted fruit juice, a sip at a time, as frequently as the patient can accept them without inducing more vomiting. The general rule is not too much food or liquid at once as the patient slowly works their way back to a normal diet.

TIP

For a home-made oral rehydration solution mix 1 teaspoon salt and 8 teaspoons sugar in 1 litre (2 pints) of cool, previously boiled water.

With infants and young children particularly, dehydration can develop very rapidly. If an infant is vomiting repeatedly, seek medical attention, and do not give the child more than a couple of teaspoons of water. Rather give a teaspoon every five minutes of half-strength formula or oral rehydration solution (keep some in the medicine cabinet – your doctor or pharmacist can advise you on a suitable product and dosages).

Since vomiting is almost always accompanied by some abdominal discomfort, generally you need be concerned only if the pain is severe.

DEHYDRATION

Suspect dehydration if a person complains of or exhibits any of the following:

· Being thirsty
· A dry mouth
· Eyes appear sunken
· Skin loses its normal elasticity
· Crying does not produce tears
· Infrequent or dark yellow urine

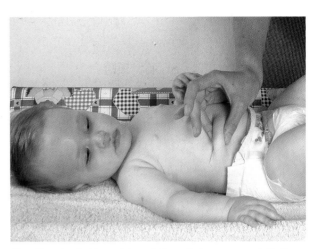

Gently pinch the side of the abdomen and if the raised skin does not return immediately to its normal position then suspect that dehydration has begun to set in.

SEEK MEDICAL HELP IF:

● You suspect that a child has taken a drug or ingested a poisonous substance.

● The patient is vomiting and also displays any of the following symptoms:

· headache and/or stiff neck.

· an adult cannot retain any fluids for 12 hours or more.

· nausea persists for a prolonged period (apart from pregnant women, who may experience long periods of 'morning sickness').

· a young child becomes dehydrated and produces less urine than normal.

· a young child is lethargic, markedly irritable, and unable to retain fluids for eight hours or more, or vomiting recurs.

MOTION SICKNESS

Some people are prone to motion sickness – either in a vehicle or at sea. Lying down will frequently help relieve the condition, as will the intake of fresh air, so open a window or get on deck. Looking ahead, at the horizon, rather than at the road or at moving water, also helps, as motion sickness occurs when the brain receives mixed messages from the eyes and the organs of balance in the inner ear. There are a number of proprietary medications aimed at preventing or reducing motion sickness. Ginger is often an effective remedy, so try ginger beer or biscuits (cookies) in small quantities.

PREVENTION

Attacks of nausea tend to occur suddenly and are very difficult to prevent, but you can reduce your susceptibility by taking the following steps:

Adults:
· Moderate your intake of rich foods and alcohol.
· Avoid eating food that appears 'off'.

Children:
· Follow normal feeding practices with infants, and avoid overfeeding.
· Guard against bacterial contamination of feeds, bottles, pacifiers and toys.

Home nursing and frail care

The cost of long-term hospitalization or frail care, coupled with the tedium and lack of intimacy and stimulation which characterize many institutions, may make home nursing an attractive option for ill, disabled or recovering elderly family members. Although the decision to nurse someone in your home is inevitably based on love and a deep sense of commitment, these sentiments alone are not enough. To succeed in practice, home nursing requires careful stocktaking of your own resources, planning, possibly some structural alterations, consultation with other family members and professionals and, of course, a budget. Here, we offer some general suggestions which should guide your decision as to whether home nursing is a viable option, and help you create the correct environment and other conditions necessary for successful home care.

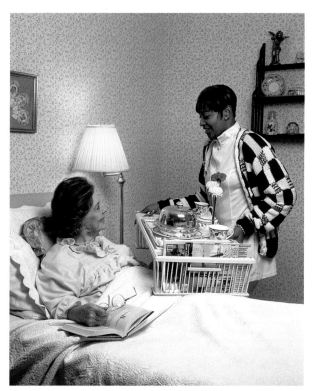

Trained nurses can be hired to take care of the elderly person at home.

FAMILY CONSULTATION

If you plan to care for a parent or grandparent, discuss your plans with members of your extended family, to confirm that you have their support, and which of them will lend a hand when needed. Raise the important subject of finances, how best to cover the costs of home care, and who will contribute to costs as and when necessary.

Consult with the elderly person's doctor and any other medical professionals who have been providing regular care, such as physiotherapists and dieticians. Establish what medical and other routines must be maintained, and whether you can do this yourself, or will need to be supported by regular visits from the relevant community health-workers.

Last, but not least establish, by means of open and frank discussion, whether you have the unqualified support of your spouse and children, particularly if you plan to provide home care to a relative for an extended or indefinite period. The decision will impact on everyone who lives in your home, so ensure that everyone appreciates the adjustments which may be necessary.

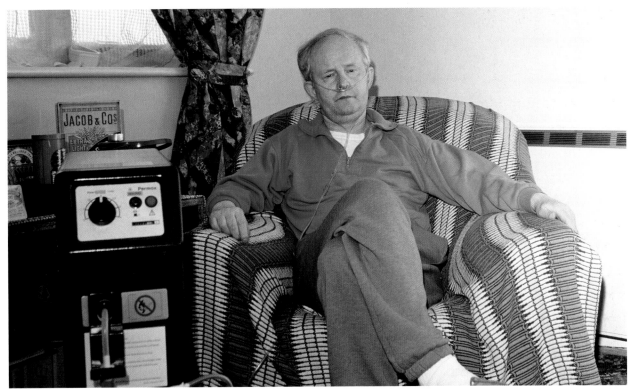

The cost of hiring special equipment must be taken into consideration when you are thinking of inviting an aged family member to come and live with you.

THE PHYSICAL ENVIRONMENT

Some hospitals or frail-care institutions may offer the services of a specially trained community nurse who does home visits and will help you decide how to adapt your home for nursing purposes. If you conduct this exercise on your own, pay attention to:

- **Overall layout**. There should be a bedroom for the sole use of the person being nursed, with easy access to a bathroom and toilet, regardless of whether they are mobile or confined to bed. If the bedroom is in a separate annex, a bell, alarm or intercom should be fitted to allow help to be summoned when necessary.
- **The toilet and bathroom** need to be spacious, so a frail person can manoeuvre themselves easily and safely, particularly if they use walking frames or wheelchairs. Handrails may have to be fitted in the shower or bathtub and alongside the toilet.
- **Staircases**, narrow doorways or poorly lit areas may create obstacles to mobility for physically dis-

abled people or those with poor eyesight. If a wheelchair is used, it is a good idea to borrow one in advance to ensure it can fit through doorways, and that there is room to turn around or manoeuvre in tight spaces.
- **Slippery tiles** and loose mats or rugs can be hazardous to a person unsteady on their feet, and should be avoided.
- **Light switches** should be easily accessible, and there should be a bedside light that can be switched on without getting out of bed.

A home environment which allows the frail person as much free movement as possible will reduce their dependence upon you, and make for a happy arrangement all round.

SPECIAL EQUIPMENT

Medical equipment can be bought or hired, according to the needs of the person you are caring for, and your budget. Items such as beds with side-railings,

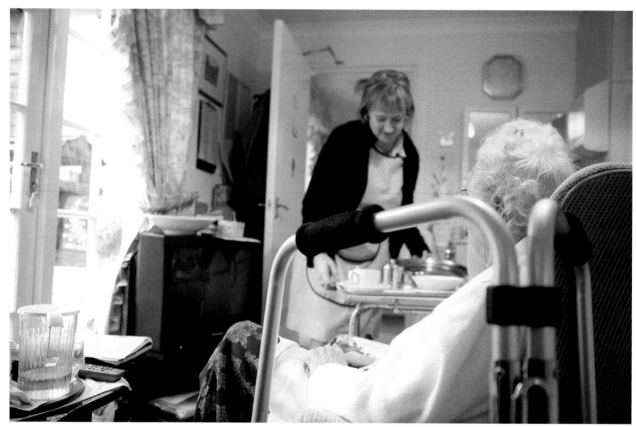

Make sure the patient is kept busy and stimulated not only mentally but also physically. Good nutrition, sunshine, moderate exercise – if possible – and frequent visits will aid their recovery.

walking frames, wheelchairs, commodes and oxygen cylinders are widely available from medical suppliers, while disposable items such as waterproof sheets, urinals and diapers can be obtained from wholesale or retail pharmacies.

Your doctor or community nurse should be able to advise on the type of equipment required for your particular situation.

LIFESTYLE AND ROUTINES

The main advantage of being at home is that it allows the frail, recovering or disabled person to move beyond the role of 'patient', and feel like a normal, dignified member of society despite their medical limitations.

Try to structure your care according to what the disabled or older person essentially needs. Even if it takes Granny two hours to get dressed in the morning, let her do it herself rather than insist on helping. At the same time, be sensitive to the fragile pride of a person who is embarrassed to ask for help. The art is to find a balance between just being available, and knowing when to intervene.

MEDICATION

If the patient is on a strict medication regime, someone must always be available to ensure the correct dosage is taken at the appropriate time. If medication has to be injected, you may require daily visits by a community nurse. Patients who suffer from respiratory illnesses often use a nebulizer throughout the day; they may also need home visits by a physiotherapist who can help relieve chest congestion.

THE BED-BOUND PERSON

A person confined to bed for whatever reason requires special care, in order to prevent the complications of immobility. The areas where you will need to assist are:

· Providing urinals or commodes when necessary, disposing of waste matter and keeping the equipment clean and germ-free.
· Having an adequate supply of fresh bedding, including waterproof undersheets, for a person who is incontinent or partially continent, and having enough hands on deck to change bedding with the person still in the bed.
· Preventing pressure (bed) sores through proper hygiene and skin care, combined with the use of synthetic sheepskins and ensuring regular changes in lying position.
· Providing a varied and interesting diet, which includes a daily portion of fibre to prevent constipation. Inactive people burn up less energy, and therefore require smaller helpings of food. However, unless a special diet is prescribed, there is no reason why they cannot share in the food cooked for the family. Fresh water should always be on hand at the bedside, and fluid intake must be encouraged to prevent the stagnation of urine and the development of bladder infections and kidney stones.
· If meals must be taken in bed, arrange for members of the family to eat with them in the room once or twice a week.

People who are confined to bed, or whose mobility is limited in any way, find that the days become long, tedious, and frustrating. If not adequately occupied during the day, they may simply sleep for long periods, and be restless or sleepless at night, creating a disruption for the whole family. To preserve a normal sleep cycle, provide mental stimulation during the day, with reading matter, radio, television and occasional visitors.

Your family doctor or a community nurse may do house visits for regular checkups.

WILL IT WORK OUT?

The outline of priorities listed in this chapter gives an indication of the substantial investment of your time, energy and money that home care requires. Still, nursing a loved one at home can be a most rewarding experience for all concerned if you have planned carefully and have support from the rest of your family as well as community services.

A person with a chronic illness or a deteriorating mental condition may become more difficult to nurse than originally anticipated, and progressively more demanding on your care. Your own circumstances may not allow you enough time to care for an invalid.

If this happens, do not feel that you are locked into an arrangement, or that you have been defeated. Instead, look carefully at what the invalid requires, discuss the situation with your family doctor, social worker or community nurse and, with their guidance, identify a suitable (and affordable) health provider or institution who can take over. Do not chide yourself for having given up. Award yourself credit for what you have done so far, and don't feel guilty about passing on increasing responsibility when you cannot cope any longer.

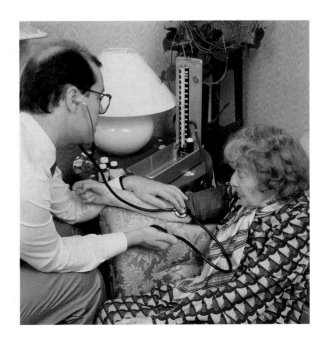

SAFETY AROUND THE HOME

We tend to regard our homes as safe havens, where we are protected from 'danger', but danger comes in many disguises. A home is only as safe as we make it, yet we often take for granted the security afforded by the sense of 'home' and forget to view our living environment in a more rational light.

An important aspect to consider when reviewing the safety of your home is who lives there. A couple with no children or pets may be at ease with open stairwells, a plunge pool and expensive artworks on occasional tables, whereas a family with inquisitive toddlers or active youngsters would be more comfortable in a home that allows the children to explore their surroundings and play freely, yet has sufficient protection to ensure that it is safe for them to do so.

Some home-based emergencies are beyond our ability to prevent, but the vast majority can be prevented. Simple precautions can make the difference between coping with a minor incident or having it turn into a crisis. In these instances, a positive outcome is often determined by your ability to find solutions and then act accordingly. Prevention is not rocket science; the key is common sense. It is also a matter of expecting the unexpected, no matter how improbable it may seem.

IN THIS SECTION

A child-friendly home

Every year thousands of children are treated for injuries sustained in their homes, most of which could have been avoided. We usually run our lives according to what is convenient but, when you have a child in the house, convenience should come after safety, so look at your home through different eyes and put safety first.

There are many things you can do to make your home safer as your child grows from that bundle of fun in the crib to an inquisitive adult in the making. Remember, as your children grow, so will their ability to reach the unreachable, and do what they are not supposed to do. As soon as they can crawl, get down on your hands and knees to see the world from their perspective to decide what he or she might be able to reach. When your child can understand simple instructions, ensure you get across loud and clear the meaning of 'No!' and 'Don't touch!'.

LIVING ROOM AND BEDROOMS

- Make electrical cords and sockets inaccessible and teach children not to touch them.
- Ensure free-standing heaters, electric blankets and hairdryers are in good condition and are used correctly at all times.
- Keep medicines out of your bedside drawer and off low shelves in the cupboard.
- Don't use tablecloths on tables that have lamps, vases or heavy ornaments on them; a child might pull the cloth off, bringing the object down as well.

Other items that could be pulled over include standing lamps and wobbly bookshelves.
- Install stair guards at the top and bottom of flights of stairs.
- Fit a fire guard in front of an open fireplace.
- Keep children away from heaters (radiators) and circulating fans.
- Buy toys that are suitable for your child's age.
- Ensure young children do not pick up or play with small items like buttons, coins, etc.

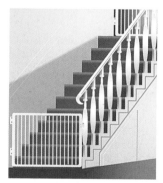

Stair guard

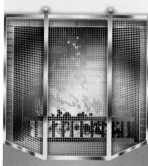

Fire guard

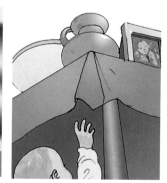

Short tablecloths

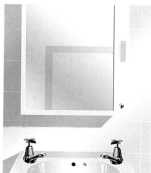

Lock up medicine

THE KITCHEN

The kitchen is not a playground; there is enormous potential for accidents, such as a bad burn or scald, which could scar a child for life.

Wherever possible, use protection devices. Stair guards, for example, not only prevent children going up or down stairs, but can be used to block doorways, to keep them out of the kitchen (a major source of mishaps), or the garage or workshop – an equally rich source of accidents, given the type of tools and chemicals often found there.

When it comes to children's safety, parents need to be consistent. For instance, if your child starts chewing on a length of electrical flex, even though it may be a short off-cut from a connection you have made, stop the child immediately and take the cord away. Why? Because this time it was safe, but next time the child might decide to chew on a wire that is live, with tragic results.

- Keep knives, skewers and other sharp objects out of the way.
- Replace the frayed or damaged electrical cords on appliances.
- Turn pot handles inwards when cooking a meal on top of the stove and ensure that hot dishes are not placed near the edge of the work-surface.
- When you need to use only one or two stove plates or burners, use the rear ones in preference to those at the front.
- If your cupboard doors do not lock, install safety latches, particularly on cupboards or drawers used to store household cleaners and detergents.

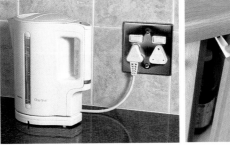
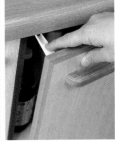

Short electrical cords prevent children from reaching appliances (left). Install child resistant latches in cupboard door (right).

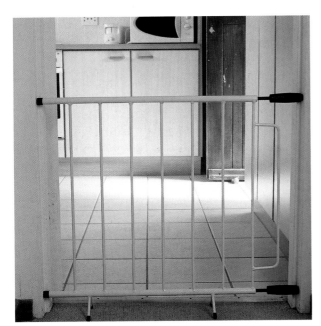

The kitchen is a major source for mishaps. To ensure your toddler's safety store dangerous goods out of reach. When you are not in the kitchen, block access to it with a gate such as the one shown above.

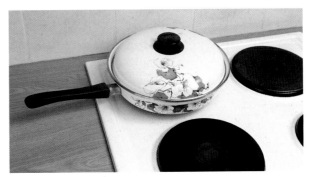

Pot handles must be turned away from the front of the stove where young hands may reach.

- Install thermostatic mixing valves in your bathroom taps to ensure that water is dispensed at a safe temperature. Water with a temperature of 60°C (140°F) can cause severe scalding.
- Always run the cold water into the bath first, and then top up with hot. Test the water temperature with your elbow, or use a thermometer.
- Supervise your toddler's visits to the toilet. A child's weight is biased towards the top half of their body, and if they overbalance head first into the toilet they could drown. For the same reason, use nappy (diaper) buckets with child-resistant lids. Remember, a child can drown in only a couple of centimetres of water.
- Keep medications and toiletries out of their reach, ideally in a lockable cabinet mounted high up against the wall. Try to purchase products stored in child- or tamper-resistant containers designed to resist being opened by small hands.
- Store sharp objects, such as razors, in wall-mounted brackets out of a child's reach.
- All cleaning products should be kept in a locked cupboard. Where possible, buy only containers with tamper-resistant caps.

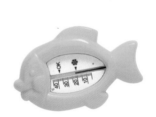

Bath thermometer

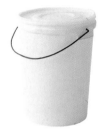

Bucket with tamper-resistant lid.

Child safety

Childproofing should not only concentrate on home and garden, but include car travel and visits to the playground. By taking precautions and adhering to standard safety regulations you can ensure the safety of your child.

SUN GLARE PROTECTION

Other simple, often overlooked, protection devices include hoods or sun visors on carry cots and push chairs, and screens on car windows, all of which help to protect a child's eyes from the sun's glare, and possible damage from UV rays, as well as from windborne dust and other pollutants.

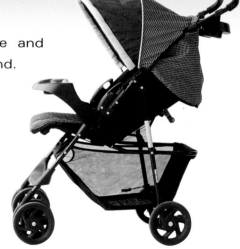

Sun visor and carry net are good ideas. Never hang bags from the handle or the pram could tip.

PLAY AREAS

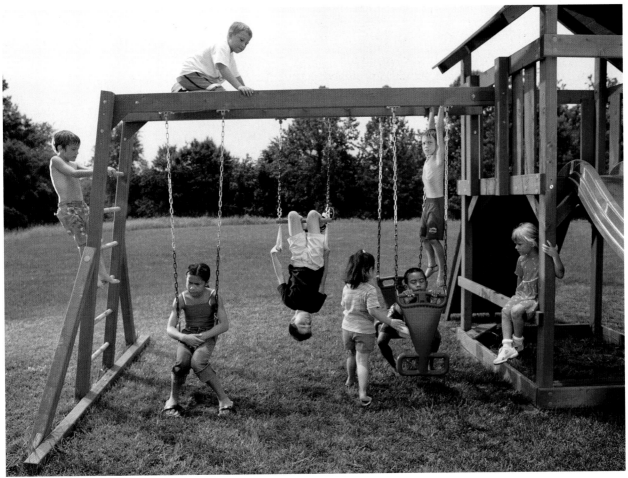

The surface underneath a play structure should be soft to protect against hard falls.

Children learn through play, but they also learn by making mistakes. Parents need to strike a happy balance between protecting their little ones from harm while allowing them enough scope to experiment – even if they end up with a few bumps and bruises, and the odd scratch.

A sturdy wooden climbing frame in the garden is a marvellous idea, not only because children love to clamber over and under things but also because these frames help the child to develop his or her hand-eye co-ordination, strength and imagination.

Do ensure, however, that the ground below the play apparatus is nice and soft – lawn or an area that doubles as a sandpit would be ideal – and that the frame structure is securely fitted into the ground and cannot topple over.

SAFE TRANSPORT

Children are particularly vulnerable in vehicles, no matter whether stationary or not. It is irresponsible and negligent to ignore the safety regulations that dictate that all children up to the approximate age of 11 or 12 should be restrained in specially designed and approved seats. Baby chairs and booster seats provide additional support and a secure safety harness that will ensure minimal injury in the event of an accident and might save your child's life.

In an accident involving a vehicle travelling along at a mere 48kph (30mph), an unrestrained child would be flung around or out of the car with a force up to 50 times greater than its body weight. It makes no difference whether the child is sitting in the back or front seat, or even on the lap of a passenger at the time – it would be crushed instantly or propelled towards the windscreen at a velocity that spells certain disaster.

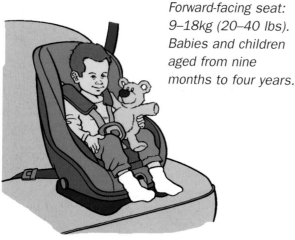

Forward-facing seat: 9–18kg (20–40 lbs). Babies and children aged from nine months to four years.

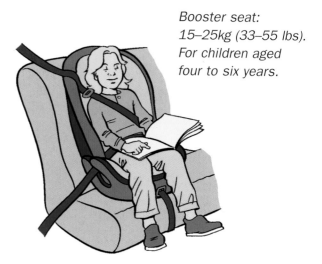

Booster seat: 15–25kg (33–55 lbs). For children aged four to six years.

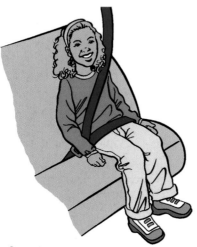

Seat belts are designed to fit around people who are 150cm (5ft) and taller. By the age of 11, your child should be big enough to discard the booster cushion and use the seat belt only.

X DO NOT

- allow a child to stand on a seat or sit on anyone's lap.
- fit a rearward-facing seat on the passenger seat if the car is fitted with front airbags.
- leave a child in the vehicle unattended – not even for a second.
- allow children to play with the vehicle's controls or the ignition key.
- allow children to play with a ball or throw toys about inside the car. The driver could easily be distracted.

Images courtesy of The Royal Society for the Prevention of Accidents (RoSPA)

Assistance for the elderly

The elderly are particularly prone to falls, which frequently result in strains and sprains. The increasing frailty and unsteadiness of old age means that even a minor fall can cause a broken wrist, while a more serious fall could result in a fractured hip.

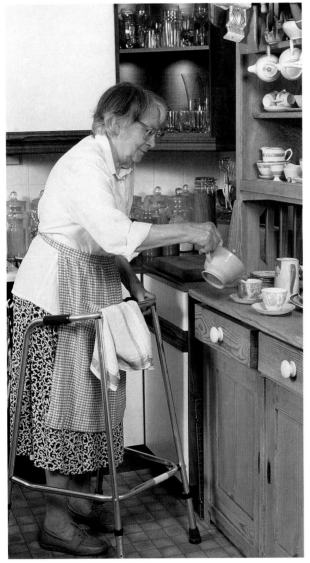

An elderly lady makes use of a zimmer frame to move about in her home.

If you have an elderly person living with you, consider making it easier for them to move around in your home. One simple remedy is to install handrails and non-slip surfaces on stairs and steps, particularly those leading into the garden or outside areas. In cases of extreme frailty, you may also have to consider putting handrails along passageways. Good lighting on stairs is essential, while some form of visual contrast, such as brightly coloured tape or paint to mark the top of each tread, makes it easier to see the edges of steps.

There are many useful aids to assist the elderly (as well as anyone suffering from arthritis or other conditions of limited mobility): scissor-grabs help to pick up anything they have dropped; a hook enables them to open and close windows; tap extensions make it easier to open and close a tap (faucet); and special chairs enable them to get in and out of the bath or shower.

If a wheelchair is going to become a necessity, you will probably have to make a number of adjustments, such as constructing a wheelchair ramp for access to and from the house, and moving furniture around to allow enough space for manoeuvring.

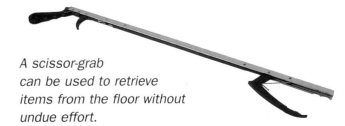

A scissor-grab can be used to retrieve items from the floor without undue effort.

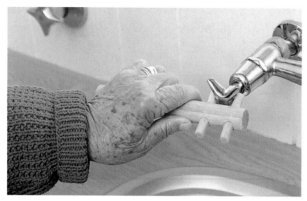

A simple tool like this makes it easier for old hands to open and close taps.

HANDY HINTS

- Position kettles, microwaves and hotplates so that the aged can reach them more easily.
- Overfull kettles are harder to lift, and may be dropped, so use just enough water.
- Remove loose mats and rugs, as it is easy to slip, or catch a foot and fall.
- Install good lighting in passageways, shaded exterior areas and stairwells. Ensure lights leading to the bathroom are accessible.
- Move obstacles such as occasional tables, large plant pots and small items of furniture, allowing a clear route to and from doorways.

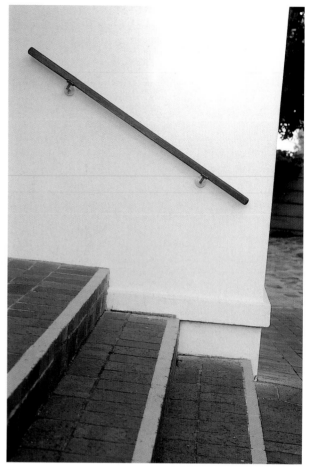

Handrails and brightly painted edges make it easier to see and negotiate a flight of steps.

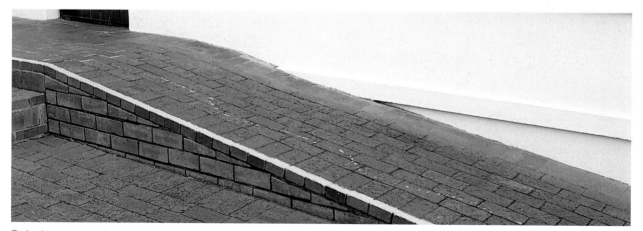

Painting a prominent yellow strip on the edge of a wheelchair ramp makes it more visible, particularly at night or in poor light. Any ramp for wheelchairs needs to have a gentle gradient (slope).

Fire precautions

Of all the disasters that can strike a home and family, fire ranks as one of the most traumatic, not only because of its danger to life and risk of injury, but also because it destroys so comprehensively. However, there are some preventative steps you can take:

- Install smoke detectors as suggested by the manufacturers. Test the alarms, and check and replace the batteries regularly.
- Buy fire extinguishers and mount them near the doorways of areas most at risk.
  - Keep a container of bicarbonate of soda close to the stove. Sprinkled on flames it will extinguish a small flare-up quickly and effectively.
  - Ensure all electrical fittings, wiring and appliances are in good order and replace as they become worn or frayed.
  - Never run electric cords under carpets or rugs. In time, foot traffic can damage their insulation, resulting in a short circuit which could cause a fire.
- Select non-flammable materials when choosing carpets, drapes (curtains) and furniture.
- Keep clothing and other flammable items well away from incandescent bar heaters (electric fires or radiators) and open flame gas heaters.
- Use a fire guard in front of an open fire.
- Use dry coal or anthracite. If coal or anthracite is wet when you add it to the fire, the moisture in it turns to steam, builds up pressure and fragments are blown off. While these can mark your carpet, they might also cause a fire, or an injury if a piece lands in someone's eye.

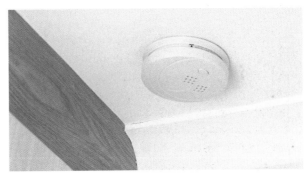

Smoke detectors are essential. Mount them outside the kitchen in the hall, on the landing, as well as in the garage and workshop.

TAKE NOTE

It is essential that you learn to use your fire extinguisher correctly and that you have it checked regularly to ensure that it won't let you down in an emergency.

 CAUTION

- Never fight a fire unless it is small and you are confident that you can get it under control safely and quickly.
- This is not the time to take risks. If the fire is too big then: **get out, stay out and call the fire brigade**.
- Never use water on a fire caused by an electrical fault. If the power is still on, you run the risk of electrocution.
- Never use water on a fire caused by liquid fuel. Most flammable liquids float on water, you will simply spread the problem.

FIGHTING FIRES

The most important point to consider is that a fire extinguisher is only as good as the person who is using it. **Let everyone in your house learn how to use the extinguisher and have it checked regularly so that it won't let you down in an emergency**.

When it comes to choosing a fire extinguisher, it is important to consider where it might be used. Dry powder (chemical) extinguishers are best as they can be used on fires fuelled by wood, paper, textiles or flammable liquids, as well as those caused by an electrical short circuit.

- Buy two small, portable extinguishers instead of a single large one that might be unwieldy. Position the extinguishers strategically in different areas of the home, such as at the entrance to the garage and near the kitchen.
- A fire blanket, which is simply dropped on to the fire to smother the flames, can be useful.

FIRE DRILL

- Turn off the power, gas line or whatever else might be fuelling the fire.
- Close all windows or doors leading to the area where the fire is, in order to avoid fanning the flames and to deprive the fire of oxygen.
- Try to smother the fire with a non-flammable material, such as a fire blanket.
- Aim a dry powder extinguisher at the base of the fire, not at the flames.
- If a frying pan ignites, cover it with a large lid or wooden board to smother the flame. Do not throw water over the fire – fat floats on water and you risk spreading the flames and causing more damage. Do not lift the lid to see whether the fire is out. Switch off the stove and leave the pan or pot in place for at least 30 minutes.

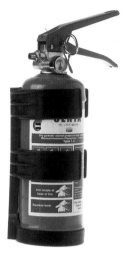

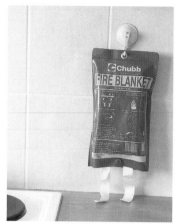

Dry powder fire extinguishers must be checked regularly.

A fire blanket is best kept near the stove area and is thrown over a fire to smother the flames.

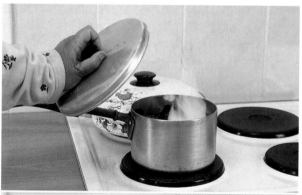

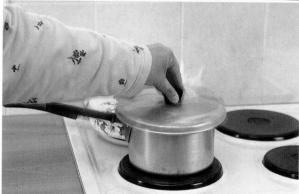

If a pot catches fire, simply smother the flames by placing a lid over the pot.

Don't be electrocuted

Electric power is a wonderful thing – right up to the second where you become the conduit between the source and the ground. Many tragic home accidents are due to accidental electrocution and there is a general call to revise the legislation governing DIY electrical work so that it must in future be inspected and passed by a qualified controller. If you are not familiar with how electricity works, get a professional to do all your installations or repairs. Assuming you are capable of carrying out simple electrical tasks, however, here are some basic rules:

HANDY HINTS

- Switch off an electrical appliance at the wall socket and unplug it before dismantling it or probing it with anything.
- As you dismantle the unit, make a careful note of what connection goes where; getting it wrong on re-assembly could turn the unit into a killer.
- Before doing any work on your home's fixed wiring (a socket for instance), let everyone in the home know what you are doing and then:

- Turn off the main power supply at the distribution board and place a large 'Do not touch' notice over the main board.
- Leave a light switched on, connected to an extension cord if necessary, and place it next to you so that, if anyone ignores your instructions, the light will come on and perhaps give you the split second warning that could save your life. An alternative is to leave a radio or TV on and turned up to full volume. You might deafen your neighbours for a minute or two, but it will be worth it.

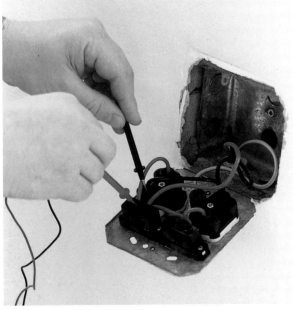

Test an electrical socket before working on it; taking two precautions too many is better than taking one too few.

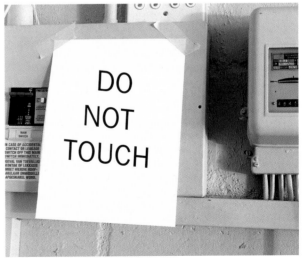

Use a large, clear sign on the distribution board to alert your family while you work on your home's electrical system, and make sure that everyone knows why the power is disconnected.

SAFETY OUTDOORS

Homes begin and end at the front gate, not at the front door, so it is important that when we focus on safety in the home, we give consideration to the exterior environment as well. Whether your backyard is only a few metres across or large and spacious, it often fulfils a variety of functions. Driveways and garages, sheds and workshops, play areas and patios all present their own set of potential dangers. Then, of course, there is the garden, which offers up a whole range of things to watch out for, from poisonous plants to the safe storage and use of insecticides and pesticides.

Home maintenance can also come under the general theme of exterior safety, as neglecting to repair or renovate in time can lead to deterioration. In the case of a rotten roof, this could necessitate costly repairs, but if a fence is left to fall apart, a child could easily slip through and wander onto a busy road. By thinking ahead and taking simple preventative steps, we can minimize the risk and ensure that our entire home environment, inside and out, is safe at all times.

IN THIS SECTION

Nonslip paved surfaces

Paved surfaces, such as paths and patios, are hard-wearing and virtually maintenance-free. There are many different surfacing materials, from rustic brick through stone chips to polished marble or travertine, all of which vary in their natural degree of unevenness and slipperyness when wet. Covered porches, patios or verandas are often given a surface treatment that blends with the internal décor, only to discover that their highly polished floor becomes treacherous when it gets wet. It can be an expensive exercise to relay a surface so, if you are installing a new path or patio, think carefully about what it will be used for. Outdoor living areas and paths leading to and from the house should be even, with a nonslip finish, whereas driveway surfaces might need to offer some traction, particularly if your area is prone to heavy rain or snowfalls.

POOL SURROUNDS

Swimming pool environments are designed for fun and play, but wet surfaces can be slippery. Apart from the bruises, sprains and other injuries that can result from falls, a major concern is someone falling into the water. The best solution is to forbid your children to run around the pool and to ensure that no one ever uses the pool alone or unsupervised.

- Ban everyone from diving or jumping into the shallow end of a swimming pool.
- When building a new pool, ensure that the coping (edge) provides an easy-to-grip handhold for even the smallest hands.
- Select a good quality, long-lasting nonslip surface for the surrounds – a pebble-dashed type of surface is worth considering. Take time to make your choice, as the right one could save you a great deal of heartache.

Pool paving should be made of nonslip material and have coping that is easy to grasp .

PATHS AND PAVING

REMOVING MILDEW AND MOSS FROM PAVING SURFACES

Mildew is a plant disease and moss a plant species, but both can cause some paving surfaces to become very slippery, particularly in wet weather or when there is dew. There are purpose-made products designed to eradicate mildew but these can take some time to work. For quick results, hire or buy a high-pressure water cleaner and blast the deposits away. Spreading coarse gravel over the worst areas will provide a temporary nonslip surface.

While velvety moss can look attractive between paving stones, for safety's sake, it is best to limit its spread to the edges of paths, or less-used parts of the garden. Gardeners tend to wear wellingtons or sturdy footwear that will not slip easily, but give mossy paths a miss when you are wearing 'everyday shoes'.

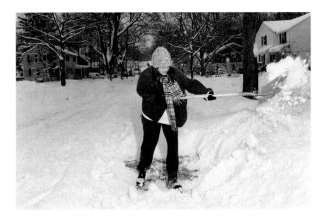

Removing snow from a pathway.

CLEARING SNOW-BOUND PATHS

The onset of winter often means having to deal with snow. If your home has a driveway or a path leading to the street, you'll have to invest in equipment to keep the path cleared and safe to walk on. A good-quality shovel is useful for clearing heavy falls of snow, and a broom will handle a light dusting. Motorized 'snowblowers' are a more costly option, but get the job done quickly.

Fresh powder snow is light and easy to clear; wet snow is always heavier. If you let snow lie in the hope that the sun will melt it, you may find that a thick layer of ice has formed underneath. The difference between day and night temperatures can lead to the formation of a thin layer of ice ('black ice'), which can lead to falls, especially if it is covered by fresh snow. Sand or fine grit scattered over your cleared path or driveway will prevent accidents and give tyres a better grip.

Salt can also be used to thaw ice and snow, but the use of salt can have negative consequences, such as salt build-up in your garden. Be sure to find out if municipal regulations in your area permit the use of salt.

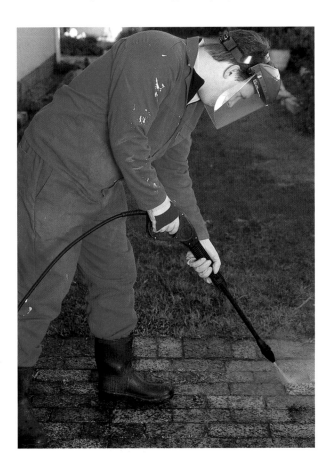

A high-pressure hose is an effective way to blast moss and mildew from paved surfaces.

Safety on the roof

The greater a roof's slope (pitch), the more dangerous it is. When in doubt, get the professionals in, and do not attempt to work on a high (double-storey) or steeply pitched roof yourself. If your roof is low, flat or has a gentle pitch, you can undertake simple repairs or maintence, providing you observe basic precautions and have a stable ladder. For more intricate work or repairs that cannot be done relatively quickly, it is safer to hire a tower scaffold so that you can stand on it and work from a fixed platform.

Tie yourself up there so that, if you do slip, the worst injury you can sustain is a graze and some wounded pride. To do this, throw a length of stout rope over the roof, more or less where you will be working, and secure it on the opposite side to a sturdy, stationary anchor, such as a large tree or patio column. Once you are on the roof, wrap the free end of the rope around your waist and secure it with a good knot. If you have a safety harness, tie it to that. Adjust the length of the rope as you work, but be careful not to trip over it or become entangled in it.

HANDY HINTS

- Begin by sweeping the work area before starting the repair job – even dry debris can be deadly and cause you to slip and fall.
- Wear nonslip footwear that fastens securely; slip-on sandals are a no-no.
- Warn others to stay away from the eaves – a dropped tool can cause a serious injury.
- When on the roof, put your tools on a nonslip mat so that they are secure.
- Use a rope to pull heavy tools up (when on a ladder, use both hands for this).
- Stay clear of overhead power or phone lines.
- If roofing material cannot take your full weight, step along the line of the roofing timbers or place boards across them to spread your weight.
- Do not go onto the roof while the surface is wet from dew or rain, or if there is any chance of rain or a storm with lightning.
- Do not work on roofs with a slope (pitch) greater than 30°.

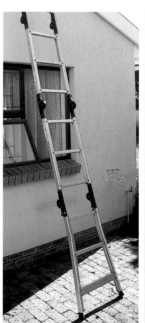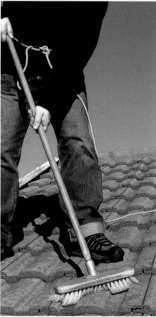

Make sure your ladder is at a safe angle (left). Sweep away any debris that may be slippery (right).

LADDER KNOW-HOW

Many gardening and DIY jobs require the use of a stepladder which should be steady, secure and in good condition. If you intend working on the roof, or have a double-storey house, there will be times when an extension ladder is required. Careless use of ladders can result in falls, with sometimes serious consequences, but taking a few simple steps before you ascend can minimize the chance of an accident.

- When using an extension ladder, keep the angle between it and the wall at about 75°.
- To stop the ladder slipping, drive a stake into the ground between the wall and the ladder's feet and tie the bottom rung to the stake. If the ground is soft, rest the ladder on a plank to provide extra support (*see* left).
- Climb the ladder a couple of rungs. If you are satisfied it will not slip backwards, continue. At the top, tie the top rungs to a secure stay, such as a roof truss. You can now climb up the ladder without the fear that it might slide away from under you, or fall away from the wall.
- Wear closed shoes, not loose or slip-on footwear when mounting a ladder.
- Don't mount a ladder if the soles of your shoes are wet due to rain or heavy dew.

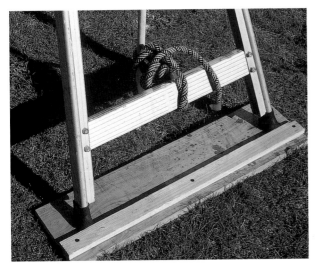

A secure base will prevent the ladder's feet from slipping away.

MAKING NONSLIP LADDER TREADS

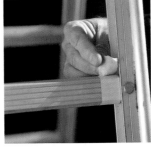
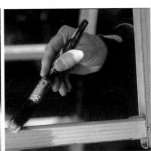

1. *Mask off areas that do not need paint.*

2. *Use bright paint for visibility.*

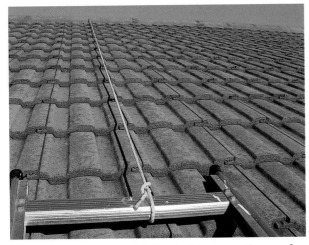

Secure the top rung of the ladder over the roof.

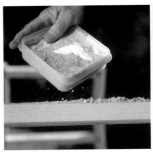
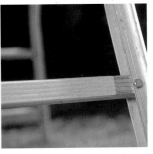

3. *Add coarse sand to wet paint.*

4. *Finish with a final coat of paint.*

Safety in the garage or workshop

The garage, shed or workshop is a place just begging for accidents to happen, filled as it is with sharp and potentially dangerous tools and materials. While regular DIYers tend to be careful and safety conscious, there are many potential hazards which can harm the uninitiated, so keep the garage or workshop securely locked when you are not using it.

HANDY HINTS

- Always wear protective gear when using cutting tools. Safety glasses or goggles are a must, and heavy-duty gloves are preferable. Depending on what you are doing, you may also require some form of ear protection.
- Use a Residual Current Device (RCD). It will cut the electricity if there is a fault or if a cable is accidentally cut.
- Wear clothing that covers most of your body and limbs (overalls). Do not wear loose-fitting garments with tassles or tie-fastenings that could catch in machinery.
- Make sure the lighting is adequate. A single, low-wattage overhead bulb can cast awkward shadows, particularly at night. If necessary, use a portable light on an extension cable to illuminate the item you are working on. If you spend a lot of time in the workshop, consider installing a decent lighting system.
- If you have long hair, tie it back. Clip back a long fringe so it can't flop in your eyes. Before you start, move into your working position to check whether your hair could get in the way.
- Keep children, pets and other distractions out of the workplace when you are busy.
- Never operate tools, power or otherwise, if you have consumed alcohol or are on a course of medication that makes you drowsy.
- Never operate power tools if you are angry or stressed as you will not be thinking straight.

- Ensure all electrical connections are sound and never overload fuses, circuits, motors or outlets. Never replace a blown fuse with one of a higher rating.
- Before using any tools or appliances, check all wiring for frayed ends or worn insulation.
- Never smoke near flammable materials or while using aerosol paints or sprays.
- If doing anything involving heat – welding for instance, do it away from where your flammable materials are stored.

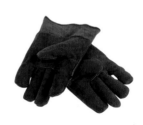
Gloves

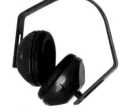
Ear protection

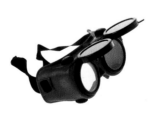
Goggles

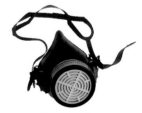
Dust mask

It is essential that you wear protective gear while working with cutting tools.

- Store flammable materials (such as paints, solvents and gas cylinders) so that you can get them out in a hurry. A handy solution is to mount a shelf, rack or storage bin on casters (an old bookshelf works well); in an emergency you can push the whole lot out of danger in one fell swoop.
- Keep your workshop tidy and clear of debris such as wood shavings, oily rags and used solvents in open containers. Contact your local authority about the proper disposal of chemicals or contaminated items, particularly those that may be harmful to the environment.
- If working with materials that produce fumes, work outside, or at least in the doorway. Using a fan to blow fumes away is an additional precaution.
- Ensure your work-piece is securely clamped into place before picking up any tool, particularly a power tool.

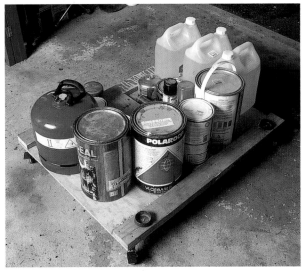

Store containers with flammable materials on an easily moveable trolley.

POWER TOOLS

Power tools such as drills, angle grinders and band saws are great labour-savers, but they can be deadly if misused. As they are designed to facilitate many DIY tasks, they make short work of any material to which they are applied, be it wood, metal, etc. The trouble is that most construction materials are much harder and more resilient than flesh and bone, which means that power tools can cut flesh like a hot knife through butter, and a great deal more painfully.

- Use power tools as intended by the manufacturers and for the purpose for which they were designed.
- Learn to use each tool before getting down to working with it.
- One basic rule is to hold a power tool properly and adopt the right stance before beginning to work – problems can arise if you stumble or trip.
- Before you begin to work,

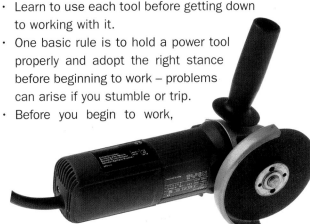

An angle grinder

clear the work area of anything that could distract you. If you get distracted, stop, and switch off the power tool. Do not work while carrying on a conversation, reprimanding the kids, or helping to decide what's for dinner.
- Don't mess about with the safety features. If a guard is provided, leave it in place; do not adapt it to keep it clear of the work piece.
- Ensure the cable is behind the machine. Work away from, never towards, the cable.
- High-quality power tools are well insulated, but don't use them outdoors in the rain, or while standing in a puddle on the floor.
- If you overload the tool and get that 'electric smell', run the machine under no load for a few seconds to allow the fan to cool down the mechanism.
- Never change an accessory, such as a blade or drill bit, without turning off and unplugging the machine.
- Secure the work-piece before you start work.
- Wear suitable protective gear for eyes, ears and face – the fine debris some tools throw out can cause health problems later in life.
- Tie-up long hair, and remove chains, bracelets or rings that could catch on parts of the power tool.
- Unplug power tools when you finish, clean and check them before putting them away.

Garden tools and equipment

In our attempts to create the perfect garden, we use a variety of pesticides, insecticides and weedkillers to combat pests or plant diseases. Many garden chemicals are poisonous and must be stored safely, out of reach of children and pets. Where possible, seek environmentally friendly alternatives and plant in such a way that natural organic defences, such as ladybirds (ladybugs), other insects and birds, reduce the need for artificial intervention.

HANDY HINTS

STORING GARDEN CHEMICALS

- Keep substances in their original containers, but check every so often to ensure that the packaging is in good condition and properly sealed. If a carton tears or breaks, transfer the contents to a new container and label it clearly. Dispose of the old one as laid down in your local ordinances.
- Some products are packed in cardboard boxes, which can deteriorate over time. Keep the contents, in the original packaging, in a larger container that seals (such as a plastic box or big zip-lock bag). Then, if the cardboard does disintegrate, there won't be any spillage.
- Treat garden chemicals as you would medicines, and discard any that have reached their expiry date, as they are likely to become less effective, and may even become unsafe.
- Store corrosive garden chemicals on lower shelves secured behind child resistant locks, rather than higher up. If one of them develops a leak, the contents will not flow over the other stored items. At best, boxes and labels might be damaged; at worst, the chemicals could combine and create a greater hazard.

Store poisons in a locked container.

USING GARDEN CHEMICALS

- When spraying plants, wear protective gear to cover your nose and mouth, and keep children and pets away from the area.
- Don't spray when there is a breeze, even a light one; as the spray will disperse and fine droplets could be carried far enough away to land in a person's or pet's eyes or food, or in a swimming pool or water feature.
- Check your garden on a regular basis and act as soon as you notice a problem with pests. Ignoring insects or pests could lead to your garden being overrun, instigating the trouble and expense of large-scale spraying.

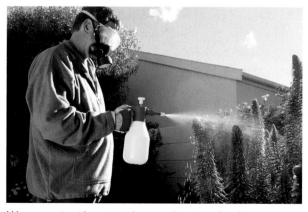

Wear protective goggles and a mask when spraying chemicals, and choose a windstill day.

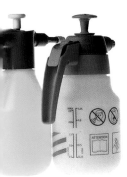

· Use the right spray. If it is not formulated for the pest in question, you'll be wasting time and money. Ensure you fully understand the instructions and keep any instruction leaflet that accompanies the product – the label on the container might not carry all the information you require.

· Always mix the formulation exactly as recommended in the instructions. Stronger is unlikely to be better and you can create more problems than you are solving.

· Mix sufficient spray solution for just a single application, as old mixtures are ineffective and could be dangerous. You might also forget what you have used, and could end up making a mistake the next time.

· Keep two clearly marked spray bottles – one for weedkillers and the other for insecticides. Clean each spray bottle thoroughly after use, as even a small chemical residue could contaminate a new solution.

· Never use empty garden sprayers for any other purpose. To discard a glass container, wrap it in a layers of newspaper and dispose of it safely. Puncture plastic containers and dispose of them safely as well.

USING GARDEN TOOLS SAFELY

Always use a Residual Current Device (RCD) when you operate power tools. Also bear in mind that the cutting parts of edge trimmers and electric or petrol-driven lawn mowers can do a lot of damage if they come loose. Spades and forks can do a fair share of damage and even small items, such as hand-shears or secateurs, can inflict a nasty wound if they are used carelessly, or dropped on a bare foot.

Never leave garden tools lying around when you have finished working with them. Take a few extra minutes to clean or oil them and put them away securely. In that way they'll be ready for the next time and you will also reduce the risk of injury in an unnecessary accident.

· When buying electric tools for use in the garden, for greater safety, select those which are double-insulated.

· Some electric mowers are designed to stop within a few seconds of being switched off, while others have blades that continue to rotate momentarily after being switched off. If you can, choose the former because, in an accident, the quicker the blades come to a standstill, the better.

· Never join two power cables to make a longer one or repair a cut by making a join. Taped joins pull apart and aren't waterproof. Buy a new cable.

· Ensure all exterior cables are bright orange or yellow, so they stand out against the green of your lawn.

· Switch off and unplug a mower, edge trimmer or bandsaw before you attempt to unclog it, or do any other work on it, such as lubricating, cleaning or adjusting.

· If you are up a ladder when using a hedge trimmer, work only within comfortable arm's reach. Rather climb down and move the ladder than risk a fall by stretching too far.

· Always use a chain saw as directed. The chain rotates away from you on the top pass, and towards you along the lower cutting edge so that if it jumps or jams, it will jump away from you rather than towards you. Never try to cut using the top pass of the chain.

· When mowing the lawn, wear shoes that cover your feet completely, with soles that minimize the risk of slipping.

· Use eye protection, as clippings and flying debris could be driven into your eyes.

· Never use an electric mower in the early morning when there is still dew present, in the rain or just after rain has fallen.

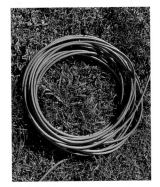

Brightly coloured extension cables stand out against the grass.

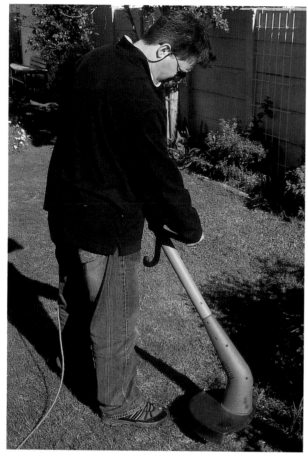

The power cable should always be behind you.

- Always work away from the cable to minimize the risk of cutting it.
- Always use a cable with a rating that is correct for the machine, or greater. Using too thin a cable could lead to it becoming overheated.
- Never bypass the safety switch on an electric tool. The switch is designed to stop the tool when it is released (for instance, if you slip).
- When checking the cutting parts of a petrol mower, switch it off and pull off the spark plug lead before turning the machine on its side. If you fail to take this precaution and turn the blades by hand, to remove grass clippings for example, the engine may start, and even one or two revolutions can result in severe injury.

- Always push a mower, never pull it, except perhaps to remove it from a confined area, such as between two flower beds. On longer runs, push – if you slip while pulling it towards you, your feet or hands could be injured.
- Work across slopes, not straight down or up; if you slip while pushing up a slope, the mower might roll down on you; if you slip down onto the mower, your feet could be injured.

STORING GARDEN TOOLS

- A safe and effective way to store large garden implements such as forks and spades is to place them 'sharp end' down in a big bin.
- Alternatively, attach a length of timber to the wall with two shorter lengths so that the beam stands clear by 15cm (6in) or so. Stack long-handled garden tools behind it. The front surface can be used to hang smaller items, such as potting trowels or secateurs.
- Keep the blades of garden shears closed by slipping a length of bicycle inner tube over the ends. This prevents the points from doing any real harm if the shears fall on anyone.

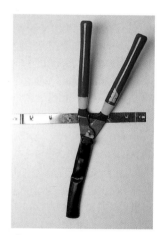

Cover the blades of unused garden shears with rubber tubing and store facing down.

- If you need to store a pitchfork or three-pronged fork with the prongs uppermost, slip lengths of old garden hose over each tine to stop the points injuring anyone.
- Never leave a rake lying on the ground with its prongs up – the experience of stepping on one and having the handle fly up into your face is something you won't forget in a hurry.

Reducing natural plant dangers

Even the best-tended garden can be a dangerous trap for the unwary. Different plants pose differing degrees of danger, from downright deadly to reasonably benign. While most of us would consider ourselves safe in our own gardens, we can get scratched by branches, prick ourselves on thorns or get sap or pollen in our eyes. Unless you are certain of your identification, it is best to assume that any unknown plant poses a risk, even if it is just of an irritating rash. On a more serious level though, while adults don't normally go around putting bits of plants into their mouths, children certainly do, and if a curious child 'investigates' poisonous leaves, berries or fruits, it is easy to have a poisoning emergency on your hands.

Every region and climate is home to common garden plants you need to watch out for. Some are widespread, others are endemic to a small area. Get to know the local plants of your region, and ask your garden centre or nursery for advice before selecting unfamiliar plants, particularly if you have toddlers or pets in the home. Some flowers and trees produce copious amounts of pollen, or have fine fibres or spores that can irritate the airway of individuals susceptible to allergies or asthma. If you are affected, getting rid of the offending plants is probably the only solution.

Many attractive garden plants are poisonous. Sometimes the whole plant is deadly, but often only one part of the plant is affected, perhaps the berries, roots, bulbs or leaves; the sap of oleander bushes for example, can cause painful inflammation if it enters the eyes. The thorns of the firethorn (*Pyracantha*) can cause blisters if the point penetrates the skin. Some plants are poisonous in their raw state but, when properly prepared, become part of dinner. Rhubarb is a good example: the leaves should not be consumed or fed to pets, but the edible stems are delicious when cooked.

Plants with thorns or spines pose a special danger. Although they may have a specific function, such as to create a secure border or hedge, they are often integrated with normal plantings. While everybody knows to keep clear of cacti or rose bushes, many plants and weeds have tiny spines or thorns that are less visible, but which can inflict a nasty scratch, sting or puncture, as experienced by anyone who has had a close encounter with stinging nettles (*Urtica dioica*).

When considering whether to plant thorny species, bear in mind their placement within the garden. A sisal plant (*Agave sisalana*), its fleshy leaves edged with thorns and tipped with a formidable spike, poses a danger at the best of times, but if it is located at the bottom of a grassy bank where children roll and play, the implications are magnified.

When it comes to safety, the best rule of thumb for gardeners is to know which plants are dangerous and where they are located, and make sure that everyone in the family, including children, is aware of them and why they should leave them alone. Ultimately if, despite doing everything you can to teach your children what not to do, you are still concerned, removing the offending plants is probably the safest route to take.

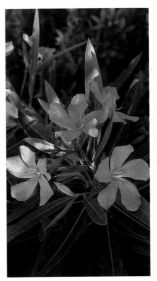

The oleander is very poisonous.

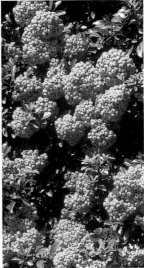

Firethorn can cause painful blisters.

WATER SAFETY

In warm climates, recreation in and on water is high on the list of preferred pastimes. When the sun is hot, we enjoy spending days at the beach, frolicking by the river or lazing around the pool. But, while many people think only in terms of swimming when it comes to safety and responsible behaviour in water, pastimes such as boating, fishing or scuba diving, also demand proper attention to safety, particularly when they take place at sea, where weather and tidal conditions come into play. Whenever you venture onto the water, pay attention to local weather and water conditions. Get out of, or off, the water at the first sign of approaching bad weather, particularly if it looks like a storm accompanied by lightning. As much as water gives us pleasure, failing to treat it with respect can prove fatal. Parents of toddlers need to be especially vigilant and maintain constant supervision anywhere near water, as drowning can occur in only a few centimetres of water. Although we consider young children to be most at risk, anyone, regardless of age, can get into trouble if basic common-sense and safety precautions are not followed in and around water.

IN THIS SECTION

Basic rules around water

SWIMMERS

- Learn to swim. Children can begin swimming lessons from a young age. If you have a pool at home, it is worth teaching your child to swim, and to respect water, as early as possible.
- Never swim alone, even in your own pool, as you never know when you might get into difficulties. At the beach or lake, swim only in areas protected by lifeguards.
- Obey all rules and posted signs regarding swimming, boating and water sports.
- Watch out for the 'dangerous too's'– too tired, too cold, too far from safety, too much sun, too much strenuous activity.
- Remember that swim aids, flotation devices and inflatable pool toys cannot replace parental supervision. Swim aids can suddenly slip or shift out of position, or an inflatable toy could lose air, leaving the child in a dangerous situation.

- Don't mix alcohol and water. Alcohol impairs your judgement, balance and coordination, affects your swimming, diving skills and motor coordination, and reduces your body's ability to stay warm.

BOATERS

- Ensure that you are familiar with the rules and regulations governing the use of powered craft, including jet skis, and obey them. Don't go boating in restricted waters, or operate your craft recklessly, or if you are under the influence of alcohol – the penalties are likely to be severe. Furthermore, if anyone is injured as a result of your negligent behaviour you may face civil action.

Water games are fun, but even the most innocent paddle in a baby pool can turn into a disaster. Be alert and on the lookout for trouble and don't rely on others to look after your child.

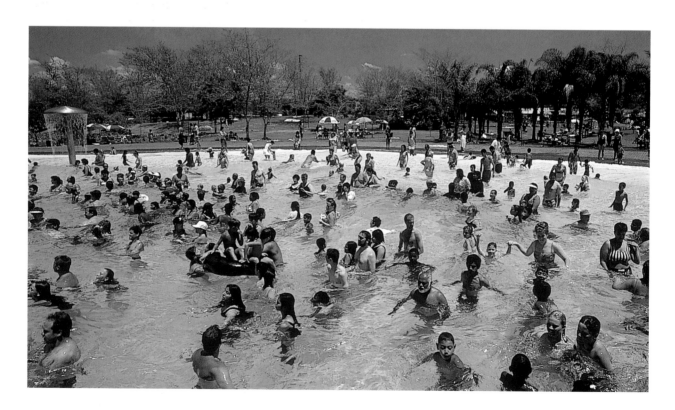

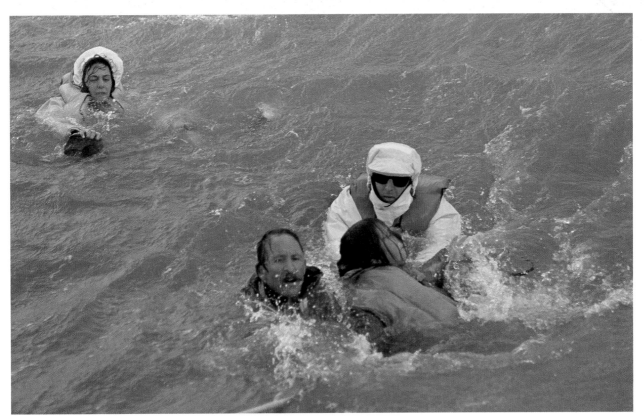
A professional rescue operation in progress.

LEGAL ASPECTS

When it comes to issues of safety, the law is usually on the side of the victim. 'What would a reasonable person be reasonably expected to think' is a question to bear in mind when considering circumstances that might cause injury, particularly if they occur as a result of negligence. Every case is different, but if you fail to take reasonable precautions with regard to the possible impact on the safety and wellbeing of others, you could be faced with criminal and/or civil actions of immense gravity. Ignorance of the law is no excuse, though it might affect whether an accused is deemed to have intended to commit the crime or not (in legal terminology this is called mens rea). But don't count on it.

THE IMPLICATIONS OF BEING RESCUED

The cost of rescuing a swimmer, sailor or anyone else in trouble on the water can be considerable. While the lifeguard who dives in and brings you to shore with little more than wounded pride may expect nothing more than a heartfelt 'thank you' and perhaps a donation to a rescue organization, in some countries, the cost of a rescue can be considerable. Rescue services are not always paid for by the state and you may be presented with a large bill, particularly if your own negligence or stupidity was the cause of the incident.

If you defy warnings and swim when conditions are hazardous and then get into difficulties, you could be held responsible for the cost of any operation required to rescue you, and face legal action for putting the lives of your rescuers at risk. Likewise, putting to sea in a small boat when a storm is approaching is foolhardy and the cost of effecting a rescue could be substantial.

Coastguard or private rescue craft, helicopters and emergency medical services all cost money to operate; if it is deemed that you are responsible for your predicament, you will have to reimburse the costs. If you spend a lot of time on the water, in whatever capacity, ask your insurance broker to amend your policy to cover any rescue services you may require.

Children and water

It is a sad global statistic that most drownings of children under the age of four occur in home swimming pools. By strictly adhering to the safety regulations and ensuring that you pay undivided attention when your youngsters are splashing around in or near the water on a hot summer's day you will be able to prevent tragedy. City and local bylaws and ordinances vary from place to place and may change from time to time. If you intend building a pool or pond, make sure that you are familiar with what is required in terms of perimeter fencing, gates and other safety devices and precautions. Although most reputable contractors will be able to advise you, remember that the onus is on you to inform yourself and then to comply. Failure to do so could lead to civil or criminal action being taken against you in the event of an accident.

PONDS AND SWIMMING POOLS

While ponds or swimming pools are undoubtedly an asset that enhances a property's value and provides a lot of enjoyment, they claim lives every year, so never leave a child unobserved anywhere near water. Adult supervision is recommended at all times when children are around water.

- Restrict access to the water by enclosing it with a secure fence and a self-locking, self-closing gate. The fence should have vertical bars with openings no more than 10cm (4in) wide. Keep the gate locked when a pool is not being used. Any doors leading directly from the house to the area should also remain locked. Add further protection with an alarm or sensor system that makes a loud noise when the gate is opened.
- A resourceful child may find a way to climb over a fence, so be careful where you leave garden furniture or other items that can be easily moved to provide a handy step.

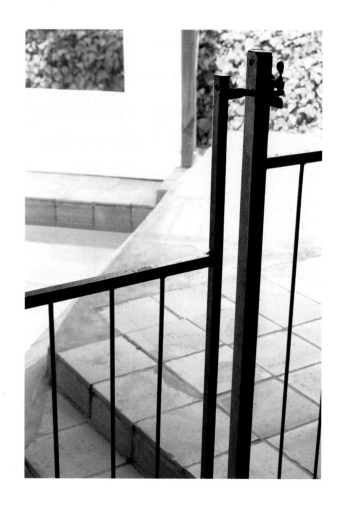

Enclose your swimming pool with a sturdy fence and ensure the gate is kept securely locked, especially when you are not around.

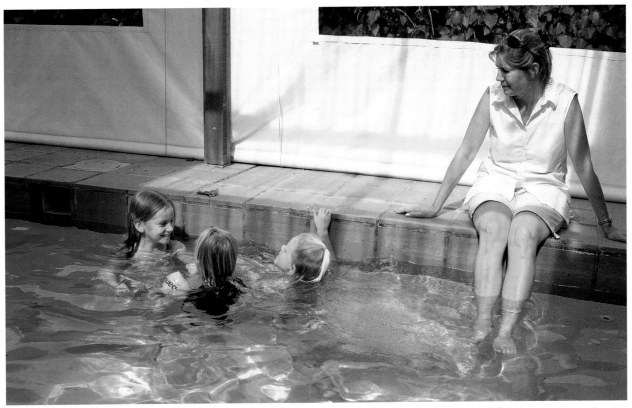

Always make sure that a competent adult is present when children are in the swimming pool.

- Keep basic lifesaving equipment near the pool. A sturdy pole, length of nylon rope and flotation devices are recommended.
- Toys can attract young children into the pool area, so pack them away after use. Floating toys are particularly dangerous as children may fall into the water while trying to retrieve them.
- Water makes some pool surrounds very slippery, so teach your children not to run around the pool. They should also not jump or dive in without checking first to see whether there is someone else on the surface or under the water.
- If a child goes missing in the home, check the pool area first. Go to the edge of the pool and scan the entire pool, bottom and surface, as well as the surrounding area. Hide-and-seek is a great game, but not around a pool.
- Buoyancy devices (swim aids) must have safety approval and must be appropriate for the age of the child. A small child is more top-heavy than an adult; if the design is faulty or the fit is wrong, the child could end up floating face-down.

- Swimming pool parties increase the risk of accidents. Ensure there are sufficient adult supervisors present, focus your attention on the children and keep a mobile (cellular) or cordless phone nearby so that you can call for assistance in an emergency.
- Learn **rescue breathing** (*see* p168) and **resuscitation** (*see* pp164–71) and insist that your children's properly trained. Display resuscitation instructions somewhere close to the pool area, and keep a list of your local emergency response numbers near the telephone.

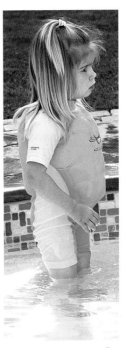

Swim aids must fit well in order to be effective.

- Store pool chemicals securely. Chlorine, pool acid and other chemicals are hazardous if mishandled and you don't want your budding scientist conducting experiments to see what might happen when they mix. The result could be severe burns, even the loss of a hand or eye.
- Make sure your pool's pump system is covered and that the power cable leading to it is buried underground and well protected from inadvertent damage by a garden fork. Ideally, sheath the cable in a conduit to protect the insulation and bury it at a depth of at least 30cm (12in). You can reinforce the safety aspect if you place bricks or paving slabs on top of the conduit before refilling the trench. For future reference, make a note of the position of the cable on your house plans, including a note stating how deep it has been buried and how it is protected.

PONDS AND WATER FEATURES

Virtually any body of water is appealing to toddlers and young children but, as they are naturally inquisitive and resourceful, in order to keep them safe, you must ensure that even the most remote chance of an accident is neutralized.

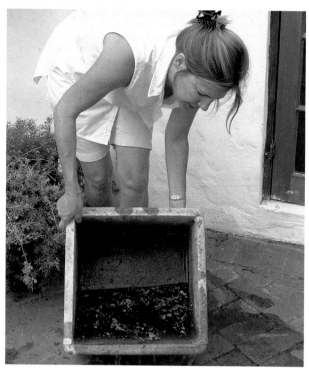

Empty rain-filled plant pots that are not in use.

- If power is required, select a pump that operates at a lower voltage than your normal mains current. In such a case, the step-down transformer will be close to the mains plug-in point, with the low-voltage cable (buried and protected as with a pool cable) going into the garden and to the pump. Electricity and water don't usually mix, nor does electricity and a garden fork, so check with your local authority beforehand to ensure that you abide by the regulations when laying the cable to the pond. When working on a pool or pond pump, switch off the power and unplug the connection before doing the job.
- If you have an external rain butt or water collection tank, make sure that the lid is securely padlocked at all times. After heavy rains, make a habit of emptying buckets, plant pots or other garden containers into which a toddler could fall.

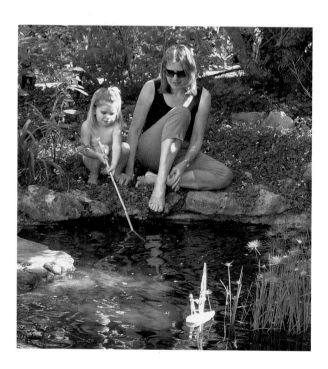

Always make sure to have an adult nearby when children are playing around a water feature.

Public waters

It is impossible to cover all aspects of safety on public waters. There are too many individual variables to take into account, not least of which is our own attitude towards safety and the behaviour and attitude of those with whom share the water. All the basic rules of water safety apply when you are swimming or boating on public waterways, but perhaps the most important one is never to get into unfamiliar water without taking the time to consider the potential dangers and assess the risks. Many local authorities demarcate specific areas for swimming, non-motorized water sports (such as surfing and sail boarding) and boating, but if there are no notices to this effect, you might find boats being launched in areas where swimmers, surfers and sailboarders play, so pick your beach or water frontage carefully. Despite regulations governing access to open water there are often grey areas when it comes to small craft. It goes without saying that responsible boat-owners comply with the relevant statutory requirements and are properly qualified to operate a vessel before they take to the water. If you take your sail-boat, powerboat or jet ski on holiday with you, ensure you observe the local rules, are familiar with the conditions, and have the local emergency numbers close at hand.

SAFETY AT SEA AND IN RIVERS

- Check surf and water conditions. If there are warning flags up (these vary from country to country), observe them.
- Select a supervised area. A lifeguard who can help in an emergency is the best safety factor.
- Even good swimmers can have an unexpected emergency in the water, so never swim alone.
- If there are no supervised areas, select a spot that has good water quality and safe conditions. Murky or churning water, hidden rocks, unexpected drop-offs, and aquatic plants are hazards. Strong tides, currents and big waves can spell tragedy. In rivers and lakes, water pollution can cause health problems for swimmers.
- Never jump or dive into water unless you are positive of its depth. Every year, many swimmers suffer serious neck and spinal cord injuries from diving headfirst into water that is too shallow.

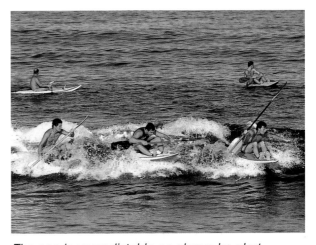

The sea is unpredictable so always be alert.

Remember that tides and wave movement can alter the depth of the water and create sand bars where there were none before.

- Don't swim too far from the shore, or too far up- or downriver, and make sure you always have enough energy to swim back, particularly if it is against a current. If you get caught in a crosscurrent, don't try to swim against it. Swim gradually out of the current by swimming across it.
- Be sure that docks and floating rafts are in good condition. A well-run open-water facility maintains its rafts and docks in good condition, with no loose boards or exposed nails. Never swim under a raft or dock. Always look before jumping off a dock or raft to be sure no one is in the way. When in the sea, stay away from piers, pilings, mooring buoys and scuba diving platforms.
- If you get caught in river rapids, keep your legs together, arms outspread and face downstream so that you can spot rocks or overhanging branches ahead and avoid them. Don't try to stand up. Rather crawl over to the nearest shore, cutting across the current. If you swim against it, you are unlikely to get anywhere very quickly.
- In lakes and rivers, drainage ditches built to handle water run-off are dangerous. After heavy rains, they can quickly change into raging rivers that can easily take a human life. Debris picked up by the rushing water adds to the danger.

- On rivers, a sharp bend tends to shelve towards the outer edge of the bend where the water is deepest and the bank is often steep and undercut. A swiftly flowing current will push you towards this deeper, outer area and you could be out of your depth very quickly.
- Whether you are going to the beach or to the shore of a lake or river, select an area that is well maintained. Clean restrooms and a litter-free environment show the management's concern for your health and safety.

BOATING AND MOTORIZED WATER ACTIVITIES

- Sign up for one of the many recognized training courses that are available. These will teach you general water safety and rescue techniques and prepare you for all eventualities.
- Before taking your boat out, sign out at the club, or give a responsible person details about the direction you plan to go in and how long you expect to be gone. If you do not have radio or cellphone contact, do not deviate from your plan – certainly not substantially anyway. This is important because if you are delayed by a change in the weather, become lost, or encounter any other problems, you want help to be able to reach you.

In rivers, follow the current feet first so that you can see obstacles in your path.

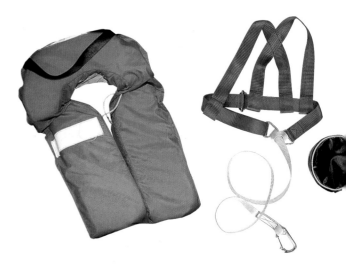

A life jacket and a harness must be worn at all times when boating or fishing.

- Approved life jackets or safety harnesses must be worn at all times, even when fishing. Children's jackets should be correct for body size and weight.
- Keep a watch for vessels or activities on and in the water. Be aware of boats that may have divers or snorkellers in the water, and of boardsailors trying to right their craft. Slow down when passing, and clear the area by a wide margin.
- Operate your craft with courtesy and common sense. Follow the traffic pattern of the waterway, keep to marked channels and adhere to the 'rules of the road' as indicated by navigation buoys and/or lights. Obey no-wake and maximum speed zones, and watch the water ahead of you at all times. Do not operate the boat at night or in restricted areas.
- Power boat operators should use extreme caution around swimmers and surfers. Maintain a slow speed until your craft is away from the shore, swimming areas and docks. Avoid passing too close to other boats, or jumping wakes.

The rules of the 'road' state that sail must give way to larger, powered vessels in a narrow channel.

- Jet skiers should always travel in groups of two or more as you never know when an emergency might occur. When you are far from shore, even running out of petrol constitutes an emergency, particularly if the wind is blowing you out to sea!
- Ensure your equipment is in good shape and operating properly before setting off.
- When water-skiing, boat operators must turn the motor off when approaching a fallen skier. Have a person aboard to watch and assist the skier, who should use proper hand signals to communicate with the boat operator. When coming in to land, skiers should run parallel to the shore and come in slowly. Sit down if you are coming in too fast.
- Alcohol and boats don't mix for the same reasons as drinking and driving (impaired judgement, lack of concentration and a greater propensity for accidents), so keep these activities separate.

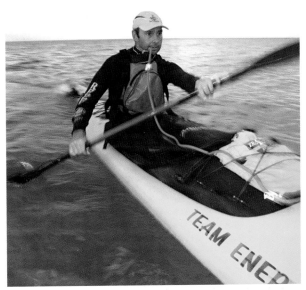

If you are planning a longer kayaking trip, ensure that you are suitably equipped.

NON-MOTORIZED WATERCRAFT

- Never go out alone. If you are new to an area, watch the locals and ask questions about the wind and wave conditions before putting to sea.
- Board sailors must always wear an approved life jacket or safety harness and check all their equipment before setting out.
- For rafting or tubing on white water a buoyancy aid, PFD and protective helmet are essential.
- In cold conditions, surfers and board sailors should wear a full wetsuit to prevent hypothermia. On sunny days, a long top and sun-block (sunscreen) will help to reduce the risk of wind- and sunburn.

Personal flotation device (PFD)

- Remember that you need good physical strength and swimming ability for most water sports. Being on a board or tube does not negate the need to be able to swim!
- Do not overload a raft or tube.
- Watch out for swimmers and other water users, particularly when coming around a bend in a river.
- Do not go rafting or boating in rivers after a heavy downpour, as flash floods may occur.

SNORKELLING AND SCUBA DIVING

- If you are new to snorkelling, practise in shallow water until you feel confident. Check your equipment carefully and know how it functions. Learn how to clear water from the snorkel and how to put your mask back on while you tread water.
- Be careful not to swim or be carried by a current too far from shore or the boat.
- Observe the 'buddy' rule and never dive alone or snorkel alone in deep waters.
- No reputable dive operator will sell, hire or refill a scuba cylinder unless you produce a valid C-card (diving licence), so there are no short-cuts to proper lessons and certification before venturing underwater. Once certified, do not dive in environments for which you are not qualified. Your dive master or boat operator should ensure that you are trained and equipped for any dive you are about to undertake.
- Responsible divers 'plan the dive and dive the plan'. When underwater, do not deviate from your agreed plan. Monitor your underwater time and remaining air, allowing for any decompression stops you may have to make on the way up.

- A common mistake novice scuba divers make is to dive when they have a cold, sinus infection or other respiratory ailment. You will not be able to equalize properly, resulting in a painful and unpleasant dive.

WATER THEME-PARKS

- Be sure the area is supervised by lifeguards. Read all posted signs, follow any directions given by the lifeguards and ask questions if you are not sure about the correct procedure.
- When you go from one attraction to another, remember that the water depth may differ.
- Before you start down a water slide, get into the correct position – face up and feet first.
- Some facilities provide life jackets at no charge. Anyone who cannot swim should wear a life jacket on all rides and attractions.

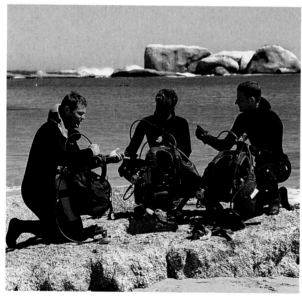

Safe diving means making sure that your equipment is in good working order before you enter the water.

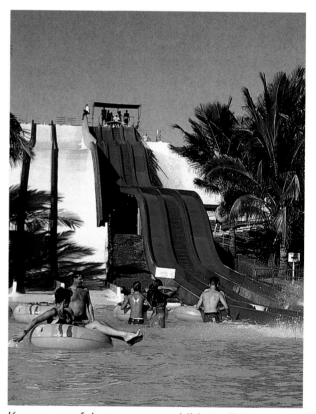

Keep a careful eye on your child at all times in a water theme-park. It could slip and fall, or be pushed into deep water – so be alert.

BASIC LIFESAVING TIPS

RESCUING YOURSELF

If you find yourself in trouble, there are steps you can take to help yourself while you wait to be rescued.

- As you fall in, hold your breath and close your mouth to avoid swallowing water. Once in the water, try to stand – some rivers and dams may not be as deep as they seem.
- If you cannot stand, and the shore is some distance away, tread water. Keep your body upright and use your hands and feet to 'pedal' towards the shore or nearest safe object.
- If you are wearing heavy or bulky clothing or shoes, see if you can remove them, and perhaps even use them as flotation devices.
- Reduce the loss of body heat by adopting a sitting position in the water, drawing your knees up and hugging them to your chest.
- If you can swim, and conditions allow it, make for the nearest shore. Go with the flow of the current and swim with a stroke that does not tire you too quickly, especially if you have some distance to cover. If you get tired, float on your back or tread water for a while.
- If someone throws you a life ring or some form of flotation device, make sure you get a firm grasp on it, so that they can tow you to shore. If the current is strong, or there are breaking waves, try to use the natural ebb and flow to assist the rescuer, but allow them to take control of the situation.

HELPING OTHERS

- Do not attempt to rescue someone else unless you have had training and know what to do.
- If you need to rescue someone else from deep water, be aware that they are likely to panic, and could force you underwater.
- Do not swim out unless there is no other means of reaching the person. Take something they can hold onto, such as a life ring, or rescue buoy. Improvise with a towel or piece of clothing if there is nothing else to hand.

MOUTH-TO-MOUTH RESUSCITATION

1. *Gently tilt the head back and lift the chin to open the airway. Ensure that nothing restricts breathing.*

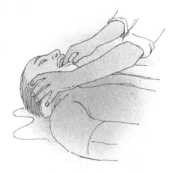

2. *Pinch the nostrils closed, take a deep breath, place your mouth firmly over his.*

3. *Exhale deeply into his mouth for two seconds and see if the chest rises. If it doesn't check the airway for blockage.*

4. *As his chest falls, breathe in again deeply and repeat. Check the pulse to see if the heart is beating. If it is, continue breathing into his mouth every five seconds until breathing is normal. Then place in the recovery position.*

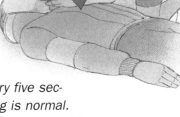

QUICK REMINDER – SAFE

In an emergency, the last thing you need is to wonder 'what should I do next?' By memorizing the well-tested sequence of actions summarized below and on the opposite page, you will be able to take effective action in those first vital minutes of an emergency situation.

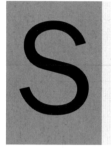

SHOUT FOR HELP
Summon medical assistance or the emergency services immediately. The ideal is to send a responsible person to make the call while you immediately begin attending to the casualty.

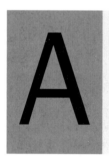

APPROACH WITH CARE
Check the surroundings for any hazard that might endanger you or the casualty. This also includes an assessment of the casualty's state of mind.

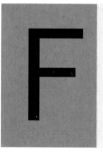

FREE FROM DANGER
Even though a casualty should not be moved until the emergency services arrive, this must be weighed against any further risk to the casualty or to yourself and any other rescuers.

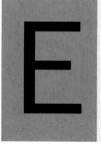

EVALUATE THE ABC
Having taken the above precautions, you are now ready to assess the level of consciousness and the casualty's vital functions (the ABC) and commence resuscitation if required.

QUICK REMINDER – ABC

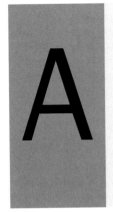

AIRWAY
An unconscious person may need to have his airway cleared to enable him to breathe on his own. Turn the casualty onto his back and use head tilt and chin lift to position the head (*see* p164). If a neck injury is suspected, support the head carefully during any movement; first try the chin lift alone.

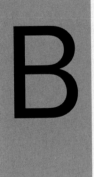

BREATHING
Having positioned and cleared the airway, you need to establish whether the casualty is breathing, by looking for chest movement, listening for sounds of breathing, and feeling for exhaled breath. If there are no signs of breathing within 10 seconds, give rescue breaths (*see* p168).

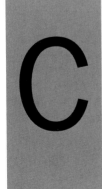

CIRCULATION
If the casualty is breathing, or has resumed breathing once the airway is cleared, check the circulation by feeling for a pulse in the carotid artery (below the jawbone) or brachial artery (at the elbow joint). If you cannot feel a pulse within 10 seconds, start chest compressions (*see* p169).

GLOSSARY

A

ABC Acronym meaning A = Airway; B = Breathing; C = Circulation.

Abdominal thrust The manual thrusts to create a pressure wave to expel an airway obstruction.

Abrasion A scraped or scratched skin wound.

Acute A condition that comes on quickly and has severe symptoms (*see* **chronic** for comparison).

Airway The route for air into and out of the lungs.

Allergens Substances which trigger an allergic reaction in the body.

Amputation Complete removal of a body part.

Anaesthetic (general) Use of injected or inhaled drugs to induce unconsciousness for surgery

Anaesthetic (local) Use of drugs to induce numbness in a specific area of the body for painless surgery

Anaphylaxis Very severe form of allergic response, usually to foods, drugs, venomous bites or stings.

Angina (pectoris) Sudden pain in the chest due to a lack of blood supply to the heart muscle.

Artery Blood vessel carrying blood from heart to organs.

Arteriosclerosis A name for several conditions that cause the walls of the arteries to become thick, hard and inelastic.

Asthma Condition causing recurrent wheezing, cough and breathing difficulty.

Atherosclerosis A form of arteriosclerosis caused by fat deposits in the arterial walls.

B

Back blows Sharp blows to the upper back, done to relieve an airway obstruction.

Bacteraemia Germs multiplying in the bloodstream

Bacteria Germs which can cause disease.

Basic life support Maintaining ABC without equipment.

Blood pressure The pressure of blood against the walls of arterial blood vessels.

Blood volume The total amount of blood in the heart and blood vessels.

Brachial pulse Pulse felt on the inner upper arm, usually taken on infants.

Bruise Broken blood vessels under the skin.

C

Capillaries Very small blood vessels that link the arteries and the veins and allow gases and nutrients to move into and out of the tissues.

Capillary refill test A test to determine whether a person is in shock: press on the casualty's finger tip for five seconds and then release. If the normal pink skin colour does not return within two seconds, the person suffers from **shock** (*see* p38).

Carbon dioxide (CO₂) A waste gas produced by the cells and breathed out via the lungs.

Carbon monoxide (CO) A dangerous, colourless and odourless gas which displaces the carrying of oxygen by the red blood cells.

Cardiovascular disease Refers to disorders of the heart and blood vessels, such as high blood pressure and arteriosclerosis.

Cardiac arrest The sudden stopping of cardiac function with no pulse, and unresponsiveness.

Carotid artery The main artery of the neck, used to assess the carotid pulse.

Cartilage A tough, rubbery tissue that covers the surfaces where bones meet, and also forms part of the nose and ears.

Central nervous system Part of the nervous system consisting of the brain and the spinal cord.

Cerebrovascular accident (CVA) A stroke, or the sudden stopping of circulation to part of the brain.

Cervical collar A device used to immobilize and support the neck.

Cervical spine Portion of spinal column located in the neck.

Chest thrusts Series of manual thrusts to the chest to relieve airway obstruction in infants and children.

Chronic A long-standing, persistent or relapsing condition or illness.

Chronic obstructive pulmonary disease (COPD) A term describing a group of chronic lung diseases that cause obstructions in the airway and lungs.

Circulation Collective term describing the blood, heart and blood vessels.

Closed wound Where the skin is intact.

Compound fracture Bone injury with associated damage to the neighbouring soft tissues.

Concussion A temporary disturbance of brain function, usually caused by a blow to the head.

Convulsions Involuntary contraction of muscles caused by head injury, poisoning, or sometimes no obvious cause, as in epilepsy.

Coronary artery Vessel which feeds the heart muscle.

Cornea The transparent front part of the eyeball.

Croup Inflammation of upper airway, resulting in harsh cough and difficulty breathing in.

Cyanosis A bluish or grey colour of the skin due to insufficient oxygen in the blood, or poor circulation.

D

Defibrillation Applying an electrical shock to a fibrillating heart (*see* Fibrillation).

Dehydration State whereby the body loses more fluid than is being replaced, with risk of damage to the brain or kidneys.

Deoxygenated blood Blood containing a low level of oxygen.

Diabetes A disease caused by lack of insulin, or insulin resistance, which causes excess blood sugar.

Diarrhoea Frequent soft or watery bowel movements.

Dislocation When bone surfaces at a joint are out of alignment.

Dysentery Infection in the large bowel, with loose stool containing blood and mucus.

E

Embedded object A foreign object stuck in the skin or impaled in body tissue.

Embolus Any foreign matter, such as a blood clot, fat clump or air bubble carried in the blood stream.

Emetic A substance which causes vomiting.

EMS Emergency Medical Services system; a community's group of services which respond to emergencies.

Emphysema A chronic lung disease characterized by overstretched alveolar walls (*see* COPD).

Epidermis The outer-most layer of skin.

Epiglottis A lid-like piece of tissue which protects the entrance to the larynx (voice-box).

Epiglottitis Infection, usually in children, resulting in a swelling of the epiglottis (may cause croup).

Epilepsy A chronic brain disorder characterized by recurrent convulsions.

Exhalation Expiration, or breathing out.

F

Fibrillation Uncoordinated ineffective contractions of the heart muscle.

Flail chest A condition in which several ribs are broken in at least two places, creating a segment that does not move normally.

First aid The help given to an injured or suddenly ill person, using readily available materials.

First responders People such as the police, fire fighters, ambulance attendants, etc. who are called first to an emergency scene.

Fontanelle The soft gaps between the bones of the skull that can be felt on babies' heads.

Fracture A cracked or broken bone.

Frostbite Tissue damage as a result of exposure to extremely cold conditions.

G

Gangrene Irreversible destruction of tissue, most commonly as a result of poor circulation.

Gastric distention A swelling of the stomach, usually with air, due to ventilating with excessive volume or force during artificial respiration.

Gauze An open mesh material used for dressings.

Glasgow Coma Scale (modified) A method of estimating the casualty's level of consciousness.

H

Haematoma (bruise) Collection of blood caused by a damaged blood vessel.

Heart attack Chest pain due to a death of a part of the heart muscle; a myocardial infarction.

Heart failure A weakened heart muscle that is unable to push blood forward; fluid backs up into the lungs, causing swelling of the ankles etc.

Heat cramps Painful muscle spasms due to excessive loss of fluid and salts by sweating.

Heat stroke A life-threatening emergency where the temperature regulation mechanism cannot cool the body and the temperature is far above normal; also called hyperthermia or sunstroke.

Heimlich manoeuvre (*see* **abdominal thrusts**).

Hernia Rupture.

History Information about the casualty's problem, symptoms, events leading up to the problem, applicable illnesses or medications, etc.

Hyperglycaemia Abnormally high blood sugar.

Hypertension High blood pressure.

Hyperthermia Too high body temperature.

Hyperventilation Too deep or rapid respirations.

Hypoglycaemia Too low blood sugar levels.

Hypothermia Too low body temperature.

Hypoxia Too low levels of oxygen in the tissues.

I

Immobilization Placing some type of restraint along a body part to prevent movement.

Immunization Artificially induced protection against certain illnesses.

Incontinence Loss of bladder or bowel control.

Infarction An area of tissue death due to lack of blood flow.

Inflammation A tissue reaction to irritation, illness or injury; shows as redness, heat, swelling or pain.

Inhalation Breathing in, inspiration.

Insulin Hormone produced by the pancreas; important in the regulation of blood sugar levels.

Insulin coma/shock Too low blood sugar levels (hypoglycaemia) due to excessive insulin.

Involuntary muscle Muscles not under conscious control, such as the heart, intestines etc.

Ischaemic Lacking sufficient oxygen; as in ischaemic heart disease.

J

Joint A place where two or more bones meet.

Joint capsule A tough covering over a joint.

L

Laceration A jagged wound from a rip or tear.

Ligament A tough cord of tissue which connects bone to bone.

Lymphatic system A system of vessels and glands which collects strayed proteins leaked from blood vessels and cleanses the body of microbes and other foreign matter.

M

Mechanism of injury The force that causes an injury and the way it is applied to the body.

Meningitis Inflammation of the membranes around the brain.

Micro-organisms Germs which can cause illness.

Mucous membrane A thin, slick, transparent lining, covering the tubes and internal organs such as the inner surface of the mouth, nose, eye, ear, intestine etc.

Musculoskeletal system All the bones, muscles and connecting tissues which allow movement.

Myocardial infarction Death of part of the cardiac (heart) muscle; heart attack.

N

Nervous system The brain, spinal cord and nerves which control the body's activities.

Nitroglycerine A drug used to ease the workload on the heart; often carried as a pill or spray by people with angina.

O

Obstructed airway A blockage in the air passageway to the lungs.

Otitis media Inflammation in the cavity behind the eardrum.

Oxygen An odourless, colourless gas essential to life. (Symbol O_2).

P

Papular (rash) Describes skin rashes where the markings are red and raised above the normal skin surface, e.g. papular urticaria.

Paralysis Inability to move, or loss of motor function in one or more parts of the body.

Peritonitis Inflammation of inner lining of abdomen.

Pertussis Whooping cough.

Physiology The study of the functions of the body.

Plasma A pale yellow fluid containing proteins, i.e. blood after the cells have been removed.

Pleural membrane A slick membrane covering the outside surface of the lungs and the inside surface of the chest cavity (thorax).

Pneumonia Inflammation of the lungs.

Pnuemothorax An accumulation of air in the pleural space. Normally the pleural space contains a negative pressure, or vacuum; the air mass (instead of a vacuum) collapses the lung under it.

Primary survey Assessing the casualty for life-threatening injuries and giving appropriate first aid.

Pulmonary artery The major artery emerging from the right ventricle; carries deoxygenated blood to the lungs.

Pulse The rhythmic expansion and relaxation of the arteries caused by the contractile force of the heart; usually felt where the vessels cross a bone near the surface.

R

Red blood cells The most numerous type of blood cells, which carry oxygen.

Respiratory arrest Stopped breathing.

Retina The lining at the back of the eyeball which converts light rays into nerve impulses.

RICE R=rest; I=ice; C=compression; E=elevation. First aid for certain bone and joint injuries.

Rule of Nines A system of estimating the amout of skin surface damaged in a burn injury.

S

Secondary survey Assessing the casualty for non-life-threatening injuries and then giving appropriate first aid.

Spontaneous pneumothorax Air in the pleural space which has leaked from a weakened area of a lung.

Sprain Supporting tissues about a joint (such as ligaments) are stretched, partly or completely torn (*see also* **strain**).

Sternum The breastbone.

Strain A stretched muscle (*see also* **sprain**).

Sucking chest wound A chest wound through which air is pulled into the chest cavity. It can cause a collapse of the lung beneath.

Suffocation Inability to obtain enough oxygen due to lack of oxygen in the atmosphere, or obstruction of the mouth and nose.

Symptom An indication of illness or injury experienced by a casualty; cannot be detected by an observer without asking.

T

Tendon A tough cord of tissue that attaches muscles to bones and other tissues.

Tetanus A type of bacteria which invades wounds and cause severe muscle spasms.

Transient ischaemic attack (TIA) Temporary signs and symptoms of a stroke due to a lack of sufficient oxygen to the brain.

Trachea Main tube through which air passes to and from lungs (windpipe).

Traction Gently but firmly pulling below a fracture to bring the limb into alignment.

Trauma Any physical or psychological injury.

Triage A system of assigning priorities for first aid and/or transportation for multiple casualties.

V

Vaccination *see* Immunization.

Vein A blood vessel carrying blood to the heart.

Ventilation Supplying air to the lungs.

Ventricles The muscular lower chambers of the heart which pump blod to the arteries.

Ventricular fibrillation A quivering action of the heart muscles so that little or no blood is pumped into the arteries.

Vital signs Signs that show the basic condition of the casualty: breaths per minute, heart rate, temperature and level of consciousness.

W

Wheezing Breathing difficulty resulting in whistling sound on breathing out.

White blood cells Blood cells which are involved in immunity and control of infection.

INDEX

Note: *italicized* page numbers refer to illustrated material.

CONTACTS AND SAFETY ORGANIZATIONS

UNITED KINGDOM
THE BRITISH RED CROSS
44 Moorfields
London EC2Y 9AL
tel: +44 (0) 870 170 7000
www.redcross.org.uk

ST JOHN AMBULANCE
27 St John's Lane
London EC1M 4BU
tel: +44 (0) 870 010 4950
www.sja.org.uk

ROYAL SOCIETY FOR THE PREVENTION OF ACCIDENTS (ROSPA)
Edgbaston Park
353 Bristol Road
Edgbaston, Birmingham B5 7ST
tel: +44 (121) 248 2000
www.rospa.com

USA
NATIONAL SAFE KIDS CAMPAIGN
1301 Pennsylvania Ave, NW
Suite 1000
Washington, DC 20004-1707
tel: +91 202 662 0600
www.safekids.org

CANADA
SAFE KIDS CANADA
Suite 2105, 180 Dundas Street West
Toronto, ON M5G 1Z8
tel: +91 416 813 7288
www.sickkids.ca/safekidscanada

GERMANY
SAFE KIDS GERMANY
Heilsbachstrasse 30
D-53123 Bonn
tel: +49 228 688 8340
www.kindersicherheit.de

FRANCE
COMMISSION DE LA SÉCURITÉ DES CONSOMMATEURS
Cité Martignac
111 rue de Grenelle
75353 Paris 07 SP
tel: +33 (1) 43 19 56 53
www.securiteconso.org

SOUTH AFRICA
CHILD ACCIDENT PREVENTION FOUNDATION OF SOUTH AFRICA (CAPFSA)
PO Box 791
Rondebosch 7701
tel: +27 (21) 685 5208
www.childsafe.org.za

AUSTRALIA
KIDSAFE CHILD ACCIDENT PREVENTION TRUST (CAPT)
PO Box 3515
Parramatta NSW 2124
tel: +61 (2) 9845 0890
www.kidsafe.com.au

NEW ZEALAND
CHILD SAFETY FOUNDATION NEW ZEALAND
15 Veronica Street
New Lynn
Auckland
tel: +64 9 827 6182
www.childsafety.co.nz

PHOTO CREDITS

14		SPL	167		BRC	252		SPL/JG
56		MS	168		BRC	253		SPL/CC
114	b	HZ	169		BRC	254		SPL/MD
116	t	SPL	171	bl	BRC	255		SPL/CP & MC
120	tr	SPL	173	t	BRC	261		PA
134		SPL	175		BRC	263		SPL/CP
136		SPL	177	tr	SPL/MT	271	tr	PA
137		SPL	196		PA	279	bl	IoA
138		SPL	206		PA		br	IoA/NG
139	r	SPL	209		IoA/JM	282		IoA
140	t	SPL	214		IoA/DvO	283		CCl
	cr	SPL	228	br	A/JA	287		IoA
141	t	SPL	232		WP/JB	288	bl	IoA/JM
142	br	SPL	235		IoA/JM	289	tr	IoA/JM
143		SPL	246		CM/H	290	bl	IoA/AJ
144		SPL	247		IoA/JM		br	IoA/SA

ACKNOWLEDGEMENTS

The publisher would like to thank everyone who participated so enthusiastically in the photo shoots, in particular: Heather Baker; Helaine Beukes; Ulla and Amber Bothe; Elroy Cameron; Amy Chaplin; Emma Charles; Lloyd Christopher; Marjory Dobell; Lexie and Gina du Toit; Jarryd and Justin Florentino; Ashleigh Hamilton; Catherine, Georgia, Joshua and Denim Haywood; Noah Innes; Carla and Robyn Kellermann; Jamie Knowles; Shirley, Hannah, Joshua and David Lim; Lee Maneveldt of St John's Ambulance for the loan of first aid kits; Tyler Miller; Kerry and Brenna Nel; Debra and Savannah Orffer-Brown; Benjamin and Claire Rideout; Dr Cleeve Robertson; Victor Tiludi; P. J. van Tonder; J.A. van Tonder; Thomas, Lilly and Ella Waterkeyn; Claudia and Elvano Willemse; D. A. Winter; Kat Ziegenhagen; Ron van Til for providing DIY props.

PERSONAL EMERGENCY RECORD

Ambulance/emergency service...

Hospital ....

Doctor ....

Paediatrician ....

Dentist ....

Pharmacy ....

Fire brigade ....

Police ....

Poison centre ....

Relative ....

Friend ....

Neighbour ....

School ....

Dad Work ....

Mom Work ....

Vet ....

Electricity ....

Gas ....

Water ....

Insurance company ....